NATIONAL INSTITUTE SOCIAL SERVICES LIBRARY

Volume 8

DAY SERVICES FOR ADULTS

T0386412

DAY SERVICES FOR ADULTS
Somewhere to Go

JAN CARTER

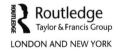

Routledge
Taylor & Francis Group

LONDON AND NEW YORK

First published in 1981 by George Allen & Unwin Ltd

This edition first published in 2022
by Routledge
4 Park Square, Milton Park, Abingdon, Oxon OX14 4RN
605 Third Avenue, New York, NY 10017

Routledge is an imprint of the Taylor & Francis Group, an informa business

British Library Cataloguing in Publication Data
A catalogue record for this book is available from the British Library

ISBN: 978-1-03-203381-5 (Set)
ISBN: 978-1-00-321681-0 (Set) (ebk)
ISBN: 978-1-03-204536-8 (Volume 8) (hbk)
ISBN: 978-1-03-204541-2 (Volume 8) (pbk)
ISBN: 978-1-00-319369-2 (Volume 8) (ebk)

DOI: 10.4324/9781003193692

Publisher's Note
The publisher has gone to great lengths to ensure the quality of this reprint but points out that some imperfections in the original copies may be apparent.

Disclaimer
The publisher has made every effort to trace copyright holders and would welcome correspondence from those they have been unable to trace.

DAY SERVICES FOR ADULTS

Somewhere To Go

JAN CARTER

London
GEORGE ALLEN & UNWIN
Boston   Sydney

First published in 1981

GEORGE ALLEN & UNWIN LTD
40 Museum Street, London WC1A 1LU

© National Institute for Social Work

British Library Cataloguing in Publication Data

Carter, Jan
Day services for adults – (National Institute for Social
    Work. Social services library; no. 40).
    1.   Day care centers for adults – Great Britain
    I. Title   II. Series
    362.1'2'0941   HV245   80–41363

ISBN 0–04–362035–3

Set in 10 on 11 point Times by Inforum Ltd, Portsmouth
and printed in Great Britain
by Lowe & Brydone Limited, Thetford, Norfolk

CONTENTS

PART THREE

PART FOUR

FOREWORD

The Board of Governors of the National Institute for Social Work first began to consider a research project into day care services in about 1972. I strongly supported the idea as I had visited several day centres a year or two earlier and had come to the conclusion that sooner or later alternatives to residential care would be forced on us by costs, shortage of trained staff and by the needs of these vulnerable people and their families. It is not possible to say categorically how many centres there were at the beginning of the 1970s, or how they were divided into the various categories, that is, for the physically handicapped, the old, the mentally handicapped, and so forth, but the numbers had probably increased threefold from 1970 to 1976 and will be much larger by now. This study, therefore, could be of considerable value to those starting up new day units, as well as to those that are already operating. I believe there is a good case for further study of the *families* where a member is a 'user' of a unit to find out what they get out of it, as there is strong evidence that the users and staff find the day unit approach satisfying for some of the problems.

As the author states, 'This book cannot provide more than the first word on day services. Predictions for the future would probably be more accurately made by an astrologer than a social researcher', but nevertheless the implication that there will be a growth in both numbers and variety is strong, and in my view such impediments to growth caused by the present financial restrictions will be temporary, as day units could prove to be cost effective as well as promoting fresh approaches to the improvement in social care.

The project was financed by the Joseph Rowntree Memorial Trust and research was much aided by the Department of Health and Social Security. Our sincere thanks go to Jan Carter, the project leader and author, and her colleague Carol Edwards, both of whom worked for long hours for nearly five years, and to many others (especially the members of the Advisory Committee) who contributed in various ways to the production of a very thorough and stimulating book which will be of considerable value to those who now have to consider 'What Next'.

LORD SEEBOHM
Chairman of the Advisory Committee

PROLOGUE

━━━━━━◆━━━━━━

'WHAT HAS COMING TO THIS PLACE DONE FOR YOU?'

Somewhere to come . . .
nowhere else to go . . .
feeling more settled in myself . . .
helped me to be with people . . .
mixing . . .
enabled me to make friends . . .
helped me a lot . . .
kept me going . . .
taught me how to go on public
    transport . . .
got me out of the house . . .
changed my life . . .
activated and even resolved some
    problems together . . .
given me the satisfaction of making
    up a contribution in work . . .
it hasn't done a lot . . .
it's done good for my son . . .
helped me make friends which I
    can't do alone . . .
this is a place I can bring my
    son . . .
made me independent and speak up
    for myself . . .
made me much better in health . . .
cheered me up a bit . . .
brightens up life, I can't wait
    till Thursdays . . .
don't know really . . .
taught me self control and
    independence . . .
everything, kept my sanity . . .
learned me to walk . . .
can't say it's done anything . . .
it brings people together and
    relaxes tension . . .
the dinners, that's the most
    important thing . . .
given me a grateful heart . . .
made me feeel much calmer . . .
I feel better . . .
it's O.K. . . . .
helps me a lot – the company . . .
opened me up a bit . . .
I feel happier in myself . . .

don't know ...
it's very intellectual, you meet
    people you would not meet otherwise ...
it's made me think of other people ...
gets me out of the house ...
cheered me up ...
met some new friends with more
    problems than I've got ...
made me realise I've got to get well
    soon ...
it's relaxing ...
I feel happy ...
made me feel I would like to go out
    and work ...
gives us a place to relax and take
    us away from ...
it's done me good in health and
    everything ...
it's helped me to occupy time ...
helped me to make friends ...
made me feel as though I'm wanted ...
helped me stop being so miserable ...
gets me up in the morning and
    occupies my time ...
given me company ...
helped my legs and arms ...
broadened my outlook and introduced
    me to my future husband ...
I get on better with people since
    coming ...
brought me forward ...
made me feel a different person ...
nothing really ...
made me easier to handle at home ...
helped me forget my troubles ...
everyone is nice to me ...
a heck of a lot to tell the truth ...
have met different people ...
it's improved my loneliness ...
taken me out of myself ...
it's eight hours talking to other
    people and it's done wonders to me ...
improved my writing ...
it hasn't done much ...
they're good to me ...
it helped me to meet more people and that
    helped me to make more friends ...
    that's it ...

(extracts from national random sample of users of day units)

INTRODUCTION

This book reports on day services for adults, a relatively recent development in health and social services in Britain – and elsewhere for that
matter. Most people assume immediately that day care is only provided
for children: this book will make it clear that many hitherto unknown
services exist by the day for adults, and in a diversity and variety which has
enormous potential for those who use them and those who work in them.

The research on which this book bases its report was funded by the
Joseph Rowntree Memorial Trust between 1974 and 1979. The research
took the form of a national survey in thirteen areas of the country selected
at random. The following were the broad terms of reference: 'To review
the present provision of day centres for persons over school age by public
authorities and voluntary agencies. This includes the groups served in day
centres and the kind of service provided (e.g. recreational or treatment).
To consider staffing and accommodation and to suggest the groups in the
community that might benefit most from day centres and to advise on
how these might contribute to the integration and development of local
services for those in need.'

More specifically, the aims of the project were these:

1 To examine current provision for day services in England and Wales
   offered by central government, local government and voluntary
   agencies. This includes an examination of
   a) The types of facilities provided (for example, day hospitals,
      rehabilitation centres, etc.)
   b) The types of users catered for (the main groups include the
      elderly, the mentally ill, the mentally handicapped, the physi-
      cally disabled, the smaller groups such as offenders, the drug
      addicted and those in family care centres). What are the rates of
      usage and the kind of activities provided?
   c) The types of service providers in relation to staffing ratios, skills
      of staff and training backgrounds.
2 To analyse the day by day practices in day services.
3 To examine the implications of day services for the training and
   organisation of staff.
4 To describe the experiences of the participants in day services:
   managers, staff and users.

The book is divided into four parts. The first part introduces the reader
to adult day services and then to the main groups of users and the bodies
which provide their services. The second part is an account of the aims of
the staff in day services and the way the aims apply to certain groups of
users. Essentially, this part of the book deals with specific user groups and

specific issues which relate to these. In the third part of the book, an attempt is made to look at day services in the round, by examining issues of the gains and losses currently attributed to day services by both users and staff. Part Four of the book is essentially a section for the technically minded. A more detailed account of the method and procedures and most of the tables from the survey are to be found in C. Edwards and J. Carter, *The Data of Day Care* (London: National Institute for Social Work, 1980).

AUTHOR'S NOTES

◆

Special Thanks

The project on which this book has been based could not have been completed without the help of Carol Edwards. Appointed as a research assistant, she exceeded her brief and made a strong contribution to the practical tasks composing a national survey. Her energy, competence and unremitting hard work made her a close and valued colleague. She contributed to this book by drafting parts of Chapters 3.1, 3.4, Chapter 15 and Appendix I and by preparing most of the tables. She had the primary responsibility for preparation of the supplement of tables companion to this text (Edwards and Carter, 1980).*

* C. Edwards and J. Carter, *The Data of Day Care* (London: National Institute for Social Work, 1980).

ACKNOWLEDGEMENTS

Nearly 3,000 people have been involved with the day care project and the purpose of this is to thank each of these for the enthusiasm and helpfulness they have shown in enabling the project to be completed.

First, there are those members of the Advisory Committee to the Joseph Rowntree Memorial Trust chaired by Lord Seebohm, who have given liberally of their time. Robin Huws Jones first had the idea of doing the project and Tilda Goldberg, the past Director of the Research Unit of the National Institute for Social Work, nurtured the research into birth and then life. The names of others on the Advisory Committee are listed at the end of this section. Since the task of steering projects inevitably falls on busy people, their contribution in terms of attending meetings, reading endless drafts and offering advice has been especially valued. Not all will find themselves equally happy with every detail of the outcome, which, in the end, has to be my responsibility.

This has been a project about people. A large debt is owed to nearly 600 heads and staff and over 900 users in the day units in the main study, as well as to the fifty staff and 200 users involved at the pilot stages. At a point in time when members of many professional groups – and the public – are fed up with researchers, their intrusiveness, their broken promises and impenetrable reports, it is pleasant to report that the project met with enthusiasm, concern and responsiveness from the outset. This, in turn, made the research team deeply aware of the obligation owed to the respondents. We hope that we have not let them down. The book which follows is critical sometimes, but so were they, usually with the honest intention of reflecting their life in day units.

Gratitude is owed to those officers in the large organisations sponsoring day services in the areas covered by the pilot project and the main survey, for the courtesy and assistance they gave us concerning our entry to their day services. This refers to area medical officers and directors of social services. Particular help in each authority was given by a 'contact person', usually the specialist in community medicine (social services) for the area health authority and the assistant director (day services) in the local authority social services departments. I cannot thank these individuals by name, having promised to protect the confidentiality of the authorities, the day units and the respondents concerned.

Thanks go to those bodies whose representatives listened to our hopes, read our protocol and then asked their membership to co-operate with us. These include, amongst others, the Association of Directors of Social Services, the Royal College of Psychiatrists, the British Geriatrics Society, the Royal College of Nursing, the Association of Area Medical Officers, the Association of Chief Health Administrators, the Department of Health and Social Security, the Home Office and the Central Council for Education and Training in Social Work.

Other people have helped by sharing their knowledge and providing technical advice. Aside from Michael Warren, Austin Heady, Tilda Goldberg and David Fruin on the Advisory Committee, these include Ed Whelan, Norma Raynes, Brendan McGuinness, Peter Gorbach, Ann Glampson and June Neill. Eileen Goddard of OPCS gave invaluable advice about drawing the national sample. Jessica Brill (London Borough of Camden), Douglas Bennett (the Maudsley Hospital) and Bob Lewis (Metropolitan District of Stockport) showed us their day services and endured long discussions on philosophy and practice. Jimmy Algie and Clive Miller at the National Institute for Social Work have given time and encouragement, so has Jackie Tombs of the Scottish Day Care Project, a replication of the survey under the auspices of the Central Research Unit, Scottish Office. Joan Warren, Ann Glampson and Brian Williams were valuable external raters on the health and depression data.

Then there was the execution of the national survey. In this connection we wish to thank the fifty or more interviewers from Research Services Limited, who worked for the project in a most committed way in different parts of the country. These people endured a number of changes to 'normal' interviewing procedures and demonstrated a flexibility and interest beyond the money they earned. For example, surviving a two-day briefing where the hosts are members of a centre for offenders and where part of the learning involves interviewing the staff and members in public is stressful, compared with doing routine interviews with housewives about preferences for soap powder! Organising and sustaining the precise military-like operation which undergirded the national interviewing schedule could not have been achieved without the patience, good humour and intelligent involvement of the Field Controllers at Research Services Limited. Our special thanks go to Dorothy Tchekemian and Therese Singleton. Yolande Benn, Maureen Richards and Joan Whitton were also helpful. Michael Warren, from Research Services Limited, liaised between us and the technical and computer staff, and presided with stoicism over requests for alterations to company procedures and numerous misadventures and difficulties in processing the data.

Others have helped by reading and commenting on chapters. Those members of the Advisory Committee who have read all of it are of primary importance here, including David Jones and Ian Sinclair. The latter suggested the helpful idea of structuring the book around the aims of day units as viewed by the staff. Others who have helped by reading individual chapters are John Keet, Douglas Bennett, Chris Arthur, Enid Levin, Inge Midforth, Stephen Hatch and Margaret Jeffery.

Over a five-year project, people come and go. Those who transformed labours of technique at the typewriter and coding frame into labours of love and commitment are numerous. I am grateful for the interest shown by Marlene Wild, Eve Gross, Janice O'Malley, Jan Anderson, Valerie

Jones, Rodney Patterson, Patricia Sloper, Margaret Jeffery, Ann Mackenzie, Hemlatta Shah, Anne Auden, Dee Bourne and Janet King. (Dee Bourne, who typed most of the final manuscript, and Patricia Sloper met on the study. They are about to start a drop-in centre for parents tempted to batter their children under the auspices of Parents Anonymous London; one unanticipated day care spin-off from the study.) Others who have been vital in getting the work done are the library, accounts, administrative and print room staff at the National Institute for Social Work.

Many friends in England and in Australia have supported and encouraged me at times when writing this book was difficult. (It is, after the experience, not difficult to see why so few research workers go on to do a second national survey!) Special thanks go to Eva Learner at the Human Resource Centre, Latrobe University, Melbourne, who provided me with space and an appropriate climate for writing between January and May 1979.

Five years is a long time to work on one project. If its results are read and discussed, I know that this will be rewarding to the many people who have contributed so generously to it.

PERMISSIONS

Thanks go to the following publishers for permission to quote copyright sources:

George Allen & Unwin ('The Tender World of Timothy Shy' by Eric Midwinter from *Education for Sale*, 1977)

Faber & Faber ('Old People's Home' by W. H. Auden from *Epistle to a Godson*, 1972)

Penguin Books ('Metroland' by John Betjeman from *The Best of Betjeman*, 1978)

Faber & Faber (*The Elder Statesman* by T. S. Eliot in *The Complete Poems and Plays of T. S. Eliot*, 1969)

Secker & Warburg (*On Margate Sands,* by Bernard Kops, 1978)

Virago (*Beyond the Glass* by Antonia White, 1979)

Oxford University Press (*Community Care for the Mentally Disabled*, edited by J. Wing and R. Olsen, 1978)

NATIONAL DAY SERVICE PROJECT
Advisory Committee to the Joseph Rowntree Memorial Trust

PART ONE

Chapter 1

---◆---

INTRODUCING ADULT DAY SERVICES

Some may feel that when Ecclesiastes declared that there was nothing new under the sun, that he had not thought of day units in the mid twentieth century. The day centre, the day hospital and those other forms of day units which constitute contemporary day services offer a different kind of personal service. Day units neither confine people to the four walls of an institution, nor do they operate on a domiciliary basis, from people's homes. Literalists might argue, in support of Ecclesiastes, that day services are nothing more but variants of each of these types of care: for example, that day services are part of a 'community care' movement, which far from being an invention of the modern age has been with us for centuries. Others will claim that day services have grown out of institutions such as hospitals, as a specific attempt to 'open up' institutional care.

But although different kinds of community care and institutional care have existed for centuries, services provided by the day in a day unit have not. We are entitled, therefore, to regard day services as 'something new under the sun'. At the same time, although day services are, *sui generis*, of their own kind, they owe parts of their current format to the practices of workers in the institution and in the community.

This book, then, is about day services for adults. Day units for adults appear to have developed after the Second World War, although a few existed beforehand, mostly as occupation centres for the mentally handicapped and sheltered workshops for the disabled. But in recent years, day services have not only expanded, but boomed. In 1959 our estimates indicate that there were just over 200 day units in England and Wales. By 1969 this number had increased fourfold, but by 1976 we estimate that there were about 2,600 day units open each weekday up and down the country. A similar growth had taken place in Scotland (Tombs and Munro, 1980).

The numbers of people attending day units seem to have increased too. In 1959 our estimates indicate that the numbers of attenders at day units represented the population of a large village, whereas by 1969 the attenders on any given weekday at day units might fill the equivalent of a market town with a population of 70,000, such as Bury St Edmunds. But by 1976 the estimated number of attenders had swollen to the dimensions of a city the size of Blackpool or Brighton, with about 138,000 people setting off on any weekday to attend a day unit. Over 17,500 paid staff members worked to these attenders and there were large numbers of unpaid volunteers.

What are day units for adults? They are organisations offering a form of personal service during the day, organised by statutory or voluntary agencies. All that these organisations have in common is that attenders and staff are present at a day unit by the day: at night they go home or elsewhere to sleep and in the morning, normally on a weekday, some or all of them reassemble. Nearly all day units are open for five days a week but a minority open for a more limited period, perhaps two or three days each week.

However, this does not distinguish a day unit from other organisations where people meet by the day. Can a pub, or a gambling club be a day unit? How does a day unit differ from an adult education centre, a community arts centre or even a university? What marks it off from the House of Lords? Further research by the broad-minded may find elements of day services in each of those settings. For the purposes of this book, however, approaches more pragmatic and pedantic have guided the definition. First, a day unit has been regarded as a day unit if its staff say it is. When in doubt a definition was applied: 'A day unit is a non-profit making personal service which offers communal care and which has care givers present in a non-domiciliary and non-residential setting for at least three days a week and which is open at least four to five hours each day.'

This definition excludes luncheon clubs and evening clubs as being open for an insufficient period of time. It also excludes pubs or cinemas, gambling clubs and betting shops as profit-making ventures. It would exclude the House of Lords because it lacks care givers offering communal care. A more serious problem is posed by adult education centres and community arts centres. The lack of inclusion of these facilities in the survey can be explained by an element in the definition which is implicit rather than explicit. This is that attenders at day services must fall into a defined administrative category, by reason of being in a certain age group, or because they suffer from a disorder. This disorder is usually a mental or physical disability and restricts, in theory, attendance at the day unit to those who share this disability. The 'care giver' works with those within a defined category of disorder or age.

This book will report on the current state of day services from the perspective of the national survey which took place between 1974 and 1978. The information collected during this time is the basis of statements made about day services and their practices. This survey discovered that most day units are called day centres or day hospitals, but there are less common names, too. Adult training centres, day training centres, workcentres, sheltered workshops, drop-in centres, family and community centres are examples. Attempts to introduce common names for day units need to be informed by common usage and professional sensitivities. For example, the term 'day care' is controversial in many day hospitals in the health service, where, for some, 'care' and 'treatment' are antipathetic concepts. For others however the overlap is a *fait accompli*.

Likewise in many work centres and sheltered workshops sponsored by voluntary and statutory agencies, the term 'day care' is unwelcome: 'care' and 'work' are considered to have nothing in common. A variety of sponsorship by both statutory and voluntary organisations provide day services for a range of user groups, from old people to the families of the very young on the one hand, or to those with a particular disability or disorder on the other.

Day units for adults are the preserve neither of a rural arcadia nor of the madding crowd. While few day units are to be found in the countryside, equally few coexist in inner cities. Most day services are to be found in areas more prosaically twentieth century: in suburbia. About four out of every ten day units are to be found in those locations where the Englishman maintains his castle, that is, in concentrations of public and private housing. About the same proportion are located in areas which are 'mixed': that is to say, they contain a mix of housing alongside commercial premises and light industry. Thus unlike many residential institutions such as asylums which during the last century were placed purposefully out of cities, or prisons which were built on their perimeter, day units are placed in dormitory areas: 'in the suburb that's thought to be commonplace' as that poet of the suburbs, John Betjeman, put it. 'Home of the gnome and the average citizen, Sketchly and Unigate, Dolcis and Walpamur'.

About four out of every ten day units are in the grounds of residential institutions. These are usually hospitals, but are sometimes residential homes or hostels. The rest are to be found outside the parameters of institutions; freestanding within the 'community' although some are alongside churches or community centres. A number occupy eccentric sites: a double-decker bus, a former police lock up, a country house, and so on.

Most day units insist that prospective attenders live within a defined area or district. They must be one of very few contemporary organisations where adults congregate regularly and routinely on a day-long basis outside a work place. Several aspects of this need comment. Although day units, like schools and hospitals, are part of larger bureaucracies, day units are relatively small when compared with other modern organisations. An average-sized day unit has forty-three places and the average ratio of staff member to users clusters at about the one to eight mark. Day units might be said to be unfashionably small. It is true that extra-large hospitals (of 2,000 beds or more) are no longer favoured, but neither are very small ones: those with fewer than fifty beds are being phased out. In contrast, the hospital which provides between 500 and 999 beds has steadily grown in the past ten years. And a decade ago, the average-sized secondary school catered for just over 400 students, but by 1974–5 the population of an average school had doubled.

Another unusual aspect of day units which cannot be disconnected from their small size is an almost unique emphasis on regular meeting and day by day assembly.[1] Given that they offer a relatively small, artificially constructed society to certain people living within the same district, they may have a certain contemporary significance. It is beyond the scope of this book to examine this, but perhaps day units, along with community centres, offer a rare but quite specific suburban alternative for some, to the 'fellowship' of church or chapel accepted by earlier generations. Day units are not separated by theological differences, but as we shall see, they are constructed by forms of twentieth-century secularism, in the shape of professional ideologies which carry some of the normative functions formerly the prerogative of church and chapel.

Who attends day services? The first point to be made about attenders (who are called the users in this book) is simple but not obvious. Users of day units are, in many respects, like other people. Most of this book will concentrate on the ways in which users of day units differ from the average man or woman, so it is legitimate to start by emphasising their commonality. Attenders at day units watch television, read newspapers and listen to the radio as regularly as anybody else. Like the general population, they are enthusiastic pet owners and occasional visitors to museums and exhibitions. There are as many users of day units who do their garden and indulge in 'do it yourself' decorating as there are addicts of these pursuits in the population at large. Users of day units are, however, slightly more frequent visitors at the cinema or theatre than the general population.[2]

Day services have slightly more women users than might be expected from the proportion in the general population and slightly more persons who live alone. The percentage of the middle-aged groups, those aged 30 to 64, who use day services is similar to those in this age group in the general population, but young people aged from 16 to 29 and those past retirement age are over-represented. Only 13 per cent of the population is aged 65 or more, but this age group represents nearly a third of those attending day units.

The most striking difference between day unit users and the general population is that all users of day services are outside the open labour market for one reason or another. All, except those few in sheltered work, are, to use the technical phrase, 'economically inactive'. This is striking once it is understood that one in every two day units see 90 per cent more of their users as 'long term' and never likely to leave the unit. By comparison, in only one out of every twenty day units are 90 per cent or more of the users thought to be likely to leave within six months of enrolling.

Most users of day services are at the unskilled, unqualified end of the scale. Half, excluding the elderly, left school at the age of 14 or before; 76 per cent have no qualifications or any type of job qualification. Only 4 per cent have a job they can return to after they leave the day unit. Users of day services start at the bottom of the skill pile. Given that most have an additional disability, by reason of labelled mental disorder or extant bodily infirmity, the combination of lack of skills plus disability leave many day unit users as difficult employment propositions.

However, while the existence of day services is a witness to the lack of jobs available for users, on the other hand, one unintended consequence is that day units offer improved employment prospects to many of their staff. Day services are evidence of the growth in jobs in the public sector and in service industries in recent years. A sizeable group of day unit staff – nearly a quarter – represent people who have transferred from blue collar manual and trades occupations into the health and personal social services. So day service staff may have accommodated to the restructuring of employment opportunities rather better than their users. In strict educational terms, however, many of the staff are as unqualified as the users: half the staff left school at the age of 15 or before. Ways in which the staff as a group differ from the general population include the rather obvious fact that they are 100 per cent 'economically active', which certainly cannot be said of the community at large. Also there is a higher proportion of women and the middle age groups to be found as staff of day units than in the general population.

Within day services, the attenders or users can be subdivided into a variety of what can be called user groups. These groups cover a broad range of the human condition. According to our estimates, the largest group catered for by day services is the elderly: 39 per cent of units, whether day hospitals and day centres, are for the elderly. The second largest group, the mentally handicapped, comprise 19 per cent of units. Then there are those services which deal with those labelled as physically handicapped. These units have 19 per cent of the overall number of units and day services for the mentally ill comprise 14 per cent of units. Next come those day units which deal with a specialist group of the elderly, the elderly mentally confused, which provide for 4 per cent. Then come a group of services called family day centres. In these day services the focus is on involving the *parents* of children, as well as often providing care for pre-school children. These services are offered from a centre, not a private home and make up 2 per cent of the sum.[3] A few centres for offenders total 1 per cent of the units. Finally, there are some units which draw a mixture of two or more of user groups called 'mixed' centres. For example, a centre may provide for two or more disability groups, such as the physically and mentally handicapped, or two or more age groups, such as the elderly and pre-school children. Mixed centres were 2 per cent of all units.[4] (Figure 1.1)

APPROACH OF THIS BOOK

Not much is known about day services. This was one motive behind the Joseph Rowntree Memorial Trust inviting the National Institute for Social Work Research Unit to undertake a national survey. It was originally envisaged that this would include Scotland but as inflation pre-

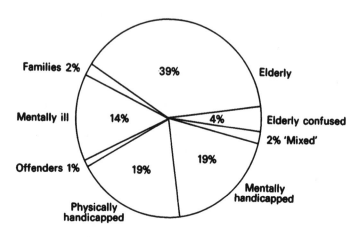

Figure 1.1 *What are the User groups?*

cluded this, a replication of the study in England and Wales has been undertaken in Scotland. This study is reported separately (Tombs and Munro, 1980).

In writing this book a number of considerations have shaped the approach. The first is the likely readers. One group might be those who have an interest in policies – or as it stands at present, perhaps the non-policies – of day services. These include politicians, national and local, senior administrators in health, social services, probation and other statutory services, as well as the voluntary agencies. Those few senior practitioners who regard policy creation and service formation as a fundamental part of their job may also be interested.

This book tries to paint a picture with a broad brush rather than a fine pen. Information about what happens, day by day, in services has been included, primarily to satisfy what is seen as a second group of readers, those who see themselves with a primary interest in practice in day services. This includes those who select and work with the staff of day services, advisers and consultants, heads of large day units, or those who teach and lecture potential day unit staff on courses. Deliberately, no effort has been made in the book to separate out so-called policy from practice issues. This is in the belief that this distinction is more academic than real: all policy has practice or anti-practice repercussions and in reverse, all practice has implicit policy outcomes.

It is hoped that the book may also offer a useful introduction to a third group, the non-specialist reader with a working interest in the health and social services field: perhaps the schoolteacher, the journalist or the trade unionist. A caution needs to be addressed to a fourth potential group, comprised of social researchers and research students. They are not the primary audience of this book and some of them may feel that the book is insubstantially documented. For those devoted to the quantitative rituals of the social sciences, a companion document has been prepared. This reviews the main results of the survey in tabular form and gives detailed accounts of method and procedures (Edwards and Carter, 1980).

There are many ways this book might have been written: the minutes of the meetings of the Advisory Committee to the Joseph Rowntree Memorial Trust about the project bear witness to this! The outcome will not suit everyone. The text of the first part of the book is an introduction to day services. In this first chapter and the next, day services are discussed as if they had a certain homogeneity. However, this useful analytical device cannot be pushed too far. By Chapter 3 when each user group is introduced separately, the account mirrors the actuality of everyday life.

The second part of the book examines what goes on in day services in a framework derived from topics nominated by staff as their view of the aims of their day unit. One reason for arranging the book around the staff's views of their aims is that it allows contrasts to be made between different groups of users, or between different sub-groups *within* a particular group of users. The second part of the book has been the most difficult section to write: complex judgements have entered into the selection of material. Not all the information of the survey seems equally relevant to understanding day services in each user group. It seemed wasteful to spend precious space discussing the obvious: it is of little consequence to confirm that parents in family day care centres can walk up and down stairs by themselves, walk a quarter of a mile outside the house alone and dress themselves. However, considerable coverage is given to these same factors in the case of the mentally handicapped where the same issues, namely the degree of mobility and the amount of self-care of a mentally handicapped person, relates to his or her facility in leading an independent existence. The third part of the book discusses the users and staff in general again. Throughout the book, names of areas, units and persons are protected and pseudonyms are used.

Another reason for discussing the findings of the project according to the aims of the staff in day units, is that heads and staff of day units are very preoccupied with this matter. The aims, as the heads and staff see them, are a mental touchstone against which to evaluate the perceptions of both staff and users about the practices of the unit. Of course, a survey of this nature has its limits: we do not know whether the reports we give of the aims, or the staff view of the ways these are made manifest, *really* happen, a matter discussed at greater length in Appendix I. In this sense, one social purpose of a survey is to point out directions and alternatives: in the opinion of the writer, a survey of this nature is less about accuracy, in the formal experimental sense, than achieving an embryonic order out of conceptual chaos.

The aims are reported as the staff see them, in descending numerical order. Thus, Chapter 4, which reports the view of those who see the unit providing straightforward, practical services, is based on a larger number of staff than Chapter 15, which reports a minority aim rarely mentioned by staff, about staff relationships with users. In the end the reader will have to decide whether the importance of the subject matter diminishes with the lack of numerical force the staff accord it. In the view of the writer, it is as important to demonstrate what people in day services are *not* thinking about as the reverse: this contains the seeds of thinking about how the day units might change. To move outside the format of reporting what 'most said' and to give covetage to minority views allows the reader to decide the validity of minority opinions. Some of these may be important in trying to change the *status quo*.

Different readers respond to different degrees of evidence and persuasion: some may consider the findings reported in this book compelling enough to promote changes in their day services. Others, more sceptical, will see this book as offering no more than a series of hypotheses as a basis for more rigorous social observation and more precise evaluation. The writer's position on this matter is that this study has been more concerned with learning than with measuring. It has attempted to find out what day units do ahead of categorising their effectiveness. The question we have been asking is not 'Does it work?' but 'What goes on?' (Weiss and Rein, 1969).

Large-scale surveys are unfashionable at present. Accused, often justifiably, of mindless empiricism and useless number-crunching in order to report breathlessly on the obvious, surveys are also considered to be antagonistic to ideas. This survey hopes to show that this convention is not inevitable. It is absurd to claim that a survey is essentially atheoretical. A theory of one sort or another guides all the practical decisions taken during a survey. Which questions should I include and which should I eliminate? How should the questions be administered and what degree of flexibility and latitude will the interviewers be encouraged to demonstrate? How can this flexibility, encouraged in the hope of obtaining valid and reliable data, be squared with requirements for standardising methods of collecting data? Those who are interested in some of the technical questions raised in this paragraph should consult Appendix I of this book and the companion document (Edwards and Carter, 1980).

Writing a book which transacts the conventional boundaries of statutory and voluntary services poses a developmental problem. More is known about some fields of day services than others. For instance, a great deal has been written on a purely descriptive basis about day hospitals for the elderly (National Day Care Project, 1978). It would be less useful to geriatric day hospitals to reiterate information already available than to enter new controversies. On the other hand very little has been written about other areas such as family day care, or 'mixed' user groups, where introductory descriptions are valuable in themselves.

The Advisory Committee to the Joseph Rowntree Memorial Trust for this project requested that his book should present the results of the survey in the first place, rather than the implications of these results. Each chapter reports survey results first, before a discussion or review. An attempt has been made to purge the book of the worst obscurities of social science jargon, although this surgery has not necessarily left the book easy to read. It is not intended as a bedtime bromide; it reflects the complexity of day services themselves.

A survey can be likened to a still photograph. More like a snapshot than a moving picture, a survey takes snapshots of day services which then become frozen at one particular point in time. In this survey, we took a number of still photographs, so as to speak, in the same day units on the same day. The results are numbers of pictures from different angles showing dissimilar poses. In outcome, this offers a different result to the more developmental process of the cine-film, which provides moving and processional accounts of its subjects. These analogies are a reminder that the tactic used by the survey, that of freezing a subject into still life, are not the only way of understanding day services. The method chosen is only a device, not an end in itself.

Charles Booth put it well, back in 1891:

The methods employed in the collection and tabulation of the information were adopted, as suited to the peculiarities of the subject and the materials with which we had to deal, but doubtless are open to criticism from many points of view. Not only is exactness in this case out of the question but even the most general results obtained are open to dispute. At every turn the subject bristles with doubtful points. For each one of these, as it has arisen . . . the best available solution has been sought, or what seemed the most reasonable course has been taken. (Booth, 1891, p. 18)

NOTES

1 Not *all* users go to day units every day, of course, as we shall see.
2 Survey data was compared with information provided by the Central Statistical Office (1976).
3 Day care for pre-school children, in the form of day nurseries, playgroups, childminding and other day provision has been excluded from the scope of this book.
4 The survey on which this book is based took place in thirteen areas of England and Wales, selected by stratified random sample. No services for drug addicts, alcoholics, the homeless or youth were found. The survey took place in 1976 and the impression is that facilities for each of these groups have developed since then.

REFERENCES

Betjeman, J. (1973) 'Metroland', in *The Best of Betjeman,* selected by John Guest (Penguin).
Booth, C. (1891) *Labour and Life of the People,* Vol. II (Williams & Norgate).
Central Statistical Office (1976) *Annual Abstract of Statistics* 1976 (HMSO).
Central Statistical Office (1976) *Social Trends,* 1976, No. 7, (HMSO).
Edwards, C. and Carter, J. (1980) *The Data of Day Care* (National Institute for Social Work, London).

National Day Care Project (1978) *Adult Day Care: Selected Readings* (National Institute for Social Work, London).

Tombs, J. and Munro, G. (1980) *Scottish Adult Day Services* (Central Research Unit, Scottish Office: in preparation).

Weiss, R. and Rein, M. (1969) 'The evaluation of broad aim programs', *Annals of American Academy of Social and Political Science*, 385, pp. 113–42.

Chapter 2

THE CONTEXT

This chapter will consider briefly the following: first, reorganisations of public services affecting day services; second, the swing in public policy from an emphasis on institutions to 'community care'; third, the organisations which provide day services and the way in which local policies reflect (or do not reflect) the push towards day services; and fourth, the question of which organisations provide what day services?

LIVING WITH REORGANISATION

Latter-day Britain has developed a reputation for cavalier redistribution of tasks and boundaries in its public sector. However, it was not a prescient hospital consultant nor a seasoned director of social services who said: 'We trained hard – but it seemed that every time we were beginning to form up in teams we would be 're-organised'. I was to learn later in life that we tend to meet any new situation by 're-organising', for creating the illusion of progress while providing confusion, inefficiency and demoralisation.' Rather, it was said to be Caius Petronius, AD 65, demonstrating again, perhaps, that there is nothing new under the sun (except a day unit!).

Many recent rearrangements of services have affected personal health and social services in Britain. But the three pertinent to day services are the reorganisations of social services, health services and local authority boundaries. These alterations are relevant as they transferred day service between service providers and authorities.

First, the restructuring of the personal social services – the Local Authority Social Services Act 1971 – followed the deliberations of the committee chaired by Lord Seebohm. This placed in one local authority social services department a composite of day services, such as those for the mentally handicapped, the physically handicapped and the elderly. Then the reorganisation of the national health service, 1974, combined the formerly separate hospital and community health services together on a geographic basis and established three administrative tiers: region, area and district. The essential point is that these two reorganisations – social services and health – resulted in a transfer of some day services from a health sponsorship to that of social services.

A third rearrangement affecting some day services was the change to local authority boundaries in 1975, after the Redcliffe-Maud report. This replaced county boroughs by large industrial conurbations, the metropolitan districts, and thus reallocated some day services between new local authorities. None of these reorganisations made the task of assessing what day services existed in a particular area in 1974 particularly easy; some authorities were barely aware of their own assets at the inception of this project.

INSTITUTIONAL TO COMMUNITY CARE

Since the Second World War there has been considerable talk in the United Kingdom about winding down residential institutions. The success of this is still a disputed matter. Although there is little evidence that there are fewer institutions, the existence of day services is some evidence of community alternatives. On the one hand, no prisons or mental hospitals have closed, although since 1960 the number of patients in mental hospitals has decreased considerably. On the other hand, the standard practice of placing aged or disabled persons in institutions when they are no longer able to manage alone or when their families cannot cope has been questioned.

The active promotion of 'community care' has been emphasised in most government statements about the future of the groups of users considered in this book. Most statements since the early 1960s have advocated a shift from the institution towards care at home, within the community: day services are usually seen as an aspect of this. For example, for the elderly the government pointed to the need to help people to live independent lives in the community and to the requirement to expand community-based services – including day services – to achieve this (DHSS, 1978). Services needed for 'mental illness related to old age' include places for day hospital treatment for elderly persons suffering from dementia (DHSS, 1972). For the mentally ill, the government proposed that day services develop as part of a strategy of community care promoted by both health and social services (DHSS, 1975). Then a number of government documents from 1971 to 1979 have promoted the merit of community care for the mentally handicapped (DHSS, 1971). A shift of resources has begun: the number of mentally handicapped people resident in hospitals has decreased since 1970 and the number of places in hostels and training centres has increased (DHSS, 1979, p. 9).

For the physically handicapped, a Minister for the Disabled now co-ordinates services and the Chronically Sick and Disabled Act 1970 obliges local authorities to meet the practical needs of the physically handicapped living at home. A recent estimate suggested that up to 30 per cent of disabled people living outside hospital use a club or day centre (Knight and Warren, 1978).

POLICIES ABOUT DAY SERVICES

In practice it is difficult to decide suddenly to develop day services at the expense of other kinds of services. When it comes to the point, few authorities (particularly health authorities) have highly developed policies about day services, implying that central government statements have not been transferred into hard local realities. Social services departments had more clearly defined management structures and planning targets for day services than area health authorities: some of the differences between the two will now be defined.

No health authority, or its area medical officer, had a written or verbal policy about day services,[1] and the question of whose job it is to start and maintain day units is vague. One authority which announced a general commitment to shift resources from inpatient to day services admitted that this was difficult in practice. Lack of money was the most common constraint; but another hurdle was overcoming adverse medical attitudes to the new multi-disciplinary Health Care Planning Teams.[2] The new area health authorities had not yet overcome the opposition of those consultants who wanted to maintain the old system of developing services by *ad hoc* initiatives (called the 'he-who-shouts-the-loudest system' in one authority). This opposition was exacerbated by diverging opinion in area health authorities about the person or committee to whom consultants in day units were accountable. Some reports indicated that consultants were responsible only to 'themselves', others that consultants were responsible only to their 'patients'. One doctor said: 'This is a difficult question. Consultants are a very isolated group and for many the reorganisation of the health service hasn't happened.'

A confusing list of people and committees in whom a secondary accountability for consultants resided was nominated: these ranged from medical executive committees and local divisions of psychiatry or geriatrics to district management teams, and area health authorities, or regional health authorities (with whom consultant contracts are made). According to one specialist in community medicine: 'There is no hierarchial system in senior medicine. The social services department have a strict hierarchy and this is constraining. It could be said that the consultant's responsibility to the authority is a moral one.'

Contrast this with the local authority social services departments, where a group of officers is aligned to a part of the organisation known as day care. Sometimes day care is allied together with residential or institutional care: at other times it stands alone.

Organising day care in the social services departments most often combines day and residential services under one assistant director. Alternatively day care is organised as one element of a package of services offered from an area office on a local district basis. Less commonly, day services are managed either by an assistant director also in charge of fieldwork services, or managed as a service of their own, or organised around the services being developed for a particular user group: so that day care services are structured – in the language of the social services – along client group lines. Whatever way, a clear line extends from the senior officer responsible to the director of social services, thence to the local politicians, the councillors composing the social services committee of the local authority council.

Between the day units themselves and the assistant director is 'middle management': the people usually known as principal officers who 'manage' day services for the assistant director. Five areas had one principal officer; four had five or more principal officers and each was responsible for managing anything from five to fifteen establishments. Chapter 17 will make the relevance of this clearer.

Little can be said about the way that day services are organised in voluntary organisations, or in 'other' statutory agencies. Voluntary agencies rarely have specific policies for developing and maintaining day care, partly because most voluntary day centres are the responsibility of local committees, making them 'one-off' ventures. Whilst this localism has many advantages, one of its main drawbacks is that many day units operate in isolation and a brand new day unit has to set about a process of 'discovering America' again.

WHO PROVIDES WHAT DAY SERVICES?

To find out which organisations sponsored what day services, we took thirteen areas of England and Wales at random and investigated the services of the local authority social services department, the area health authority, the various voluntary organisations and any other statutory services. On this basis we are able to estimate that local authority social services departments in England and Wales are the largest sponsors of day services, offering 47 per cent of the total number of day units.

Second largest providers are the various area health authorities, which combine to support 26 per cent of adult day units. The third sector, 23 per cent of the total, are the province of voluntary agencies such as Age Concern, the Spastics Society or MIND (the National Association of Mental Health). Finally came a residual group of statutory authorities which are responsible for a mere 4 per cent of units: the probation service, for instance, the Employment Services Agency and the occasional local educational authority.

The local authority social services departments have a virtual monopoly of day services for the mentally handicapped and sponsor about 95 per cent of these day units, called adult training centres. This is a great change, since much early day care for the adult mentally handicapped commenced as voluntary initiatives. Aside from this, the major commitments of local authority social services departments are to provide over half the day units for the physically handicapped, one-third of the units for the elderly and one-fifth of the day units for the mentally ill. As well, there are small numbers of day units for the elderly confused, for family day care and for a mix of user groups. Few local authority day care staff came from residential or institutional backgrounds and three-quarters of

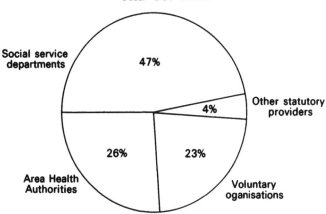

Figure 2.1 *Who Provides Day units?*

the local authority social services day units were found outside institutions, that is, in 'the community'.

In the area health authorities, less than 10 per cent of the day units
stand in the community and so most day units are based within an
institution. Half the staff have spent the longest period of their work life
in institutions. Area health authorities have fewer day services than social
services departments. They provide three-quarters of the units for the
mentally ill – the day hospitals. Day hospitals for the elderly represent
just over a quarter of all day units for the elderly. Most of the units for the
elderly confused (usually known as psychogeriatric day hospitals) are
provided by health authorities.

The sector with the highest proportion of day units outside a residential
or hospital setting are the voluntary agencies. Currently, the main commitment of the voluntary agencies is to the elderly. A number of
voluntary agencies, principally Age Concern, the Women's Royal
Voluntary Service and Help the Aged, sponsor one out of every three day
units for old people: sometimes with some financial aid from local
authorities. Three out of ten units for the physically handicapped are
voluntary sponsored; in the small field of family day centres, two or three
centres are voluntary. There is also a recent trend by voluntary agencies
towards offering 'mixed' services for a combination of age groups such as
the elderly and pre-schoolers, and some day units for offenders are
sponsored by voluntary organisations. There is a minute amount of
voluntary-inspired provision for the mentally ill and the mentally handicapped, but nothing at all for the elderly confused.

The remainder are those services provided by 'other' statutory
services. The largest is the group called Remploy, which has for many
years run sheltered workshops for the disabled. The Employment
Services Agency operates employment rehabilitation centres, which provides a short pre-job preparation course. The probation service entered

day care recently by opening four experimental, 'compulsory' day training centres and other voluntary follow-up centres. Then the Department
of Health and Social Security operates 'reestablishment centres'.
(Intended to 're-establish' long-term holders of statutory benefits in the
'work habit', the one unit of this type in the sample refused permission for
the project to study its practices.) Finally, an occasional education authority operates a 'special care' service for young multiply handicapped
people, too old to be at school and excluded by virtue of multiple physical
and mental disability from adult training centres. (In other areas, this
function is undertaken either in 'special care' units run by social services
departments or an exceptional day hospital sponsored by a health authority.)

Has flesh started to grow on the dry bones of community care? The
very existence of day units implies this. During the 1960s, the term
'community care' was a synonym for rhetoric and enthusiasm, neither of
which needed to be trammelled by the evidence of practical services. But
during the 1970s central government has put forward more substantive
notions about what services are needed for each group and in some cases
there has been a small degree of progress. Tracing the exact relationship
between the decline of the institution and the rise of day services is
therefore more complex than is usually acknowledged by commentators
who pronounce on the decline of the institution and the complete absence
of community care (for example, Scull, 1977). What evidence is there for
the growth of day services and does this service affect many potential
users in a given user group? The next chapter considers these matters.

NOTES

1 We interviewed the specialist in community medicine (social services) in each of the
  thirteen area health authorities.
2 Under a recent system of funding it was possible to arrange 'joint funding' of day services
  between health and social services. By 1977, joint funding of new day unit(s) had been
  approved in five areas, and discussed in a further five areas. This arrangement commenced after the conclusion of fieldwork in this study.

REFERENCES

Department of Health and Social Security (1971) *Better Services for the Men-
    tally Handicapped*, Cmnd 4683 (HMSO).
Department of Health and Social Security (1972) *Services for Mental Illness
    Related to Old Age* (HMSO).
Department of Health and Social Security (1975) *Better Services for the Men-
    tally Ill*, Cmnd 6233 (HMSO).
Department of Health and Social Security (1978) *A Happier Old Age*
    (HMSO).
Department of Health and Social Security (1979) *Report of the Committee of
    Inquiry into Mental Handicap Nursing and Care*, Cmnd 7468 (HMSO).

Knight, R. and Warren, M. (1978) *Physically Disabled People Living at Home: A study of numbers and needs* (HMSO).
Scull, A. (1977) *Decarceration* (Prentice Hall).

Chapter 3

THE ANATOMY OF DAY SERVICES

Growth

Only one of ten of the day units in existence in 1976 was open by the end of the 1950s. The golden years of growth for day care, 1960–76, saw established services undergoing apparently rampant extension and whole new varieties of service flowered. For example, in 1959, only one in twenty of the day units currently available for the elderly existed: and provision for other groups was almost as scant. None of the day units for families, offenders or 'mixed' user groups had existed before 1970. (Table 3 in Appendix II at the back of the book is relevant.)

But despite this expansion, at a guess, the numbers of places provided by day units is trifling, when compared to the national estimates of the numbers of people in any one disability group who might be considered as the pool of potential users. Nevertheless, the numbers of persons in any national aggregate are not necessarily a reliable guide to preparing a local service. In fact, the doctrine that national guidelines can be a reliable basis for local planning – a notion which clearly contains at least one seed of truth – may have unwittingly diminished the utility of day services. Unlike residential care or hospitals, day care needs to be accessible on a daily basis to the homes of incapacitated people. This means that the site of a day unit, the number of places and the back up services, particularly transport – public and unit-sponsored – need to be chosen with clarity and planned precisely with respect to the prevalence, the geographical distribution and the living situations of the potential users and their supporters.

Reliance on national guidelines, not local information, may relate to the relative lack of pressure reported by most day units. Day unit places are in general under-utilised. Few have waiting lists of any length and apart from the geriatric day hospitals, and a few 'fixed time' units reported in Chapter 9, turnover is sluggish. Nor are all available places filled, as Appendix II, Tables 4–5 indicate.

More informed choices of sites and decisions about the number of places a unit should carry should not only relate to intelligence about the local need. There has been a tendency in day services to over-invest in new buildings at the expense of considering the staffing and facilities required to maintain the number of places the building can support. If reductions in public expenditure introduce more rational questioning into the commissioning and planning process, all will not be lost. The common bureaucratic practice of separating out the functions of 'research/planning' and development as opposed to 'operations' in day services has, at times, led to a lack of integrated thought between those who commission the buildings (the development group) and those who eventually provide and sustain its facilities (the operational staff).

GROWTH IN BUILDING

As reported, much of the energy – as measured by the cost – in establishing new day services has been devoted to the building in which the service is contained.[1] There are exceptions: for families, offenders, the elderly confused and for 'mixes' of user groups, smart new buildings are rare. In local authority social services departments, new edifices have, more often than not, gone to the mentally handicapped rather than the mentally ill. Of about equal numbers of centres established during the 1970s, two-thirds of the buildings for the physically handicapped and half those for the elderly were tailor made. In all, six out of every ten day units sponsored by social services departments are purpose built.

Within the health service, authorities have been slower to embark on capital programs. For instance, before the 1970s four day hospitals for the mentally ill were purpose built, but this changed in the 1970s. Three-quarters of the day hospitals opened in this period have been newly built. Overall, four out of ten day hospitals for the elderly, the elderly confused and the mentally ill are purpose built.

In the voluntary sector, a third of those centres established for the elderly are in new buildings, and those few incursions into day services for the mentally ill and the mentally handicapped by voluntary organisations have taken place under the roofs of old buildings, often older houses. In all, four out of ten day units sponsored by the voluntary sector are purpose built.

What has happened to growth of day units since 1976? That story awaits another investigation: this one was completed before public spending reductions began to 'bite'. But there are buildings due to open in 1977 left vacant, many plans left on drawing boards; units placed in metaphorical cold storage, by protracting their cycle of development. Planned as expanding services during years of confident growth, day services now exist in a new set of political and economic conditions. The increase in unemployment is unlikely to diminish at least for a decade. Inflation increases. Cuts in public expenditure have reduced current services. And against these economic realities must be set certain demographic facts: particularly the predicted rise in numbers of old people, especially the very old, those aged 80 or more in a decade. There are also increased social and economic expectations of services by certain minority groups, for example disabled people, fostered in part by changes in legislation such as the Chronically Sick and Disabled Persons Act 1970.

This altered society means a set of changed conditions for day services in the future. These issues will be returned to at the end of the book but they are mentioned here so that the reader may bear them in mind. They were not the context in which this investigation was prepared and expedited, but the facts of adult day services now need to be appraised in a revised political and economic context.

Plan of Chapter

The rest of this chapter introduces readers to the users of day services. Starting from the group with the largest number of places, the elderly, and ending with the smallest groups, those of offenders and mixed user groups, each section will commence with an introduction to the growth of the service. Then some people, either staff or users, are introduced to the reader and a table follows about the sample on which the section is based. Each section reviews the service providers and the activities of the day unit and gives some basic facts and figures about the staff and users. Each of the eight sections closes with a comment which raises problems or provides a bridge for the reader to other issues discussing the same user group in other chapters. Then a route 'map' is provided to relevant chapters on a particular user group, as some readers will be less interested in learning about day services in general than in the application of day services to a particular user group.

Chapter 3, which concludes the first part of the book, also introduces the reader to certain conventions of terminology adopted throughout the rest of the book. When a statement says '98 per cent of users' or '46 per cent of staff' or 'two-thirds of the day units' this is a shorthand way of writing '98 per cent of users interviewed from the interviewing sample' or '48 per cent of staff interviewed from the interviewing sample' or 'two-thirds of the heads of the day units who responded to the postal questionnaire'. In the belief that the reader will find such repetitions tedious because it induces the language of the book to stutter, the reader is invited to take the sampling basis on which assertions are made 'as read'. This will not please everyone, but it is possible to refer to a table in each section which reminds one of the dimensions of the sample.

Briefly, the census sample is the postal questionnaire collected from all the heads of 291 day units found in thirteen areas of the country (276 heads of day units responded to this giving a return of 95 per cent). The interview sample, however, refers to these people – heads, staff and users – interviewed in a stratified sample of 155 day units. The head was always interviewed along with three members of staff and six users, all selected at random. In effect this represents talks with 559 heads and staff and 888 users of day units. Appendix I outlines this in more detail.

The technically minded reader should know that it was found that on a large number of tested indicators the day units in the 'interview' sample were representative of the larger 'census' sample (Edwards and Carter, 1980). Despite this, a number of caveats stems from the nature of the methods. First, by randomly sampling for a fixed quota of six users and four staff including the head in each day unit, we overstate the opinions of those in small day units and understate the views of those in large ones.[2] Second, this method of sampling in the interview sample entitles us to talk about users or staff across the national sample, but does not allow us to discuss day units. The rule is relaxed in units where at least half the staff and half the users of the day unit were interviewed. Third, another limitation results from sampling staff and users at the day unit on a randomly selected day of interview. This over-represents the views of the one-day-a-week-attender at the expense of the week-long adherent. Finally, although some chapters lend themselves to statistically based comparisons (and in fact, statistical tests – usually the chi-squared test – have been undertaken) they are rarely reported in this volume.

Words and phrases invented for the study of day services are listed in a short glossary at the end of the book. In the interim it is worth noting that the phrase 'health sponsored' refers to those day services in area health authorities, while the term 'social services' needs to be understood as a contraction of 'local authority social services departments'.

NOTES

1 An investigation of the relative costs of day care for the elderly (capital : maintenance : staffing costs) is being undertaken by the University of Kent Personal Social Services Unit. Comparison of health, social services and voluntary day units will be provided.
2 The sample of units, the census sample, is accurate and representative, but in a strict statistical sense the interview sample of staff and users as analysed is not a random sample of 'all' staff and 'all' users of day services. User characteristics associated with unit size are over- or under-represented in the sample. For example, from analyses specifically on day services for the elderly, the size of the day units was found to be associated with some important characteristics, most notably whether the unit does or does not provide transport for its users. This relates in turn to the degree of disability found amongst the users. The results relevant to elderly day units in the next section, Chapter 3.1, and subsequent chapters should therefore be treated as tentative and exploratory. Day units for the elderly have a larger variation in size than units for other user groups, so the results for other user groups may be more representative. This problem is being explored further and will be reported elsewhere (Edwards and Carter, 1980).

REFERENCE

Edwards, C. and Carter, J. (1980) *The Data of Day Care* (National Institute for Social Work, London).

CHAPTER 3.1

——◆——

THE ELDERLY

INTRODUCTION

According to T. S. Eliot, 'to make an end is to make a beginning. The end is where we start from.' So we start with the elderly. By numbers of units and numbers of places available, day services for the elderly are the largest user group in day services. Yet this was not always the case: three out of every four day units for old people have been established during 1970–6. The aspect of services for the elderly which is perhaps the most recent growth point is the feature of developing a day centre inside a local authority old people's home. Almost all these services have been established in the 1970s:[1] so were other local authority social services day centres for the elderly, those centres we will call community-based. There has also been an expansion of services run by voluntary agencies for the elderly: three out of four units are new in the sense that they have been established since 1970. The best-known day service for the elderly is perhaps the geriatric day hospital and it is also the most established service, for one-third of these units were established during the 1960s. Services for the elderly confused, the so-called psychogeriatric day services are reported in Chapter 3.5.

INTRODUCING THE PEOPLE

This introduces four heads of day units for the elderly. As we shall see, each has a different view of the job and a different workload to master to get through the day. The way each approaches his or her workload made a difference to what might be termed the 'atmosphere' of the unit. These differences are familiar territory to people who work with old people but others may enjoy a less formal introduction to a selection of day units before reviewing the information which follows. The units described were all visited by the writer. None were selected 'at random' in a statistical sense; each was selected for its features in common with units of the same type. Where a unit – or a head's – practices seemed unusual in a statistical sense, as in the geriatric day hospital, this is mentioned.

A DAY CENTRE SPONSORED BY A VOLUNTARY ORGANISATION

This day centre is in an outer borough of London and is sponsored by the

Outerborough Old People's Welfare Association. An annual grant given by the local authority social services department is spent in paying the two part-time organisers of the day centre. Since 1961 there has been a day centre in this hall from 11 a.m. to 5 p.m. each Monday through to Saturday. At present the centre is used by about a hundred old people each day, of whom about forty have a hot lunch. All these old people must be active enough to make their own way to the centre, but once a week volunteers bring in about ten 'housebound' to spend the day at the centre.

Mrs Henderson is the 'morning' warden, and she arrives at the day centre at 10.30 with four plastic bags full of cabbages and carrots. Each day she stops at the market to buy the vegetables for lunch. She buys enough for forty: the first forty old folk in the centre get the lunch. Yesterday over forty-three were refused lunch, but they could buy tea, homemade cakes, and sandwiches and bread and butter – 'all priced very cheap'. After she arrives, she discusses the lunch with the three volunteer helpers of that day and often stays to give them a hand to peel the potatoes.

She spends most of her week organising the voluntary workers. She says: 'My job is to ensure the smooth running of the centre. To achieve this you have to be a tough nut. The most important thing I do in my job is keeping the voluntary helpers happy. Without them we wouldn't be here. You do have to be a diplomat. Each one has to be treated with kid gloves.' She sees the purpose of this centre for the elderly as 'providing comfort and company, and reasonably priced refreshments', and views her job as 'largely common sense and experience'. She does not think a qualification would be any help. She used to run a pub and she thinks that gave her sufficient experience with organising food and dealing with the public.

Mrs Henderson herself gets no time to talk to the old people who use the centre, although she considers their main characteristic is loneliness. But she does think the centre makes some contribution to keeping them in touch. 'They come to read notices on our board, they don't buy the paper these days because of the price. So the council make their announcements here and our posters help the old folk keep in touch.' However, although Mrs Henderson and the volunteers don't talk to the users or organise any activities for them, she says they talk a great deal to each other. Mrs Henderson does not encourage the users to be involved in any way in helping to run the centre: 'They're not capable. There is a lot of jealousy if one does a job and another doesn't.' She gets her personal satisfaction from the job in feeling that it is well done: 'If people say "I've had a lovely lunch", that is a reward. One can only give of one's best, one's dedication and loyalty.'

A DAY HOSPITAL RUN BY AN AREA HEALTH AUTHORITY

This day hospital in a north-west city called Cottontown is not really an average day hospital, because it has more patients each day than the usual run of day hospitals. It also has fewer staff to cope with them. The ratio of staff to the seventy patients who come each morning to the day hospital is 1 : 9 (much lower than the national average of one staff member to every three day patients). The workload is heavy too: for example, fourteen of the seventy elderly patients cannot get to the toilet by themselves, and almost the same number need to be fed their lunch by the staff. The most common condition suffered by the patients is the stroke, but as there are no speech therapy, physiotherapy or occupational therapy staff attached to this day hospital, strokes go untreated in the conventional way.

'Getting through the day' for the sister in charge is a task a long way from the traditional bedside nursing she was taught. Only half her time is taken up with looking after the patients' physical needs or in practising her traditional nursing skills. Sister defines her primary task as 'supervisory'. By this she means that she is the antennae of an information system, the central task of which is to ingest every conceivable type of information about patients from all staff, including the doctors and ambulance men. To achieve this, she encourages certain attitudes in her staff:

> As the patients only spend a certain time here, the staff need to be observant in a special kind of way. They need to be involved but not too involved. I expect that attitude from everyone from the ambulance man up. If a nurse baths a patient who chats to her I want to be told everything of significance: I want them to hear what the patients eat at home, so I can persuade them to eat here what they miss out on at home. You have to be very observant here and it takes above average skills to communicate with the cross-section of the community we get here. A nurse needs to have an ability to evaluate.

Apart from being at the centre of an intelligence network, getting through the day in the day hospital also requires that the sister be able to deal with negotiations between the staff of the day hospital. This is rather less complex a matter in this particular day hospital, where the only other professional discipline caring for the patients is medicine and where all staff other than doctors are answerable to the sister in charge. Nevertheless, the heavy human workload will not be processed without fairly refined co-operation from all staff. 'I like to get across this idea that it is the staff's job to help the patients, first and foremost.'

The sister has a meeting with her staff nurse, her two nursing auxiliaries, the three therapy aides and the domestics each morning to discuss the logistics of the day. This may involve role-swapping. 'I may need to help my domestics out with the washing up, and my nurses might make coffee. We have learned we all have to help each other.'

However, this day hospital provides more than just a forum for the intelligence system for the elderly ill of the town and a venue for staff negotiation about getting through the work. The sister has determined views about how to maintain, as opposed to undermine, an elderly patient's dignity. Unable to fall back on a highly technical conception of treatment for the patients, her own approach stresses the common touch. The day hospital, a prefabricated building on the periphery of a gaunt district hospital, formerly the town's workhouse, is decorated with huge collages of crepe paper. The day hospital is locally famous for this craft. The aged infirm sit in chartreuse easy chairs, crocheting or knitting under six foot high paper collages: one, an Easter bonnet papered with spring flowers, hangs skittishly overhead. At the end of the huge room are small tables, each laid with a gingham cloth, a vase of fresh flowers, a coffee pot, a milk jug and a sugar bowl. There are no pre-sugared, pre-milked hot drinks in this day hospital. 'Of course, it makes more work', admits the sister. 'All those tablecloths have to be washed each day, and so do the pots and jugs. But a day hospital should make them feel like a person and help them to know somebody cares.'

Although sister finds achieving any kind of change – from unblocking the drains to achieving a new member of staff – 'slow and dreadfully frustrating', she is basically satisfied with her job. Her success is 'making the patients happy. Not only the patients but the staff too. If I've done that I've achieved something.'

A COMMUNITY-BASED CENTRE SPONSORED BY A SOCIAL SERVICES DEPARTMENT

Although in theory this centre sponsored by a county council social services department can cater for a hundred each day, there are usually about seventy old people each day at the centre. The centre is an attractive new building set in a new garden. Defined as a community centre, it opened last year on new housing development on the fringe of a city in Welshire. Most old people walk to the unit, but about a quarter come each day on a special minibus. There is an active entertainment programme, there are outings during the summer, and of course bingo. Knitting, toy-making and making nail and thread pictures are available for those who want this, as well as a hot lunch. The building holds adult education classes in the evenings and acts as a community centre at weekends.

Mrs Davies, the 50-year-old officer in charge, came to this centre from a job as an education welfare officer. Because the centre is new, she finds she spends more time with architects and workmen than with staff and users. Despite this she interprets her obligations as those of providing a happy atmosphere at the centre: 'to have a staff working well together and making each member feel well cared for, and to make sure that someone can listen always to their problems. And to provide them with a varied and interesting programme.' In principle, Mrs Davies is keen on involving the old people themselves in the running of the centre, although she is a bit vague on how to achieve this. 'Well, I don't know really: partly we use them as voluntary help and largely we value their personality and friendliness. They make suggestions. Also they do organise their own evening outings to clubs and things, which means they can carry on their friendships outside.' The centre has both a waiting list (twenty-five old people wait to join) and a staff shortage (a post of driver has been 'frozen' in the local authority financial cuts, thus limiting the number of old people who can be transported to the centre).

Mrs Davies finds that the most frustrating aspects of her job are those of dealing with the problems of the building, and also 'the fact that with the elderly you have to repeat everything every day ten times over: this needs infinite patience'. (Like most heads of similar centres, she has no special training on what might be expected from elderly people.) Despite this, she counts her work as satisfying: 'I always tell people how lucky I am in my work, because I see results. After coming here, people look fitter and happier. They come out of their shells, and their friendliness towards me and the staff is a reward.'

DAY CARE PROVIDED IN A LOCAL AUTHORITY SOCIAL SERVICES' RESIDENTIAL HOME

Fifteen old people are transported each weekday to an old people's home in Cartown, a metropolitan district in the midlands. They sit in two gloomy sitting rooms devoid of any furnishing other than a low table and chairs backing against the walls.[2] The only decoration in the public rooms of this home is a bowl of artificial flowers under the plaque beside the front door. The warden, Mr Poulter, has been at the job for nearly two years, and his wife is employed as matron. A former stores officer in the NHS, Mr Poulter had been unable to find work in the NHS on his return from abroad. He finds this present job very congenial. He now sees this job as split between the care of the residents of the home ('We provide a good home and care – feeding and comfortable quarters') and day care ('We provide a haven for them: we give them contact with other people to help with their loneliness').

Mr Poulter finds that half his week is taken up in administration and clerical activities – I'd like to spend as much time as possible with them, but it's not enough, I'm afraid.' He does, however, need to spend time sorting out problems between the residents and the users: 'It's difficult when you are a combined centre [day and residential]. Residents tend to resent the day people. We have to discourage quarrelling. Basically we are *residential*, and the place is geared to them.' For this reason he would not encourage users to have any part in helping to run the place.

His two biggest job problems, as he sees them, are a lack of reliable staff, and the relatives of his residents ('usually they have a guilt complex'). Despite this, he finds his work gratifying and he defines 'success' in this way: 'Success is a first-class home with contented and well cared for

Checklist: Vital Statistics

Day Units for the Elderly

	Sample as a whole	Sponsored by: Voluntary Organisations	Area Health Authorities	Local Authority Social Services Departments Community-based	Based in Residential Homes
Number of units in national census	109[a]	43	31	19	16
Number where interviewing took place	35	13	10	9	3
Number of heads and staff interviewed	105	48	40	27	
Number of users interviewed	168	79	73	57	
Average size of unit (user places)		51[b]	30	56[b]	12
Range of size of units (user places)		12–200[b]	10–70	12–120[b]	6–14[c]
Average ratio of staff to users		1:11[b]	1:3	1:27[b]	1:6

[a] Three units did not participate ($N = 112$).
[b] The number of users attending the day unit was used as an estimate for the established number of places in units where this information was not available.
[c] In homes with 24–55 places for residents.

residents – residents who will reflect my success in their happiness.'

No particular activities are provided for the users. As we spoke, the day users, slumped around the darkened room, slumbered on.

DAY UNITS FOR THE ELDERLY SPONSORED BY VOLUNTARY ORGANISATIONS

As these introductions to four heads of day units for the elderly imply, there are four distinctive brands of day services for elderly people in England and Wales. First we will discuss the forty-three centres sponsored by voluntary organisations[3] who provide the bulk of day care places for the elderly – 57 per cent.[4] Most of these voluntary centres are supported financially by a combination of voluntary and statutory sources and administered by a local old people's welfare association. These arrangements vary a great deal locally:

> Our finance is assisted by donations from various bodies. Grants for the rent come from the county council. Rotary clubs and the Catholic Church help us out. Also we get a donation from employees of ICI: though not perhaps more than £10, this is greatly appreciated. But mostly we are self-supporting.

> The local Age Concern provides the transport costs and the building. Social services subsidises the meals.

> The Old People's Welfare Council provides equipment, for example, a sewing machine, stereo equipment and tools for carpentry. The county council and the district council pay loan charges, maintenance, heating, lighting, cleaning, the wages of the cook and the warden.

As these comments imply, many of the heads of voluntary centres, variously known as 'organiser' or 'warden', were paid a salary or at least an honorarium, but there was no payment for their 'staff' of volunteers. In the day hospitals sponsored by area health authorities and the day centres run by social services departments, heads and staff were, of course, all salaried.

Although about half the day hospitals, social services centres and day centres in residential homes used volunteers, they were never considered to be 'staff' in the same way as they were in the voluntary units.

Local authorities often play some part in the financing of the day services for old people offered by voluntary organisations. Two patterns in particular emerge. In the first, local authority social services departments collaborate with voluntary organisations to provide day care. The local authority may provide the building and some service, such as transport to the centre for the users, while a voluntary organisation 'staffs' the centre with volunteers. In the second pattern the local authority turns over a grant to a voluntary organisation which then offers an independent service to the elderly. Chapter 5 gives more information about these services.

DAY HOSPITALS FOR THE ELDERLY

There were thirty-one day hospitals for the elderly in the sample, and they operated quite differently from voluntary and social services centres in terms of their turnover. On average, the day hospitals claimed a discharge rate roughly eleven times as great as that claimed by social services day centres and seventeen times as great as that claimed in the voluntary sector. Whilst this suggests that day hospitals and day centres do not substitute for each other, there was a considerable amount of variation between day hospitals, as Chapter 8 points out in more detail.

Their heads – and their staff too if it comes to that – represent the most 'professionalised' sector of day services for the elderly. Very few of those working in social services or voluntary centres – paid or unpaid – had any kind of academic or vocational qualifications. But this was not the case in the day hospitals. In the day hospitals, we have chosen to regard the head as the person who was in charge of day by day activities in the unit: the person or persons responsible for ensuring that the day hospital personnel and patients got through the day. This person was never a doctor, and was rarely anyone but the nurse, as the example of the day hospital in Cottontown implies. In five of the thirty-one day hospitals the head was an occupational therapist and in three other day hospitals, leadership had a collective meaning, for a management team of equals – occupational therapist, physiotherapist and nurse – collaborated to administer the day hospital. These three different kinds of leadership – nurse, occupational therapist and the collective – need further comparison.

SOCIAL SERVICES DAY CARE IN RESIDENTIAL HOMES

Altogether there were thirty-five social services day centres in the sample. Of this number, nineteen were community-based centres: that is, they were separate from any other kind of establishment. Aside from the community-based centres a further sixteen centres were held within local authority residential homes for old people. (To be included within the survey, these centres in homes had to cater for at least one day attender to every four residents. Homes which catered for fewer day attenders to users – perhaps one day attender to, say, twelve users – did not get included in the survey.) The day centres conducted in residential homes are perhaps the most straightforward centres to describe, since they cater more or less exclusively for the more disabled elderly who need to come to the centre on special transport. These centres are discussed at greater length in two papers (Edwards and Sinclair, 1980; Edwards *et al*., 1980), and are touched on briefly in Chapter 15.

Day centres in residential homes have developed along two quite different patterns. One of these patterns might be described as 'segre-tated' and the other as 'integrated'. In the 'segregated' day centre, day care attenders have separate facilities (such as their own dining room, common room, toilets) from the residents living in the home. Most of the segregated day centres had a separate staff to look after the day users, even though one head usually continued to be responsible for both day attenders and residents. In the integrated homes, however, the reverse applied: the day attenders shared their facilities and the staff with the residents.

The evidence from both the staff and the day attenders was that 'integrating' day attenders and residents produced some conflicts amongst the staff about where their priorities lay. It also led to conflicts between the residents and the day attenders about who should have the territory. Unfortunately the residents were not interviewed but these issues were thought serious enough to require further investigation. The evidence points in the same direction as the information given by users and staff in mixed centres (Chapter 3.8) and suggests a similar implica-tion: that mixing two groups of people perceived as 'different' creates more difficulties than allowing each group to have its own territory.

These residentially based day centres did not always form a discrete group. For example, one puzzle centres around wide variations in the number of old people they discharged. It is hard to explain why one residentially based centre of twelve places should report discharging in the previous year fifty-seven users, of whom thirty-two went into hospital or residential home and twenty died, while another of similar size should discharge only two users. This survey was unable to explain these differ-ences but such findings have clear importance for practice. 'A day centre with no turnover must provide a very different environment for its clients to one provided by a unit with a turnover resembling that of a transit camp' (Edwards and Sinclair, 1980).

Another important issue arising out of the use of day care in residential homes is that the practice appeared to be confined to a small number of authorities. In only three of the thirteen areas did local authorities pro-vide day care in residential homes for a substantial number of their day care users. These three authorities relied on day care in residential homes as their only form of direct provision for the elderly (unless they were classified as 'confused'). They were also the three areas with the *least* day care provision for the elderly in the thirteen in the sample. Given that fewer day places were available for old people these three authorities seemed to have decided to use them for the 'heavy end' of day care for the elderly. Other aspects of day care in residential homes are mentioned in Chapter 15.

SOCIAL SERVICES DAY CENTRES – COMMUNITY-BASED

In the nineteen community-based centres, the kinds of elderly users coming to centres was not as straightforward as in the residentially based centres. In effect, there were three kinds of social services day centres for the elderly based in the community: comparatively large day centres with few staff, to which the elderly made their own way; smaller, more highly-staffed centres which brought in more disabled users by special transport; and centres which had a mixture of these patterns – large centres where the great majority of users made their own way but a small proportion (often called the 'housebound') were brought in by special transport.

One other interesting matter about social services day centres was that they appeared to be under-used. Most centres were able to quote an 'established number of places' on a daily basis, but when this was compared with the actual number of old people who came along on the day of the census, the occupancy rate of community-based social service centres was found to be only 70 per cent. Whether this was because of the users' illness, a lack of transport or a lack of demand is not known. What is apparent, however, is that an increase in occupancy rate, say from 70 per cent to 90 per cent, would represent a 20 per cent increase in the number of day places available for old people in any one district. Chapter 5 deals with other aspects of day care in these kinds of centres.

DEVELOPING NEW SERVICES

The growth of day services for the elderly has been mentioned already and a great deal of money was spent on building programmes. About two-thirds of the nineteen community-based social services units are now housed in buildings built especially for their purpose, compared with about half the day hospitals and just over a third of the voluntary centres. But the social services units (leaving aside those situated within the orbit of a residential home) appear to get more community use out of their buildings than either the day hospitals or the voluntary day centres: for instance, two-thirds of the community-based social services centres allowed the use of the buildings in the evenings by outside groups: such as community or neighbourhood groups, or special clubs for the handicapped. At the same time, there is a paradox built into this, for it also seemed that purpose-built buildings tend to become more self-contained as far as their own users and staff are concerned. This is because fewer of the community-based social services units used facilities outside the day centre, such as local clubs, exhibitions, adult education or shops than the more *ad hoc* voluntary day centres.

The expense of building new units has led some of the voluntary agencies to search for less costly alternatives. In one of the areas of the study, a consortium between the local authority social services department and two voluntary agencies – Age Concern and Help the Aged – set up a mobile day centre, staffed by volunteers. The 'caravan', parked on a different road each day, was patronised by rather frail elderly people who could not walk far to a conventional day centre. This mobile development has future possibilities in both urban and rural areas (Kaim Caudle, 1977).

STAFFING DAY SERVICES FOR THE ELDERLY[5]

The *modus operandi* of four heads of day services, three of them women, began this section. Leadership of day units for the elderly is nearly always women's work, for nearly all heads – nine out of ten – are women. Three-quarters of staff working with old people are women too, but this was not so in day services as a whole, where the overall balance between the sexes is close to 1 : 1.

Money and kudos are rarely given as consequential reasons for working with the elderly. In common with the four heads introduced already, the factor which brought the heads and staff together was a special interest in the field of ageing. Making the users happy, comfortable or contented emerged as the most critical factor in denoting job satisfaction and in defining success on the job.

The predominance of women working with the elderly has been noted. Over two-thirds of the staff working with the elderly were married, but widowhood was the second most common marital status. This was particularly so amongst those in the voluntary sector, where the biggest age band of volunteers belonged to those aged over 65 years: a quarter of the volunteers interviewed were aged over 70. The largest age band of those working in the social services centres were people in their 50s, whereas in the day hospitals it was people in their 40s.

As we have already noted, very few heads, staff or volunteers outside the day hospitals bring to their job any kind of professional qualification. In the day hospitals, the most common qualification is that of the state registered nurse, followed by the state enrolled nurse (a two-year practical nursing qualification). One other large group associated with the day hospitals for the elderly are the doctors. Although one, two or even three medical consultants might be in titular control of patients at a day hospital, in practice consultants spend very little time in the day hospital itself apart from seeing patients in clinics. In some day hospitals even this task was delegated to junior staff or, more often, to clinical assistants, often visiting general practitioners.

Apart from doctors and nurses, the existence of other professional staff was patchy. The other main group of staff in geriatric day hospitals, the physical and occupational therapy staff, were, as Chapter 8 indicates, by no means distributed equally throughout the country. Some day units have no occupational or physiotherapists at all (14 per cent), and under half (45 per cent) had what might be termed an 'adequate' supply of therapists. This left four of every ten day hospitals with an adequate supply of therapists.[6] For other therapy staff there was much the same picture: only just over half the day hospitals had at least the services of even a part-time speech therapist.[7] The supply of chiropodists was similarly sparse, for only four out of every ten day hospitals had the services of at least a part-time chiropodist.

The day hospitals had the most favourable staff ratio, with an average of one staff member to every three patients. In the day care provided by residential homes the ratio of staff to users was 1 : 7. In the voluntary day centres there was, on average, one volunteer for every eleven attenders, whilst the community-based social services centres made do with, on average, one staff member to every twenty-seven elderly members. These members reflect the physical workload of the units; as we shall later see it is the day hospital patients who are also the most physically helpless group, while the community-based social services day centre users are the fittest.

GETTING INTO DAY SERVICES

Who recommends that old people get day services? Predictably, the day hospitals nominated their hospital doctors, general practitioners and hospital social workers, in that order, as the most common referees. The voluntary centres viewed the local authority social worker as their main formal recruiting agent, but a high proportion of old people had heard about the centre from informal sources, and were either referred themselves or came alone on the advice of friends or neighbours. For both types of social services centres – those in residential homes and those community based – those who most commonly referred were reported to be the local authority social worker, the general practitioner and the hospital social worker.

All day units had 'eligibility' qualifications: a series of hurdles to be surmounted which might well put a service beyond a potential applicant. The implication of these is that the greater the need, the harder it is for an old person to get a place. For example, two-thirds of the day hospitals and the community-based social services centres defined aggressive or disruptive behaviour on the part of the elderly user as a disqualification. Fewer voluntary centres and day centres in residential homes debarred users for such behaviour. More voluntary and social services centres were intolerant of incontinence in their users than either the day hospitals or the residential homes. But although being unable to walk was not a bar to getting to a day hospital for the elderly, about a quarter of each of the other types of services for the elderly would automatically exclude the immobile user. (One head of a day hospital for the mentally ill reported her satisfaction that the day hospital was placed at the top of a long narrow stairway, thus excluding the elderly user who could not walk!) Outside the special day centres for 'confusion', a confused mental state was tolerated by more day centres in residential homes than by either day hospitals, voluntary centres or the social services centres.

Once an old person actually got inside the unit, relatively little attention was paid to introducing him (or more likely her) into the practices of the place. Few offered any kind of special induction to their users. Perhaps the extended length of time the users were expected to stay decreased the pressure on centres to provide any kind of orientation. Apart from the day hospitals, most users were expected to stay on. None of the users were considered to be short term and likely to leave within six months in three-quarters or more of the voluntary units, the community-based social services units and the day care in residential homes. In contrast, just under half of the day hospitals said than none of their users were long stayers and all were likely to leave within six months.

Many of the ground rules which prescribed the margins of behaviour which the day unit defined as tolerable related in part to the sheer difficulty of getting some old persons to the units. The importance of transport for day services for old people has already been hinted at. Nearly all of the patients at day hospitals or in day care in residential homes came on special transport. Only half the users in voluntary and community-based social services centres came on transport offered by the centre. Of the rest, nearly a third of the elderly users walked to the unit, and a further fifth came by bus or by train.

Transport to the day hospital was usually organised centrally, through the NHS ambulance service. The consequence of this was that affairs of transport loomed large on the day hospitals' agenda of problems. As might be expected from a centrally organised service which was set up primarily to provide an emergency service to hospitals, the three main transport problems, as seen by the heads, were as follows. First, the poor *timing* of the service (patients sometimes arrived and went home within one hour). Second, the large *distance* that patients were expected to travel (sometimes some ten to fifteen miles: although this was never reported as a problem by the patients themselves). Third, the interruptions to service caused by industrial problems within the ambulance service itself.

By contrast, the voluntary units with no access to much transport at all saw their main transport problems as a lack of it, and its prohibitive cost. Social services units had rather fewer grumbles about transport than the other sectors. Some possible factors behind this are discussed in the Appendix at the end of this section.

THE USERS OF DAY SERVICES FOR THE ELDERLY[8]

Old people are to be found in all types of day services. A granny aged 64 was found in a family day centre because she cared for two pre-school grandchildren, and two 'old lags' aged 63 had recently joined centres for offenders where the average age was under 29. Five mentally handicapped people aged between 60 and 64 years were interviewed, and 16 per cent of those in units for the mentally ill were aged 60 or more. But, more substantially, four in every ten users of social services and voluntary units for the physically handicapped were elderly. In the centres with a 'mix' of users, described in Chapter 3.8, nearly half the users were over retiring age. So although this section deals only with those in centres *officially* designated as units for the elderly, it is clear that some day care for the elderly is provided outside those units designated for them (and for the elderly confused too, a group dealt with separately in Chapter 3.5).

Within the units for the elderly, the oldest groups are to be found in the social services day centres provided in residential homes – a third of the day attenders interviewed were over 80 – and in the voluntary centres where just under a third of the old people are over 80. (A quarter of the day hospital users, and a fifth of the community-based social services users, are octogenarians.) Elderly women users outnumber the men by two to one. The gulf between the numbers of men and women is widest in the social services centres, where there were three women to every man; in the day hospitals there were three women to two men. As the users got older, the proportion of women increased too, for example, eight out of ten of the users aged over 80 were women, whereas only six out of ten of the users still in their sixties were women. This is scarcely surprising, since it reflects the general population where women account for three-fifths of all people aged over 65 and three-quarters of those over 80.

The physical dependence of those in geriatric day hospitals is the most extreme of any group in any day service. According to the day hospital heads, a third of the users either need the help of the staff to walk at all, or are confined to a wheelchair. (Fewer than one in ten of the users in voluntary and community-based social services units need this help, and slightly more than one in ten of those in day care provided in residential homes.) Further, four out of every ten of the day hospital users either needed help to go to the toilet or were incontinent, compared to only one in twenty of the users of voluntary centres. And one in ten of the day hospital users needed to be fed by staff, whereas all the users at voluntary centres could feed themselves.

The users had clear views of their disabilities. In the day hospitals, the most common disorders reported were diseases of the central nervous system, of which the stroke was the most common. In fact, half the patients in the geriatric day hospitals were stroke victims,[9] and strokes also accounted for a third of the disabilities reported by the elderly in day care associated with residential homes. It was, however, a relatively minor condition in both the voluntary and the social services centres, where complaints connected with ageing bones and joints – particularly arthritis – were complained of most by the users. These disorders extend themselves into the users' views of what it was and was not possible to achieve by self-care. For example, where only just over one in ten of the users in geriatric day hospital considered that they could walk a quarter of a mile down the road unaided and unaccompanied, three out of ten of the voluntary users thought they could do so. Less than one in ten of the day hospitals' patients could travel alone, but five of every ten users in voluntary centres said they could do this. Again, whereas only a fifth of the day hospital patients could get up a flight of stairs by themselves, well over half the voluntary users could do so. It was therefore perhaps a paradox that the most physically infirm users, those in the day hospitals or in day care provided by residential homes, came to the units less often than their more active counterparts. At the same time, it was these more physically infirm users who indicated that they were less able to compensate by finding themselves busy in activities at home. Almost half of the geriatric day hospitals' users confessed that when not at the day hospital they would spend most time at home 'doing mostly nothing'. When not 'doing nothing', they watched television or listened to the radio. Their more physically active counterparts in centres run by voluntary agencies or social services would spend most of their time outside the centre divided between jobs in the house (like washing up) or devoting themselves to indoor hobbies – things like playing cards or knitting.

The depression of those with physical ailments will be discussed in detail in Chapter 8. Overall, half the users of units for the elderly – whatever the type of unit – confessed to being depressed. Fewer were depressed than either the mentally ill or those in family day care, but slightly more elderly people were depressed than the physically handicapped (of whom a third were elderly anyway). It was not only the burden of physical infirmity that was associated with depression, since nearly as many users amongst the more physically active users of voluntary and community-based social services centres were as depressed as their frailer counterparts.[10] As Chapter 4 will demonstrate, more users of social services community-based centres live alone, and most are widowed or single rather than married. So factors aside from physical infirmity relate to depression for old people in day services.

More of the day hospitals experienced trouble in getting their patients to leave the unit than the other units for the elderly (a matter which is discussed in more detail in Chapter 8, along with an analysis of where old people go after the day hospital). Of course, it is the day hospitals who actively discharge old people: 6.34 old people per year per place are likely to be discharged, compared with a ratio of 0.59 for users of voluntary centres. More surprising is the fact that more elderly people than other users leave day units because they don't like them. So although on the one hand, those interviewed in centres for the elderly professed themselves to be the most satisfied group in day care,[11] it needs to be remembered that we did not meet the 108 users said to have left the units in the past year because they did not like it.[12]

ACTIVITIES IN DAY UNITS FOR THE ELDERLY

What packages of activities are offered to users of day units for the elderly? Not surprisingly, very few units went in for outdoor games. But very few units (one in twenty units) offered users any kind of educational programme either. This possible deficiency will be discussed at greater length in Chapter 5. Meetings and discussion groups were also offered parsimoniously. Only one in every seven units offered meetings and discussion groups: these were most rare in the day hospitals where – as Chapter 7 will argue – meetings and groups have potentially their greatest use.

The subject of old age and employment is also introduced in Chapter 5. One in twenty of the voluntary and social services units offered very simple work subcontracted from outside the unit to their users, and they also paid their users a minimal rate for this. Activities dispensed in most of the programmes for the elderly most often amounted to social activities, arts and crafts, and a variety of treatments. Of these, social activities were the most frequent: bingo triumphed in all sectors, being most common in the day hospitals, who also went in for more cerebral memory games and quizzes, while their counterparts in the voluntary centres were swept away on outings to the seaside and country. While the day hospital patients listened to records, the users in voluntary centres played whist. Bingo, whist and cards were the social cements of the community-based social services centre, whereas in day care in residential homes, users got a bit of visiting entertainment and some outings to the sea along with their bingo, perhaps because they were invited to join in with the residents in the home. Visits out to art or craft exhibitions or to local entertainment were rare in all units. So was play-reading, dancing and swimming. In other words, the social activities offered to elderly users tended to emphasise those activities which demanded very little in terms of a user's skill or which required a minimum in terms of his relationships with other users.[13] Chapter 17 expands on this.

Next to the social programme, various arts or crafts took place as the next most frequent activity. A sex bias in these activities was implied by the iteration of knitting, sewing and embroidery in all sectors, whereas the less sexist crafts of painting, pottery, weaving, canework and woodwork were offered only with any seriousness within the day hospitals.

It was, of course, the same with treatments: day hospitals had this cornered. Inevitably, almost all day hospitals offered both general nursing care, specialised nursing procedures and drug maintenance. Nine out of ten offered what was called individual physiotherapy, and seven out of ten occupational therapy (although neither of these activities was necessarily associated with the presence on the staff of a trained therapist). The same caveats apply to speech therapy and chiropody provided by about two-thirds of the day hospitals. Half the residential homes offered nursing care to their users, and over a quarter took care of users' drugs and offered chiropody. These services were offered by a few community-based social services centres too, but by proportionately fewer than in residential homes. The voluntary centres offered next to nothing in the way of physical care – not even chiropody or keep fit classes.[14]

The users' nominations of the activities at which they spent the most time dislocate assumptions about the predictable nature of the activities offered to the elderly. For example, it appeared that more time in the day hospitals was spent on arts and crafts than treatments. Less than a quarter of the day hospital users said they spent 'most time' the previous week on treatments (23 per cent), and marginally more than a quarter claimed to have spent most time on arts and crafts (26 per cent). Then again, there were almost as many users claiming to spend most of their time at the day hospital 'doing mostly nothing' (16 per cent) as those loquacious users who claimed that they spent most of the day chatting to others (20 per cent). In the voluntary day centres and social services centres, more users – a third – spent more time chatting to each other than doing anything else, while just over a quarter claimed to have persisted for most of the time at social activities. But while more users in day centres provided in residential homes spent more time chatting than doing nothing, other activities did not appear to assume any temporal importance at all – not even eating dinner or drinking tea.

PLACES FOR THE ELDERLY

Places for the elderly are not only found in centres for the elderly. For 8 per cent of those interviewed in day units for the mentally ill, 19 per cent of those in units for the physically handicapped and 45 per cent of those in units for a mix of user groups were 65 years or more.

Taking all sectors of day care together, rather obvious points can be made. First, there are wide variations between areas in the number of day places they provide for old people. Second, at a national level there are wide variations between the different service providers in what they offer old people. To take the question of differences between the thirteen areas first, this can be illustrated by pointing out that the area with the most provision for the elderly on a population basis (an outer London borough) had almost thirty times as many places as the area with least provision for the elderly (a metropolitan district in the midlands). These variations could not be explained by the number of old people catered for in centres primarily designed for other user groups (such as the physically handicapped or mentally ill). Nor could it be explained by the provision of alternative services such as home helps or by variations in the amount of 'need' in the area. Table 3.1.1 describes the variation between these authorities in more detail.

The second point is that wide differences exist between the varying service providers on a national basis. On the basis of the number of places provided, voluntary centres are the largest sector and the health services day hospitals the smallest (Table 3.1.2 on page 40).

Table 3.1.1   *Estimated day place provision per 1,000 people over 65, by authority and sector, in thirteen areas* (Edwards *et al.*, 1980)

	SSD Residential	SSD Community	Voluntary	AHA	Total
Westborough [a]	—	—	24·4	1·4	25·8
Northborough [a]	—	3·2	12·4	—	15·6
Welshire [b]	—	8·2	1·1	2·3	11·6
Cottontown [c]	—	7·5	1·0	2·3	10·8
Innerborough [a]	—	8·2	2·5	—	10·7
Coaltown [c]	—	—	4·8	2·2	7·0
Southshire [b]	—	—	5·2	1·4	6·6
Eastshire [b]	—	—	4·1	1·8	5·9
Midshire [b]	—	0·8	2·3	1·9	5·0
Outerborough [a]	—	0·6	4·1	—	4·7
Northshire [b]	1·1	—	2·5	0·7	4·3
Steeltown [c]	0·9	—	0·4	1·2	2·5
Cartown [c]	0·8	—	—	—	0·8

[a] London borough   [b] County council   [c] Metropolitan district

Table 3.1.1 reveals a startling variation in the total quantity of day care provided for the elderly in different authorities, with the authorities where residentially based day care was used as the three lowest providers. Examination of other data from this study suggests that these variations cannot be explained by assuming that the low providers are placing the elderly in day care centres designated for other client groups. Although the order of authorities would change slightly if, for example, centres for the elderly mentally infirm were included, the size of the variation between authorities would remain essentially unchanged.

DISCUSSION

The public care and treatment of the elderly in this country has made enormous strides since the Second World War, if one compares the accounts of grim stoicism in the back wards of hospitals (Thomson, 1949) with the day services of the 1970s. Nor does the development of day services for the elderly in this country seem to have been accompanied by the definitional problems, demarcation disputes and procedural wrangles described by commentators in the USA (Weiler and Rathbone-McCuan, 1978) and France (Attias-Donfut, 1977). These indicate that much time and energy is being spent on pursuing definitions of a day hospital compared to a day centre, whereas in Britain these procedural matters have really been confined to the interest of a few geriatricians (Brocklehurst, 1970; Hildick Smith, 1977). The new structure of services in Britain – on the one hand health, and on the other hand social services – may have pre-empted semantic academicism by allocating broad responsibilities to each sector. Chapter 7 points out that pragmatic local

Table 3.1.2　*Provision of day services for the elderly in thirteen areas* (Edwards *et al.*, 1980)

	SSD Resi-dential	SSD Com-munity	Volun-tary	AHA	Total
Number of units	16 (15%)	19 (17%)	43 (39%)	31 (28%)	109 (100%)
Estimated number of places	184 (4%)	1,080 (21%)	2,942 (57%)	927 (18%)	5,133 (100%)
Estimated number of attenders on each day open	157 (4%)	753 (19%)	2,291 (57%)	784 (20%)	3,985 (100%)

The need to estimate numbers of places and attenders arose specifically in relation to voluntary units, eight of which recorded neither the number of attenders nor the number of places, and a further eleven of which did not record number of places. Among the other units, only two SSD community centres failed to give number of places, and one AHA unit to give number of attenders. The estimates were made taking account of number of attenders, size of unit (that is, number of places), occupancy rates and, where significant, the relationship between them. In all but the voluntary sector, the margin of error can be assumed to be small. If all missing information was excluded, voluntary day centres would have 38 per cent of places and 52 per cent of attenders. Voluntary units with above-average numbers of attenders were less likely to report the number of places, and this has been allowed for in the estimation.

adaptations have sometimes made a day hospital more like a day centre, and a day centre in a residential home more akin to a day hospital, but on the whole there appears to be a reasonably well-understood agenda of priorities for each service. This is despite the fact that in practice it is rare to find more than one service provider serving the same district and therefore the same group of elderly people. For this reason it is possible to argue that not all these places can be used rationally. On the other hand, given the dominance of day care for the elderly by the voluntary agencies who have sponsored units on a local *ad hoc* basis, it is possible to argue that some of this provision, at least, might not be there if planning for day care had awaited the deliberations of a co-ordinated working party!

A third issue for discussion is that the more disabled old people attend day care less often than their more sprightly peers. One wonders how much use such day care can be to relatives who are trying to share the heavy load. For example, if a user only attends a unit for three days a week, will the person looking after him be able to go out to work or lead a life which in any way is not centred around the care of the old person? (Edwards *et al.*, 1980). It is clear that the problem of providing day services for the most frail elderly is not only consequent on finding places in day centres for one or two days a week for them. At any rate this is less of a problem than finding adequate transport to day centres for the frail elderly. Many old people, of course, need specially adapted transport, which volunteers and private cars cannot provide. However, it is unrealistic to expect that the mere presence of day centres will do a great deal to substitute for the entry of old people to residential and hospital care until the linkage between the kind of day service, its number of places and adequate transport is explored more thoroughly.

ROUTES

Other chapters in this book which discuss day services for the elderly in particular are:

Chapter 5:   'Meeting Other People, Having Cups of Tea': Giving Practical Services
Chapter 8:   'Back to Life': Aiming at Clinical Assessment and Treatment
Chapter 10:   'I'm Just a Nuisance': Aiming To Relieve Relatives
Chapter 15:   'Life in a Home': Preparing Users for Institutions.

NOTES

1 To constitute a day unit in an old people's home there needed to be one day attender for every four residents.
2 On the day that these observations were made, the blinds were pulled low in these two day rooms, and there was a pronounced smell of urine. No activities were provided for users, and a bell was rung to inform slumbering users of tea and meal times. Residents and day users proceeded to a queue in the dining room and were handed pre-milked, pre-sugared tea from a servery hatch.
3 These centres did not include that substantial form of provision for old people which operates purely as luncheon clubs. Only units open at least three to four hours per day, at least three days per week, with defined 'care givers' present, were included in the study. A pilot study indicated that the number of places available for old people in luncheon clubs far exceeded the number available in day centres, but we do not have the definitive figures on this.
4 This finding needs to be treated with some caution, because the definition of 'a place' in a voluntary centre was less precise than in centres run by social services departments.
5 The sample of heads interviewed included thirteen heads in voluntary centres, the heads of ten day hospitals, those in charge of eight social services centres, and three day centres in residential homes. Aside from the heads, we interviewed forty-eight volunteers in voluntary centres, forty staff in geriatric day hospitals, twenty-seven in community-based social services centres, and twelve in residential homes.
6 For definitions of 'adequacy' see Chapter 8.
7 Only one fifty-place day hospital had the services of a full-time speech therapist. The same unit was also the only one with a full-time chiropodist.
8 The information which follows comes from seventy-nine users interviewed in voluntary centres, sixty-one in geriatric day hospitals, fifty-seven in community-based social services centres and eighteen in day care in residential homes.
9 Interviewers reported that twelve (20 per cent) of the patients interviewed in geriatric day hospitals suffered from speech disorders which affected the interview. Of these, half were able to complete about seven-eighths of the interview and deal with 'open'

questions in full sentences. Most of the rest were able to deal with 'closed' questions (with yes/no answers), but had trouble with answering open questions in full sentences.

10 Users were asked whether they had felt depressed – 'unhappy, in low spirits, downcast or gloomy' in the past month, and then *how often* they had felt depressed and *how long* the depression lasted. Their responses were rated by two independent workers (Ann Glampson and Dr B. Williams, a research psychiatrist) on a four-point scale: no depression, slight, moderate, or severe depression.

11 Ninety-eight per cent of the 215 elderly users were 'satisfied' with the centre.

12 Leaving because a user did not like the unit was a little more common in the day units run by the voluntary agencies and the health authorities than the social services units. For another account of this, see Hildick Smith (1977), who found that 12 per cent of the patients in three day hospitals in Kent were 'refusers'. Tunstall (1966) has also interviewed old people who were critical of voluntary day centres.

13 In the chapter on the programmes in the companion volume to this book this point is discussed in more detail (Edwards and Carter, 1980). Activities were classified by the amount of *interchange* between people they created, and also according to whether or not a *skill* was required. Two-thirds of the social activities in units for the elderly required neither interchange nor skill.

14 This is in contrast to centres for the elderly in Belgium, France and Switzerland, where the core activity seems to be 'les gymnastiques'. For example, every small village in the Vaud region of Switzerland has a weekly gym class for old people.

REFERENCES

Attias-Donfut, C. (1977) *Les Centres de Jour: Note de Synthèse* (Le Ministère de la Santé et La Caisse Nationale de l'Assurance Vieillesse).

Brocklehurst, J. C. (1970) *The Geriatric Day Hospital* (King Edward Hospital Fund).

Edwards, C. and Sinclair, I. A. C. (1980) Debate: Segregation versus integration, *Social Work Today*, Vol. 11, No 40, pp. 19–21.

Edwards, C., Sinclair, I. A. C. and Gorbach, P. D. (1980) Day Centres for the Elderly: Variations in Type, Provision and User Response *Br. J. Social Work*, Vol. 10, pp. 419–30.

Edwards, C. and Carter, J. (1980) *The Data of Day Care* (National Institute for Social Work, London).

Eliot, T. S. (1969) 'The Four Quartets', in *The Complete Poems and Plays of T. S. Eliot* (Faber).

Hildick Smith, M. (1974) 'A typical journey to and from the day hospital', *Gerontologica Clinica*, 16 (5–6), pp. 263–9.

Hildick Smith, M. (1977) *Study of Day Hospitals,* Dissertation for the degree of MD, University of Cambridge School of Clinical Medicine.

Kaim Caudle, P. (1977) *The Sunderland Mobile Day Centre* (Help the Aged).

National Corporation for the Care of Old People (1978) *Outpatient Ambulance Transport* (National Corporation for the Care of Old People).

Thomson, A. P. (1949) Problems of ageing and chronic sickness, *British Medical Journal*, 30 July, pp. 243–50.

Tunstall, J. (1966) *Old and Alone: A Sociological Study of Old People* (Routledge & Kegan Paul).

Weiler, P. G. and Rathbone-McCuan, E. (1978) *Adult Day Care: Community Work with the Elderly* (Springer).

Day Hospitals and Transport
Patients who attend day hospitals are often *very* elderly (half those in the survey were over 75 years) and immobile (only an eighth of patients could walk outdoors unaccompanied). So the task of transporting such frail folk to the day hospital is daunting. Add to this the fact that only a couple of patients attended five days a week, while half came two days a week, and this gives the day hospital staff a massive planning exercise. In fact this job was often undertaken by the charge nurse or sister-in-charge of the day hospital, as evident from the relatively large proportion of her working week spent on administration.

Most day hospitals relied on NHS ambulance services, and since ambulance drivers were required to do other duties, as well as meeting emergencies, this was a predictable recipe for frustration. Two-thirds of the day hospitals complained of problems in timing the service to meet their units' timetable and the patients' convenience. Other common difficulties were the length of collection routes, necessitating a very long trip for some patients (two-fifths complained of this), and industrial problems – particularly drivers' strikes and 'work to rule' (a fifth). However, a sixth of day hospitals experienced no difficulties with transport, and when transport works well the patients are clearly grateful and feel the drivers play an important part in their treatment. For example: 'I was sick on the ambulance today, but the driver was very kind', 'I'm very satisfied, the drivers are very kind and cheerful'. Some of the difficulties of providing services from the point of view of the ambulance service are outlined by NCCOP (1978).

Problems in dealing with the ambulance service figured prominently in the discussions of two-fifths of staff in geriatric day hospitals when talking of the frustrations they experienced in their jobs. In social services departments and voluntary day centres, where transport services were very rarely centrally based as in the NHS, significantly fewer staff mentioned transport problems as a frustration in their jobs. The frustration amongst day hospital staff was not matched by users – only a couple of users felt any improvements were necessary to the transport service they were offered. So clearly, the relationship between the day hospital and the ambulance service needs attention if tensions are to be reduced. An experiment with a unit-based driver, working perhaps on a part-time basis or within the day hospital itself, may be helpful in reducing timetabling difficulties and industrial problems. The length of collection routes will persist as a problem, particularly in rural areas (Hildick Smith, 1974).

CHAPTER 3.2

THE MENTALLY HANDICAPPED

INTRODUCTION

Three out of every five centres for the mentally handicapped have opened since 1970. The size of centres is on the increase too: whereas the size of the average centre opened since 1973 is 120 places, the average centre opened in the 1960s had eighty-five places.

This section begins with a report of a visit to a centre. The intention is to convey the impact of the centre on a visitor by detailing some of the relations between the staff and users observed in the visit. One centre can hardly represent a 'typical' centre; although a number of ways in which the Brightways centre is similar to others will be mentioned during the text which follows.

A VISIT TO BRIGHTWAYS

At midday at Brightways adult training centre, the first 'dinner' sitting feeds about eighty. Mentally handicapped users, called 'trainees' at this centre, are mostly young people, although the oldest, aged 55, has been a 'trainee' in three or four centres for the past twenty-five years. They wait in the lunch queue for the servery hatch in the cafeteria to bang open and when it does, the queue, which trails out of the cafeteria along the corridor, lunges forward. The trainees are noisy; chatter and laughter is contrapuntal to the undertones of woodwork machines. There is a scuffle here, a quick snog there. Doors to the corridor open and close as people emerge from workshops and lavatories to join the queue; a few disappear behind a door marked 'Private – Staff Only'.

In some training centres, men and women still queue separately for lunch and sit at different tables, but not here. There is a choice of menu: fish fingers, or steak and kidney pudding, chocolate mousse or roly-poly. Food is paid for at a cash register, and cutlery is selected from a tray. The cafeteria is a functional modern room with eight large formica-topped tables. At the table closest to the door, two middle-aged women hover between wheelchairs and spoon chocolate mousse into receptive dribbling mouths. These are the 'special care' cases: eight multiply-handicapped young people, all immobile, incontinent and unable to speak. Not all training centres have special care units, and very few go to the effort of bringing such people down to the dining room for lunch. Now they process in a formation of wheelchairs pushed by staff to their room, a cheerful place decorated with mobiles and painted egg cartons. Part of the floor is massed protectively with banks of foam rubber to avoid damaging uncontrolled, banging heads.

Back at the dining room, trainees return plates to the servery and make their way along the corridor. At the stairs, four of them turn and go upstairs to the sitting room, presumably to watch television. Three young men, all rather overweight, perhaps mongols, make for the entrance foyer. Ignoring the discreet sign which reads 'Visitors Only', they sit in a small glassed ante-room protruding into the garden. They read tabloid newspapers, peering through their spectacles with intent conscientiousness.

Two girls arm-in-arm leave the centre and the front door slams behind them. The royal family, postered above the door, shiver from side to side as a blast of cold air pours through the heated foyer. The leaves of the logbook on the reception desk blow over. The most recent entry reads 'Marie and Sally. 12.40. Gone for icecream.' In this centre, unusually, trainees can leave the centre at lunchtime, unaccompanied and without seeking permission, as long as they are able to record their absence in the logbook. 'In case of fire', explains the receptionist cryptically.

Back in the recreation room, a space divided by movable dividers from the dining room, there is a lunchtime record session cum discotheque. The music is very loud Manfred Mann, the dancers are flushed, excited and energetic. Most of the first 'dinner' sitting are now there, although if it were not raining outside some of the young men would probably be outside kicking a football.

Back in the 'workshops' a group of workers await second 'dinner'. 'Workshops' are, in reality, one large concreted space, separated by glassed room dividers. Intended by the architects to 'creatively divide space in a spontaneous way', the dividers are now fixed permanently. 'Head Office' regulations: the manager shrugs: he does not know why. Each workshop has enough space for about a dozen workers sitting at benches beside two long trestle tables. This particular workshop has about eight trainees, the 'highfliers' who are thought likely to leave the centre soon for outside jobs. Dust-coated, they screw the parts of electric plugs together. A young woman of about 25, presumably an instructor, sits alone at the table at the top of the room, engrossed in a novel. She puts down her book when we arrive and explains the value of the work the trainees are doing for habit formation and personal discipline. She also considers (in their hearing) that these trainees, like most, do not want to leave the centre for jobs outside. Why should they? They get a bus ride to the centre each day and their girlfriends are here. They get taken swimming once a fortnight. The manager added, 'Some of our more capable people have too soft a life here. They need a more demanding environment.'

Trainees showing 'potential' spend every fourth week in the domestic training flatlet. They cannot stay overnight, but they learn to make the beds and look after the place. Preparing food is important: mostly pretty basic stuff like opening cans of baked beans, making toast and tea. Last night the instructors roughed up the room as if a burglary had taken place: this morning's exercise was to put the room together again. The trainees put the room together again – inserted the lampshade on the base, collected all the forks from the floor and replaced them (washed) in the cutlery drawer.

Next door is the centre's 'shop'. The nearest supermarket is 2 miles away, and not on a bus route from the centre, so 'shopping classes' take place *in situ*. The idea is to teach the trainees how to use money by demonstration rather than by formal classroom teaching. 'Further education' in this centre results from a policy of selective 'creaming' rather than a trainee's universal right: for example, only 2 per cent take part in a literacy class. The manager considers it sensible to conserve his limited staff resources by concentrating education and social training on the 10 per cent of trainees whom he believes will 'progress'.

Checklist: Vital Statistics
The Mentally Handicapped

Number of units in national census	50
Number of units sponsored by social services departments	47
Number of heads and staff interviewed	105[a]
Number of users approached for interview	193
Average size of unit (user places)	97[a]
Range of size of units (user places)	23–175[a]
Average ratio of staff to users	1 : 9

[a] These figures apply only to social services department adult training centres.

Most centres for the mentally handicapped are adult training centres run by local authority social services departments. Practically all of the fifty centres for the mentally handicapped were sponsored by social services departments; of the rest, two were special care units, one run by a local spastics society and the other by an education authority. The third was a day centre 'club' run for prospective trainees of adult training centres by another set of unemployed school leavers, as part of a job creation project.

All centres, including Brightways, are open for five days a week. More users come to centres for the mentally handicapped on each weekday than in other forms of day service, where attendance is more likely to be rotated or confined selectively to particular days of the week. To start the day at the centre, most users come on transport provided by the day unit. In the forty-seven training centres themselves, for example, about 70 per cent of users arrive at the centre on special transport. Only 7 per cent of the users walk, and 16 per cent come on public transport – the local bus service or a train.

Once at the centre, the question is how the day should be organised. Usually the day starts at about 9.30. Trainees alight from transport and leave their belongings in a locker room. Very few centres provide individual hanging space which users can call their own.[1] Then most users move to the workshops. Sometimes a small group uses a small room provided as an education centre. At about 11 a.m. the morning is punctuated by a coffee break in the dining room. Hot drinks are usually served by ancillary staff, and trainees have little involvement – or choice – in this process. (In some centres for instance, users queue for coffee which is already 'milked and sugared'.)[2]

After morning coffee, most trainees in most centres work in the workshops until lunchtime: lunch is almost always served in the centre; cafeteria-style lunches with a choice of menu, and a pay desk as at Brightways, would appear to be unusual. Although nearly all of the centres charge users for their food, collecting the 'dinner money' is often a clerical transaction, once a week, so the user is unable to relate the matter of buying lunch to personal income and expenditure. A choice of menu is also rare. In many centres lunch is transported to the centre from large kitchens which may prepare meals for institutions and meals-on-wheels in the area.

Most units, like Brightways, have separate lunch rooms for the staff, which means that staff rarely eat with users. Separate lunch and – if it comes to that – separate toilet facilities in centres are a feature of the building design of many centres. Thus users and staff have minimal social contact in the human processes of eating and toileting. For example, in five of the eight centres observed, staff ate separately from the users, in separate lunch rooms. In one centre they ate at separate tables but in the same dining room. Only two centres modified the 'separate eating' routines. At Brightways the staff are rostered for a week about, to eat with users at the same tables. In another centre those users 'on duty' in the 'flat' cook lunch once a week and invite some staff to a lunch party. Similarly seven of the eight centres observed had separate toilet facilities. Only half the centres offered users toilets with doors that locked, thus enabling privacy. Two units had users' toilets with all doors which were unlocked. Two units had doors with and without locks. Users' toilets were usually in a reasonable condition of cleanliness.[3]

Returning to the results of the survey, we can confirm that two-thirds of the fifty centres were purpose built.[4] Over a half were in mixed areas of housing and industry or business. A fifth were located in areas of private housing and less than a tenth were found in solidly industrial areas. Most managers were satisfied with their building. Only 14 per cent saw their building as 'unsuitable'.

Two-thirds of managers and instructors (as heads and staff are called in such centres), including those at Brightways, considered that *most* users had spent most time at contract or industrial work in the centre in the previous week. Of those users able to answer the question according to definitions discussed later in the chapter, over half claimed to have spent *most* of their time on contract and industrial work in the centre in the previous week. Contract and industrial work is known to be the staple activity of centres for the mentally handicapped.

In nearly all centres, including Brightways, the simplest kind of work was done without any tools at all, or with the very simplest handtools. For the sake of simplicity we have referred to this as 'simple work'. Three out of five users, on average, were estimated by the managers to do the simplest type of 'simple' work, that without the use of handtools. The most common of these jobs are packing, labelling or assembly work.[5] Packing could involve slotting paint blocks into trays, putting together literature kits for charity appeals, packing bin liners or even bulbs. Labelling was often a straightforward matter of sticking a label to a consignment of aerosol sprays or to hacksaws. A common assembly job involved putting together the pieces of ballpoint pens, or perhaps connecting pieces of the headphones used by airline passengers on intercontinental flights.

Simple work was often part of a contract or sub-contract job from a local industry or from a public sector agency like the area health authority. At many centres like Brightways, handtools were used for sub-contract work: for example, staplers might be used to assemble magazines or to fix packets of string to paper, screwdrivers to screw plugs or cassette cases.

What has been defined as 'simple' work is not the complete work schedule, for some of the centres, although not Brightways, had facilities for providing work with powered tools and machines. Very few centres had their own product on which users could work. One centre manufactured fibreglass canoes for commercial sale, but there was very little attempt to gear work to a marketable product. There was a lot of variation in the actual numbers of users who worked with machines. At one extreme in one centre, for example, only 2 per cent of the users ever used the machines, while at another extreme 80 per cent of the users had spent some time on machine work in the previous week. Machine work most commonly involved using powered handtools like electric drills or wood or metal work machines. It is impossible to judge whether machine work necessarily involves more complex work than the simplest hand-work done by users, but some user opinions about using machines in the case of the sheltered workshops are reviewed in Chapter 12.

Other than simple work and machine work, some 'service' or 'domestic' work was available in some units, although not at Brightways.

This included 'out-of-doors work' like gardening, provided in one-third of centres for very few users, on average. 'Indoors work' using laundry machines was provided in nearly one-fifth of units and domestic work around the centre was offered in a quarter.

'Wages for work' is a central issue at most centres, including Brightways. Users were 'paid' a weekly 'wage' for contract and industrial work which ranged from 4 pence to £1. In all centres the average 'wage' according to the managers was £1.05 weekly; the users interviewed grossed an average weekly 'income' of £1.22. Since users always paid for lunch, and usually for tea, it is not surprising that only a quarter found the system 'very fair'.[6] A woman aged 31 at Brightways asserted: 'We should be paid more – at least £5. My friends and I all say this. I've asked my MP, and he's asked the council, and they said they can't afford more. It would help with my clothes.'

The amount that centres can pay their users is constrained by the fact that once earnings go above a certain minimum then users' supplementary benefits are reduced. At the time of the survey the amount in excess of supplementary benefits that might be earned was £2 per week: but this has now risen to £4 per week. No information is available on how many users actually claim these benefits. (One centre was setting up an advice centre to give information to users and families about welfare rights.) Bonuses were awarded to some users under a number of systems in half the centres: there was some dispute as to whether 'wages' and 'bonuses' should be awarded for effort or for actual production. Some centres also paid bonuses to get rid of cash surplus: 'Once a year each trainee is given two weeks' extra payment when our income exceeds payments.' More often both 'pay' and 'bonuses' were used as mechanisms of control of users' behaviour,[7] as these randomly selected comments make clear.

Payments are based on attendance, hygiene and work performance. (A centre paying a range of 'wages' between £0.80 and £2.00 per week)

We pay no bonus, but deductions can be made from pay for a specified amount as a disciplinary measure. (Centre paying a flat £1.00 per week for trainees under 21, £1.50 for those over 21)

The bonus scheme grades the trainees on the following: time-keeping, effort, behaviour, response to authority, cleanliness. (Centre paying a range between nothing and a top limit of £2.00 per week)

The significance of work for the users in centres for the mentally handicapped discussed in Chapter 6 indicates that some users were far from neutral about the work they were expected to do in the centre. When criticisms and suggestions about improvements to the centres were made it was the activities that came in for strongest reproach. Most laments of those one-third of users with complaints or suggestions for improvements were about the work programme. This is detailed in Chapter 6 and 17, but meanwhile one example comes from a young woman who said: 'They could teach us more workwise, more about other jobs and how to do them. It's bad not having a change of work. I was in the workshop until I was transferred to the kitchen, but it was too noisy there so I asked for the workshop again, because I got headaches.'

Industrial contract work programmes were also a matter of contention amongst staff. A minority of one in seven managers and instructors wanted to jettison the work altogether and a further fifth made it clear that in their view, the amount of contract and industrial work in the programme should be reduced. The lobby to reduce the work programme is given some significance by its uniqueness, for no one wanted to *reduce other* activities in the centres at all. What is more, work ranked at the bottom of the list of activities thought to be a critical 'priority' in the centres. In other words, there was no opinion that work should be increased, but heightened enthusiasm for more educational classes, more arts and crafts, increased social activities, frequent treatment, and even more meetings and discussion groups, in that order. Those were seen by managers and instructors as more pertinent to the programme they would like to develop than industrial and contract work programmes.

Both staff and users were interested in the impact of education classes. Staff wanted more education classes, and Chapter 6 discusses the 'education-consciousness' of some users, for nearly a quarter claimed that educational classes were an important achievement of the centre. But although managers said that they offered education classes almost as often as work programmes, in practice far fewer users got educational than work programmes. For example, three-quarters of the centres offered literacy classes. In three centres every single user was said to have been at a literacy class in the previous week. But this was rare: in over a third of the centres less than a third of the users were in literacy programmes. In fact, across the board, a user in a mental handicap centre stood about a 1 : 4 chance of getting into a literacy class. One of the 2 per cent of users at Brightways who took part in a literacy class, a 23-year-old man at the centre for six months, said: 'I've come on quite a lot in the education part. Reading and arithmetic. I couldn't get on with it at all before I came here.'

Educational classes as at present offered to mentally handicapped people might be conceived in two ways. First, there are what might be termed 'survival' classes – those classes carefully transmitting information basic to an individual's survival in the outside world. Examples are literacy and numeracy classes, the shopping groups and cookery classes at Brightways, and also the self-care classes. 'Social competence' classes, which include training in how to use transport, and so on, could be included here too. On the other hand, extras which – whilst scarcely educational 'frills' – add dimensions to a quality of life rather than ensuring basic survival, include the drama classes, the music groups and the current affairs teaching.

These groups (of which there were none at Brightways, and in general very few in centres for mental handicap) are rather less fundamental than the 'survival' classes. Paradoxically, very few centres encourage users to become members of further education facilities in their local community and, as already noted, education is conceived as a formally run didactic programme, rather than as an ethos which integrates the routines of the centre.

Social activities are available in most units. Most popular are record sessions (as at Brightways) and outdoor sports, particularly cricket and football. Four of every five centres offer arts and crafts to users, but only one unit in every four has a trained art teacher, which may account for the prevalence of the more prosaic painting, sewing and knitting over the more esoteric media of weaving, pottery and mosaics. Physical treatments can be found in just over half the centres. Brightways is unique in having a sessional speech therapist, but most treatments actually constitute the administration of users' drugs. (About one in eight users were estimated to be 'on drugs' dispensed but not prescribed by the centre.) General nursing care (bathing, toileting, feeding) is viewed as 'treatment' in over a third of the centres, while keep fit classes are run by about a fifth of the centres for under half the users.

Although meetings and discussion groups are not held at Brightways, just over a third of the centres say they sponsor discussion groups for half of the users, while a small number of centres – one in twelve – claimed to run a 'therapy' group orientated to discussing personal problems of users.

GETTING INTO THE CENTRE

Most users arrive literally at the centre on special transport, as they do at Brightways. But by what symbolic road do they travel to the centre? In two of the thirteen areas, assessment centres have been developed recently to channel school leavers to the 'right' placement, which may or may not be a training centre. (But these centres only cater for a fraction of users, aged between 16 and 19 years.) The three most common obstacles likely to debar a potential user's admission to the centre were cited by managers as aggressive or disruptive behaviour, incontinence and inability to walk.

The symbolic 'gatekeepers' to centres for the mentally handicapped (that is, those who are quoted most consistently by managers as the initiators of referrals) are in this order: the local authority social worker, the hospital social worker, the family of the trainee, the hospital doctor, the disablement resettlement officer, and the education authority. As Chapter 6 makes clear, at present the decision to admit a person to a centre for mental handicap is a critical one, for once in the training centre most users are unlikely to leave it. In nearly three-quarters of the units, managers predict that 90 per cent or more of the users will stay in the centre for the rest of their lives. As two-thirds of the centres had no one at all on their waiting lists, this implies that the route into the training centre is taken rather more easily than the road out of it. (The most common reason for leaving a centre is to move to another one.) In fact managers say that less than one in ten of the users leaving the centre go into open employment, and only one in every twenty-five leavers go into sheltered work. (It is worth noting too that one in five of the mentally handicapped people able to answer questions on this study claimed to have had jobs outside the centre at some time in the recent past, before their present time in the training centre. However, there is no way of checking this.)

The increasing size of centres for the mentally handicapped has been made clear already. On average, there is one direct service staff member for every nine trainees.[8] But there was a wide range of staff offering a direct service to users: for instance, to take the two extremes, in an assessment unit there was a 1 : 1 correspondence between staff and trainee, while in another centre there were twenty-four trainees for every staff member.

PEOPLE IN CENTRES FOR THE MENTALLY HANDICAPPED: (1) THE USERS

So far this chapter has mentioned that information was solicited directly from mentally handicapped users. For instance, at Brightways, although we met many of the trainees, we interviewed only six users. Their names were drawn at random from the register. One of these names came from the special care unit, and this lad could answer no questions at all. Another 22-year-old enjoyed the attention of the interview, although he was only able to answer the 'factual' questions about where he lived and how old he was. The other four interviewees responded keenly to being interviewed, as it offered an opportunity to talk over their activities, friends and staff at the centre. Interviewing mentally handicapped – or more correctly those people labelled as mentally handicapped – about their experiences of health or social services is a rare research practice.[9] Usually the family, or the teacher or manager, mediates a view of a mentally handicapped person to administrators or researchers (Bayley, 1973; Whelan and Speake, 1977). In fact researchers are sometimes positively dissuaded from talking to mentally handicapped people directly. Findings of other projects report 'questionable comprehension' or 'limited span of attention' as well as 'difficulties in verbal expression', and suggest that talking to the mentally handicapped is an unrewarding task for busy researchers interested in reliable and valid findings.[10]

On the other hand, there is a less well-documented viewpoint which coincides with our own point of view: that these cautions are based solely on the deficits of the mentally handicapped, and that more research effort could be put into finding out about their abilities.[11] We had been impressed by the competence and liveliness of some of the mentally handicapped users we met during the pilot phase of the project: we saw no rational reason for excluding them, as a group of users of day services, from the national survey. Further, we thought that it might be useful to see how people labelled as 'mentally handicapped' managed when asked to respond to an interview devised for a wider group of people. How many people within training centres could actually manage to cope with a research interview at least an hour long, and deal with a mixture of concrete and abstract questions and probes?

The assumption underlying our research interview was that it was more akin to a conversation with a purpose, than a test which almost by definition, the mentally handicapped were bound to fail. The assumption was that the order of the interview should remain fairly fixed, but that the language of the questions could be adapted by interviewers to get a response from individual users. No preconceptions should be made about the user's ability to deal with each question. In this way it was hoped that the user's view of the service would be obtained.[12] Rationally, it did not seem that obtaining information about attitudes on this basis could be seen as any less reliable or valid than interviewing other people such as parents or instructors on the users' behalf.

With some trepidation, nevertheless, we selected at random the names of 193 users in twenty-seven day units. These names included even those users which common sense or the opinion of staff debarred from interview: for example, there were those 'special care cases': people who could not speak and who sometimes did not respond either. Nevertheless, it was a rule that all potential respondents had to be approached by an interviewer. In the end 154 users of the 193 (80 per cent) were able to contribute in some way to the interview, leaving 20 per cent of the interviews as 'abandoned'.

Contributions 'in some way' need to be defined more carefully. For example, fifty-four users (25 per cent) were able to complete the interview in so competent a way that they were indistinguishable from users in other groups who took part in the survey. For instance, these mentally handicapped (or so labelled) users understood all (or a minimum of seven-eighths) of the questions put to them. They gave purposeful answers to 'open-ended' questions.[13] They composed their answers in sentences. When the interviewer 'probed', they were able to 'extend' their answer by giving more detail relevant to the question. A number of examples are provided in Chapter 6.

A further forty (21 per cent) of the users understood most of the questions put to them (at least seven-eighths), but they answered the 'open' questions in short phrases or by one- or two-word replies. These phrases implied that the user understood the *gist* of the question but lacked either the language ability or the opinions, or both, to expand answers beyond a phrase.

Then there were sixty users (31 per cent) who struggled through the interview, understanding some questions but not others. Questions of 'fact' in the interview – for example, inquiries about the user's age, where he lived and with whom – were answered more readily than matters of 'opinion', of which more were 'not understood' by the user. For example, when asked by one interviewer if he helped to run the centre, a 20-year-old reported enthusiastically, 'Oh yes, I run and run and run.' Replying with careful dignity to what must have seemed an idiotic query which asked if she 'had meals on wheels', one girl said, 'No, I have my meals right here, on the table.' It would be premature to conclude that these young people lacked ability to think in abstract terms alone, for one – unquantifiable – impression left after these interviews was that many mentally handicapped users in day centres come from extremely protected social backgrounds. Home and centre may fail to expose mentally handicapped users to many of the routine understandings by which the rest of us make sense of and run our lives. In the absence of exposure to such matters, why should the young people mentioned above know much about worker participation or about the operation of welfare domiciliary services? The environment in which mentally handicapped children develop is unlike that of normal children, and the relevant studies to produce norms for the development of the mentally handicapped have not been done. Thus it is impossible to say whether gaps in understanding and language are 'real' deficits or socially induced by the differences in upbringing, social circumstances and schooling of children with assessed mental handicaps (Ryan, 1973).

The detail which follows comes from those 154 users who were interviewed.[14] Although these users ranged in age from 16 to 64, nearly three-quarters were under the age of 35. Ninety-eight per cent were single, and four out of five live at home with parents or with other relatives. The rest lived in hostels, hospitals or residential care. Fifty-seven per cent of the users were male. In response to a direct question, nearly half the users denied suffering from either a physical or a mental handicap. But of the half who did confess to suffering from a handicap, the largest group reported 'bad nerves' or 'being unable to cope with pressure'. Some users volunteered information about their mental handicap in discussion separate to their views of their health. This implies that mental handicap may be perceived less as a health deficit and more as a social characteristic by those who bear this label. This deserves further exploration.

When it came to looking after themselves, the mentally handicapped are, perhaps, the most socially dependent group in day services. While 85 per cent[15] say that they can climb a stairway without help, only 70 per cent say they can walk a short distance down the road unaccompanied. Only four out of ten can travel on public transport alone whenever necessary. And although nearly all claim to be able to feed themselves and dress themselves, a few more said they needed help with bathing. But only a quarter said they went shopping without help, a fifth could do their washing on their own, and one in seven thought they could cook a hot meal without help.

PEOPLE IN CENTRES FOR THE MENTALLY HANDICAPPED: (2) MANAGERS AND INSTRUCTORS

There is a clear dividing line between those who work in the centres for the mentally handicapped and those who attend them, compared to some other user groups. But the divide between the centre and the community is wider. For as the managers and instructors see it, the most important outstanding requirement that mentally handicapped people lack from the community is acceptance and tolerance.[16] But the gulf between community and centre is not the only one the managers and instructors mentioned. More people working in centres for the mentally handicapped spoke of a gulf in understanding and communication between themselves and their headquarters (usually a social services department). Fewer workers than in other user groups considered that they had enough understanding and information on the day care policies of their employing body. Fewer considered that they had sufficient support and advice on the problems they encountered in the job. This matter is taken up in Chapter 17.

1964 is often considered to be a landmark in the care of the mentally handicapped, because a special form of training was started for their teachers. Before the development of the Diploma of the Training Council for Teachers of the Mentally Handicapped, there was no special training prescribed (apart from one pioneer course run by the National Association for Mental Health). Since 1964 these one-year courses have continued in colleges of further education, but they are shortly to be discontinued in favour of a new form of training for all residential and day services workers, the Certificate in Social Services (CSS).

Over a third of the 500 who worked directly in the fifty centres with the mentally handicapped were trained, and almost nine out of ten managers had undergone this special training, including the man at Brightways. Of the rest of those working with mental handicap, one-third have trades qualifications and a quarter have no training at all. But the number of staff trained in other disciplines such as speech therapy, psychology or social work is minute, as Chapter 6 points out.

What reasons did the managers and instructors give for working with the mentally handicapped? For nearly half the instructors, the motivation expressed was a strong interest in the field of mental handicap. For example, a deputy manager, a former secretary, said, 'I became interested in these people. I wanted to transfer to instructing, and applied for the first vacancy.' Of a second group, a quarter had been bored and fed up with previous work and wanted a complete change of field and scene: 'I wanted to work with people', said a 46-year-old former insurance cashier. 'I got dissatisfied with all the computerising of insurance work, and I wanted a job that was worthwhile, rather than dealing with figures and pieces of paper'.

More instructors working with the mentally handicapped than any of the other groups, nominated a personal knowledge of mental handicap as the reason precipitating their move into the field. For example, one 60-year-old instructor, a former clerk at the gas board, still untrained, said, 'The main thing is that I have a mentally handicapped sister, and in some way I thought I could help the handicapped.' Among managers, the 'personal advantages of the job' were mentioned more frequently than a pressing interest in mental handicap as predominant reasons for taking on the present job. 'It was mainly the money', said a 36-year-old former ambulance driver, now the head of a centre with seventy-five places. 'It was a higher-grade job in a forward-looking authority.'

Qualified and unqualified instructors are really of much the same range of age, but one way in which they differ is in their views on training. Twice as many of the qualified staff (those who had achieved the one-year Diploma for Teachers of the Mentally Handicapped) wanted further full-time training as did their unqualified colleagues. Unqualified instructors, less positive than the qualified about wanting training, said, when pressed, that in their view the strongest rationale for getting qualified was the status or promotion it would provide. Even though rather more than half left school at age 15 or earlier, they rarely wanted qualifications for their own personal development. Shorter 'in-service' training was more attractive to both qualified and unqualified instructors than extended vocational qualifications. Half affirmed that no in-service training had been proffered them – not even a seminar – in the previous twelve months.

For the trained staff the proposed new form of training, the Certificate in Social Services (CSS), was not seen as a satisfactory substitute.[17] Training additional to the one-year diploma – particularly more teaching and education skills – was requested because most instructors assessed their diploma to have been helpful so far as it went, but to be basically inadequate. 'The educational aspects of the course were inadequate', said one instructor. 'We were supposed to come out and teach reading and writing and numbering, but they didn't dwell on it long enough for us to teach it well to mentally handicapped people.'

Are those who become managers more ambitious, and does climbing the ladder imply a 'cool out' of idealistic motivations? This is unclear, but certainly the leadership of training centres is in the hands of a well-established group: over half the managers had been in their current jobs for five years or more, and nearly one-third had been in their post for eight years or more.[18]

By contrast, over half the instructors had been in their present post for less than two years, and when one compares the backgrounds of the particular group of instructors who have been at their jobs for less than two years there are more who are women and more who are untrained.[19]

At Brightways, as in other centres, this group does not hold the relevant diplomas, or any other qualification, for that matter. They have come, on the whole, from occupations[20] classified as skilled non-manual or clerical, such as secretarial or accounting jobs. But those instructors who have been at their posts for five years or more are more likely to be men than women. More of them are trained (in that they hold the diploma), but more are recruited from skilled manual jobs. There appears to be a tendency for the number of men coming from skilled manual jobs to have decreased, but then, this particular group has also shrunk in the workforce at large. Likewise, the increase in the number of untrained women from skilled clerical jobs working with the mentally handicapped may mirror the increased presence of women in the workforce in general, rather than a conscious shift in recruitment policies in mental handicap from men to women. So if women from skilled clerical backgrounds comprise the the largest group of recent entrants to the workforce in mental handicap centres, skilled clerical jobs supply a third of the staff of centres.

Of the qualified heads and instructors, nearly three-quarters left school at the age of 15 or earlier, so it is not surprising that a one-year course was judged to be inadequate. (This is a younger school-leaving age than that of most trainees in ATCs: in other words, many instructors have a shorter period of formal education than the trainees they teach). 'I wish I had taken some "O" levels before doing this course', said a 41-year-old former housemother in a children's home, who left school at 15. 'When I took the diploma course I had not been to school for seventeen years, and was a bit rusty.'

COMMENT

The growth of adult training centres needs to pause to ask the question 'growth for what?'. Unlike other forms of day services, day services for the mentally handicapped are a virtual monopoly – nearly all provided by social services departments.[21] By contrast, as we have seen, services for the elderly, which are offered by health authorities and voluntary agencies as well as social services departments, often lack a rational plan to their provision. One question is: to what extent is monopoly combined with expertise? This problem will be discussed in Chapter 6.

Centres themselves are nearly always organised in a hierarchy. There are so few staff trained in other disciplines to incorporate into the running of the centre, and instructors (either untrained or trained to the one-year diploma) form a hierarchy which extends from the most junior member of the centre to the manager, then through the principal officer(s) to the Director of Social Services. Within the centre itself there is some evidence to suggest that the staff are unhappy about aspects of this hierarchy, finding the extensions outside the centre remote and alienated from their day-to-day task. This may not be unconnected from the 'distance' the managers and staff feel obliged to maintain from the users, together with their reluctance – and perhaps inability – to get users more involved in the day-to-day running of the centre.

This could relate to the background from which managers and instructors are recruited. Coming as they do from the factory, or from positions in the office, most managers and instructors are used already to working in hierarchies. The transfer from the factory or office to working to ill-defined objectives about people – which include developing both coherent policies for the centre and detailed individualised plans for users – is a formidable task of thinking and practicality. The truncated training offered the staff, the relative lack of in-service development and the gaps in local consultative back-up and support services are apparent.

There is little pressure on waiting lists and not much turnover in the centres. Yet all thirteen areas have under-provided places for the mentally handicapped in terms of the interim target number of places for people in centres recommended by the government. (In fact, two-thirds of the areas would need to double their provision overnight to achieve interim government targets of 1.5 places per 1,000.) The question is: does the relative lack of pressure on training centre places, and the expected lifelong stay of most of the users, reduce pressure to get some users out of the centre and back into the outside world?

Associated with this is the trend to building bigger training centres. There is a very wide range of people labelled as mentally handicapped; yet most centres treat the mentally handicapped as homogeneous. Separate programmes and outlets for each user need to be developed: Chapter 18 gives an example. Otherwise, day services for mental handicap may become little more than big buildings in which the mentally handicapped are protected from the outside world – an outcome which is a long way from their intention.

ROUTES

Chapter 6 discusses issues related specifically to the centres for the mentally handicapped at greater length.

NOTES

1 The information which follows came from observations carried out by researchers in eight adult training centres. These centres were not a random sample. Most personal belongings are left in shared locker or hanging space. Only one unit had space for individual lockers. (See also Curtis and Edwards, 1977.)

2 These observations and those which follow were made in eight ATCs (not a random sample). In the one centre where users helped to prepare tea or coffee, their role was restricted to washing up the staff teacups. Usually staff took their tea or coffee separately, in a separate room.

3 But in one centre the observation notes read: 'Staff toilet is locked to users, but inside is very clean and hygienic. But users' toilets have no locks on the door. The basins are cracked and dirty and dusty, the floors are covered with debris and pools of urine.'

4 The building 'type' of the ATC relates to the programme the centre offers. See Curtis and Edwards (1977), who examine three different building types of ATCs. The first type, built to the specifications of the DHSS Building Note No. 5 ATCs 1972 (DHSS, 1972) is a single-storey building dominated by a workshop and also reinforcing divisions between users and staff by provision of separate facilities. The second type is a one-off architect-designed centre, like Brightways. The third type is usually a conversion, often where staff and users are forced to share facilities and make more use of outside eating and recreational facilities.

5 The classification of work activities which follows is derived from the work of Whelan and Speake (1977).

6 By contrast, half the managers and instructors thought *their* own pay was 'about right'. A third thought it was too little, considering the work they did.

7 For a comprehensive critique of the content of work offered to adult mentally handicapped people and methods of payment, see Grant *et al.* (1973), Coulter (1977).

8 These figures, based on the number of direct service staff (those who deal directly with users), include managers but do not include the support staff such as clerks, drivers or domestics. A recent survey of ATCs (Whelan and Speake, 1977) found a ratio of staff to trainees of 1 : 9. Guidelines issued in *Better Services for the Mentally Handicapped* (DHSS, 1971) recommend 1.5 places per 1,000 population 'as an interim target'. As there were about 4,670 places in the thirteen areas, another 3,600 places would need to be provided to meet these targets. The long-term future should include a target of 2.4 places per 1,000 to cater for 'substantial numbers of adults coming by day from hospital'. In this study, only 2 per cent of trainees say they live in hospital, while 14 per cent live in hostels or residential homes. This information parallels Whelan's estimate (Whelan and Speake, 1977).

9 Two exceptions are described by Birenbaum and Seiffer (1976) and London Borough of Wandsworth Social Services Department (1977).

10 Studies which summarise this point of view are outlined by Hogg (1973).

11 In fact, one possible effect of studies such as those reported by Hogg (1973) is to reinforce the label of mental handicap itself. In other words, the label (not the intrinsic handicap) implies that key characteristics are standard to all mentally handicapped individuals. These characteristics become stereotypes which become more powerful factors in predicting the attitudes and behaviour of the mentally handicapped than the actual behaviour itself.

12 See, for example, Richardson *et al.* (1965). In their terms, a 'schedule standardised interview' was prepared, the question wording and sequence being determined in advance. However, the interviewers were taught what information was required from respondents, and allowed to vary parts of the interview wording and sequence to ensure maximal effectiveness with each respondent.
    A brief version of the preparation and training of interviewers is in Appendix I and a detailed account is given in Edwards and Carter (1980). Briefly, attempts were made to break a defined question down into small components to get an answer. If the question 'What kind of accommodation do you live in at present?' met no response, the interviewer was asked to adapt the question wording, for example:
    Q. Where do you live?
    A. With my mum and dad.
    Q. So you all live in a house, or a flat, or what?
    Using this tactic, 90 per cent of mentally handicapped users were able to answer this question. The interviewer discussed the reply with the interviewee until satisfied that she and the interviewee were both clear about the answer. If an answer was not forthcoming finally, the interviewer coded the question 'not understood'. We are clear that this code refers to the *outcome* of the discussion between the interviewer and interviewee, and does not imply a label about the interviewee.

13 The user interview contained twenty-four 'open' questions (that is largely 'attitude' or 'opinion' questions where the range of possible responses was not specified or precoded in advance). There were seventy-six 'closed' questions (that is, questions with precoded

answers). Both questions probed issues of 'fact', beliefs about facts, feelings and behaviour, and reasons for beliefs and behaviour.

14 As already discussed, the proportion of users responding to each question varied, so to deal with this the proportions reported in this section are calculated according to the responses of the users answering a particular question.

15 On average, twenty users of 168 could not answer any of the following questions. The percentages quoted are calculated on a base of 168 users.

16 More of those staffing centres for the mentally handicapped (56 per cent) and for offenders (50 per cent) stated this. The next most frequent requesters of 'acceptance' for their users were those working with the mentally ill (33 per cent).

17 Those already qualified, particularly the managers, were a little less enthusiastic than their untrained colleagues about 'progressing' to the CSS qualification. Their criticisms related to the slender amount of time devoted to teaching educational practice, the 'generality' of the course, and its lack of specificity for mental handicap.

> I don't have a high opinion of the new course because it's too short. It would appear not to provide a sufficient range of experiences, and there's not enough emphasis on educational practices.
>
> For me personally, an extension of the [present] course would be more valid. The CSS as I see it embraces other disciplines, which in itself is not bad, but that will result in a dilution of what is presently being undertaken, as opposed to a development of it.

18 Long service also characterised the heads of units for the physically handicapped, mentally ill and elderly, where 37–47 per cent had served for over five years.

19 In order to compare the trained and untrained groups it is assumed that the more recently appointed staff are new entrants to day services for mental handicap. This assumption cannot be checked, so this evidence should be treated with some caution: there is no information about the mobility of staff *between* day centres. The average length of service in day centres for the mentally handicapped was three-and-a-half years per staff member.

20 The job which the respondent had for the longest period in the past was coded according to a modification of the Registrar General's Scale on Social Classes. Skilled non-manual occupations are equivalent broadly to Social Class 3a of this scale.

21 There are a few day hospitals for the mentally handicapped sponsored by area health authorities, but very few. For a listing consult the Hospital & Health Services Year Book (Institute of Health Administrators).

REFERENCES

Bayley, M. (1973) *Mental Handicap and Community Care: A Study of Mentally Handicapped People in Sheffield* (Routledge & Kegan Paul).

Birenbaum, A. and Seiffer, S. (1976) *Resettling Retarded Adults in a Managed Community* (Martin Robertson).

Coulter, R. (1977) *No Longer a Child* (Campaign for the Mentally Handicapped).

Curtis, J. and Edwards, C. (1977) *The Environment of the Adult Training Centre: A Critical Appraisal* (Medical Architecture Research Unit, The Polytechnic of North London).

Department of Health and Social Security (1971) *Better Services for the Mentally Handicapped*, Cmnd 4683 (HMSO).

Department of Health and Social Security (1972) *Local Authority Building Note No. 5 Adult Training Centres*, (HMSO).

Edwards, C. and Carter, J. (1980) *The Data of Day Care* (National Institute for Social Work, London).

Grant, G. W. B., Moores, B. and Whelan, E. (1973) 'Assessing the work needs and work performance of mentally handicapped adults', *British Journal of Mental Subnormality*, 19, pp. 71–9.

Hogg, J. (1973) 'Personality assessment as the study of learning processes', in P. Mittler (ed.), *Assessment for Learning in the Mentally Handicapped*, Study Group No. 5, Institute for Research into Mental Retardation (Churchill Livingstone).

Richardson, S. A., Dohrenwend, B. S. and Klein, D. (1965) *Interviewing: Its Forms and Functions* (Basic Books).

Ryan, J. (1973) 'When is an apparent deficit a real defect – language assessment in the subnormal', in P. Mittler (ed.), *Assessment for Learning in the Mentally Handicapped*, op. cit.

Wandsworth, London Borough of (1977) 'Project 74: A research study in which the mentally handicapped speak for themselves', *Clearing House for Local Authority Research*, University of Birmingham, No. 1.

Whelan, E. and Speake, B. (1977) *Adult Training Centres in England and Wales: Report of the First National Survey* (National Association of Teachers of the Mentally Handicapped).

CHAPTER 3.3

———◆———

THE PHYSICALLY HANDICAPPED

INTRODUCTION

Day services for the physically handicapped are difficult to classify neatly. A rational visitor arriving from another planet might assume that day services for people with physical handicaps might, at least in part, be the responsibility of the health agency of that country. But this is not the case. Most day units for the physically handicapped, aside from the elderly, are provided by social services departments or voluntary agencies. Such medical rehabilitation as exists is, it seems, rarely carried out on a day basis but confined to residential medical rehabilitation centres in rural or semi-rural settings away from the large population areas and unrelated to local catchment areas (Mattingley, 1977).

The 'body' of physical rehabilitation in day services is fractured between its medical, psychological, social and industrial limbs. The health service has been slow to enter the fields of both day services and physical rehabilitation for age groups other than children and the elderly. The social aspects of rehabilitation are carried out without reference to the medical and industrial aspects; in local authority social services department day centres, no clear distinction is made between physical and industrial rehabilitation, as opposed to the long-term maintenance needs of the physically handicapped user. Then the industrial aspects of rehabilitation are the responsibility of Employment Rehabilitation Centres which have no automatic liaison with either health or social services. The psychological aspects of rehabilitation and the impact of such factors as the morale or self-esteem of the patient and his motivation are not the official, systematic concern of any agency. The pathway of a user who needs to be linked to each of these services is not a smooth one (Blaxter, 1975) and the recommendations of numerous committees which have reported on the lack of co-ordination of rehabilitation services have been largely ignored (Tunbridge, 1972; Mair, 1972).

This background is given because otherwise day services for the physically handicapped are confusing. In this chapter the reader is introduced in turn to four users of day services who talk about their physical condition and their limitations, the household from which each comes, and what the unit contributes to each user and vice versa.

Florence: Day Centre for Physically Disabled (Social Services)

I had sleepy sickness, I don't remember the date when. I can't walk and

I can't get up stairs. I've also got arthritis. I'm 69 now but I've got my husband, I'm very fortunate. Some people who don't come here moan a lot and it would do them good to come here to see others that suffer worse than they do. Coming here has given me a grateful heart. I've got twenty-four grandchildren and nine great-grandchildren and they're all normal.

Last week here I stuffed teddy bears and sewed pyjama buttons on. We talked. Drank tea and coffee and had a good dinner, we ran the raffle for the outing. We're all a happy lot here and the driver is very kind.

Peter: Work Centre for the Cerebral Palsied (Voluntary)

I'm physically disabled, it started at birth. I can't walk but I can pull myself up and down stairs on my seat with support from the banisters. I can just about feed myself with the meat cut up and I need help with my shoelaces. I have a speech problem.

I'm thirty, I live with my mum and dad. Dad works in an office in town. I can't say what he does. But he travels. Something to do with maths. It's a boiler-making company.

This place tries to get you out in the world, makes you stand on your own feet. I work a press in the industrial section, that's all I do; except talk to the others. I get paid £1.50 per week, quite fair. I've come for ten years. I can remember things I didn't do before. I didn't walk before I came here, now I do a bit in a walking frame.

John: Day Hospital for the Young Chronic Sick (Health)

I have multiple sclerosis, it started in 1972 when I was 27. I used to be a clerk with the county council but I've come here to the day hospital for nearly two years. I do physiotherapy and occupational therapy – it's helped my depression. They've shown me how to make a tray in occupational therapy and a basket and an ashtray and make little bits of ceramics. They've done all they can – I wish they had a swimming pool though.

I have a rapport with a young patient here who can't talk. I can understand her and help her. Patience, giving love and compassion are the most important things in the staff here. They need to have the right temperament before they even start this work.

David: Sheltered Workshop sponsored by a social services department

I'm 50 now. I've been blind and deaf for thirty years, since 1946. I've got a hiatus hernia and bronchitis and arthritis in my feet and back. And my shoulders. I can get around my own area with the use of some aids and I can manage stairs at home. I only travel with another chap from here who has partial sight. I often feel sick through the hernia and my memory is patchy. I'm easily upset when the hiatus hernia troubles me, when I feel ill I find I'm easily aroused. It is partly the management, the set up is wrong to start with and you have difficulty in getting about the place.

The depression lasts until I get started with my work. Too often we are waiting for supplies and the time hangs heavy when we are waiting about all day – like being in a detention centre.

I'm a bedding maker and uphosterer. I did nothing at all Monday, Tuesday and Wednesday as we were waiting for covers. The management here just don't know how to order – I worked Thursday and Friday but the first three days were so long and time hung very heavy.

I like my trade. I was pleased to have a job here and get back to work and have some independence. Outside employers won't have me because I have a double disability. I am left without any option. I have even tried recently to get a job in a factory, but they won't entertain me. I feel I have lost my independence here, it's the travelling [to get here], I have to rely on someone else. I like to keep my independence as much as possible. It is better than lying around and doing nothing and if the place was improved it could be quite O.K. The first thing they should do is sack the manager. He won't listen to our ideas. Some of his staff are frightened of him and he puts them in their place. He often refuses to see the union committee. Some of the staff here don't know how to handle blind people, they are shy of blind and disabled people – they need some training to help them to cope and then they could do their job better.

SOCIAL SERVICES CENTRES

These introductions imply that there are wide ranges in users classified as 'physically handicapped'. For a start, the largest single group of units, over half, are sponsored by non-health agencies – the local authority social services departments. These twenty-five centres deal with users who are young, middle-aged and old but there are a preponderance of people who, like Florence, are at the ageing end of the scale. A quarter of the users interviewed in social services centres were under 40, but nearly half were older people aged 60 or more. This means that some centres labelled as venues for the physically handicapped could equally be classified as centres for the elderly.

Disorders of the central nervous system, particularly the stroke, figured prominently in the accounts given by users of social services centres, about their disabilities. Disorders of bones and joints

Checklist: Vital Statistics
Physical Handicap

Number of units in national census			54[a]
Number of units sponsored by social services departments (SSD)			25
Number of units sponsored by voluntary agencies (Vol.)			11
Number of sheltered workshops sponsored by all agencies (Sh.Wk.)			14
Number of units sponsored by Employment Services Agency (ESA)			3
Number of units sponsored by area health authority (AHA)			1

	SSD	Vol.	Sh.Wk.	Other
Number of heads and staff interviewed	46	24	35	12
Number of users interviewed	71	44	53	18
Average size of unit (user) places	61	38	68	—
Range of size of units (user places)	15–200	11–80	15–150	20–100
Average ratio of staff to users	1 : 12	1 : 12	1 : 9	1 : 6[b]

[a] Three units refused to participate, including one sponsored by the ESA.
[b] No information from one unit (AHA).

(particularly arthritis) are the second most frequent group of conditions. Yet, over three-quarters of the social services centres had no visit from a hospital consultant and almost as many had not seen a general practitioner on the premises in the previous twelve months. None reported visits from therapists such as a physiotherapist or speech therapist.

The health-based worker who visited social service centres most often was the health visitor. The relative absence of contact between physically handicapped users and staff in the health service might imply that either health-trained workers were employed on the staff of the social services department, or that the users of social services centres made frequent visits to doctors or hospitals away from the centre. But no evidence for either proposition existed.[1] More likely, no co-ordinated treatment services exist for those physically handicapped people. The extent to which their disability is affected by their lack of treatment is an open question.

What mechanisms exist for liaison between staff of social services department day centres for the physically handicapped and the health authorities? At a clinical level, as we have already discussed, the answer is practically none. And at an administrative level visits to the social services day centres by health administrators were not all that much more frequent. Fewer than one in five social services units had seen the health-based specialist in community medicine (social services) or the area medical officer a couple of times in the preceding year. Social services centres for the physically handicapped have a long way to go before the skills of the health service make any impact in assessment or treatment of users' conditions. The commonest disorder reported by users in the health-based geriatric day hospital is the stroke, yet this is also the clinical earmark denoted by more users in social services department day centres for the physically handicapped. Although the extent to which the two groups are strictly comparable is not known, Chapter 8 indicates that a considerable number of 'strokes' being treated in geriatric day hospitals are not new ones, which implies that local policies – or chance – decide whether a user gets into a health day hospital (with the chance of treatment at least sometimes) or into a social services centre (with no treatment).

VOLUNTARY AGENCIES

The second cluster of centres for the physically handicapped are seventeen units sponsored by voluntary agencies, one-third of the total. Some sponsors are local spastics societies, others are 'one-off' ventures by local agencies. Generally, these centres concentrate on serving either the young or the old but have very few users in the middle age range. (As some of the sheltered workshops are voluntary agencies which serve the middle-aged this statement is not quite true, but for a number of reasons, sheltered workshops are being treated as a separate group.) Even though their services are not, strictly speaking, sheltered workshops, for the younger age groups the voluntary agencies usually offer a work programme which pays a modicum of cash to supplement the user's statutory benefit. The cash ranged from a few pence to £2 per week.

What disorders were reported by the users interviewed in voluntary agencies day centres? Amongst the older users only, arthritis was more common than strokes; amongst the younger users the commonest central nervous system malfunction was cerebral palsy.

Staff from the area health authority did not visit voluntary units more often than they visited social services units. But it did appear that the voluntary centres were marginally better served for remedial therapists than the social services centres. On the other hand, three of the heads of social services centres were occupational therapists.

OTHER SERVICES FOR THE PHYSICALLY HANDICAPPED

Other services provided for the physically handicapped do not slot into tidy categories. The next largest sponsoring agency (by omitting for a moment the sheltered workshops) become the employment rehabilitation centres. ERCs are provided by the Employment Services Agency (ESA) – part of the Manpower Services Commission. Although ERCs made up only 6 per cent of the units for the physically handicapped, three immediate qualifications concerning them need to be made. First, the ERCs do not cater solely for the physically handicapped. They might factually be regarded as mixed centres, since their heads considered that 79 per cent of their population was physically handicapped, with 19 per cent regarded as mentally ill (and none as mentally handicapped). Second, although the number of ERCs, relative to the number of other units for physical handicap, is small, ERCs are very large centres compared to the rest. At 100 places each they provide, on average, many more places than other types of centres. Third, the Employment Services Agency do not wish the ERCs to be regarded as 'day services' in the sense of the term conceived by this project. They consider that this concept of day services is the responsibility of departments other than their own and has little to do with their brief which is to prepare people for work. In fact officials at the ESA preferred that information about ERCs be withdrawn from the study. Considerable thought was given to this but in the interests of providing a more authentic national picture of services for the handicapped some information about ERCs remains in this section. (Even then, this picture is still not complete, for the ESA asked the third ERC in the sample not to co-operate with this project. Thus, information about ERCs is based on two rather than three centres.) This in itself is a working demonstration of the absence of liaison between medical and social rehabilitation on the one hand and industrial rehabilitation on the other, which is discussed in Chapter 8 and which occurs again in Chapter 17, when users express disappointment that their day units are apparently unable to help them find jobs.

ERCs were simultaneously more multi-disciplinary and more consciously diagnostic a service than all those offered to the physically handicapped. Employing medical, nursing, psychological and social work staff for assessment purposes, the ERCs nevertheless retain no treatment staff. The orientation of the centres is assessment for work purposes and this focused the activities. Factory, trade and clerical work tasks were the programmes for users. The staff-to-user ratio was more favourable in ERCs than in other forms of centre for the physically handicapped: one staff member to six users compares with one staff member to twelve users in the social services and voluntary centres.

Although it has a base of professional staff, the ERCs operated in an automatous fashion. That is to say, very few outside visitors called at the unit, unless they were visiting disablement resettlement officers. The disablement resettlement officer, regarded as a specialist in job placement, was also one of the more frequent visitors in the social services and voluntary centres. This is not to imply that he or she was a *regular* visitor: in fact the DRO never visited more than half the centres and the rest he had visited less than once a month in the previous twelve months.

ERCs were those units for the physically handicapped which specialised in admission and discharge of users. Few users stayed longer than three months. So while ERCs have, in theory, a 100 per cent turnover of users at least every twelve months, the turnover of users in the voluntary and social services units is very slow.

Just under half the ERC users who left were referred to jobs in open employment and a modest few (4 per cent) went to sheltered employment. Thirty-five per cent were referred to other day units but this figure is not particularly informative as it may have included referral to work retraining schemes as well as the social services and voluntary centres with which we are now acquainted. By comparison, very few of the users who left voluntary and social services units (6 and 4 per cent respectively) went to open employment or sheltered employment (2 per cent each).

It is not really possible to compare the users of ERCs with those of social services and voluntary centres since the percentage of users interviewed in the ERCs was miniscule and the centres very large, when compared with those of the social services and voluntary agencies. But turning to the way that heads of ERCs regarded users, we learn that the ERC users were regarded as more physically competent than the users of other day resources for the physically handicapped. For example, almost all users in ERCs could walk independently, whereas only half the users in the voluntary and social services centres could do so. And whereas only three in four social services users and two in three voluntary users could toilet themselves completely alone, all the ERC users could. ERCs did not provide transport to the centre for their users, whereas the social services and voluntary agencies did so. (Less than a third of users in both these centres got themselves there alone by walking, public transport or private means.)

AREA HEALTH AUTHORITIES

The fourth – and most recent – service provider to the field of day services for the physically handicapped are area health authorities. Although for many years the health services have provided a small number of places for what are called the younger chronic sick in geriatric day hospitals, very little provision has existed for these people in their own right. Further, very few places in geriatric day hospitals are occupied by people under 60 years of age.

The history to the commencement of day provision for the young chronic sick is the view that 'some younger chronic sick patients were being cared for unsuitably in geriatric wards' (Ministry of Health, 1968) combined with the prediction that the numbers of younger chronic sick would continue to rise due to falling mortality and the increased number of post-accident cases. Thus it was recommended that special residential units be instituted in each health region for this group, particularly those who were incontinent, needed nursing care at night, paralysed, and in need of continuous nursing care. It was also stated that 'provision of day care can be to the mutual advantage of inpatients and day patients' (Ministry of Health, 1968, p. 5).

The one day hospital existing in the health authority sample for the young chronic sick was opened in 1976 and it was part of a residential unit. Only a fifth of the social services centres were opened in the 1970s, and well below a tenth of voluntary centres and sheltered work units. As we have already seen, the growth of services for the physically handicapped in the 1970s has not been as fast as that of some other sectors. Although day hospitals for the young chronic sick represent minute provision, they are a growth point for services for the younger physically handicapped, even though by actual age, more of the users interviewed in the day hospital were middle-aged rather than young. This group of users were very incapacitated. In the head's opinion, three out of every four of the users of the day hospital were unable to walk (that is, they were confined at least to a wheelchair) and the same percentage could go to the toilet only with the help of staff.

SHELTERED WORKSHOPS

The final group of services for physical handicap – and a group not strictly representing any one service provider – are the sheltered workshops. Like the ERCs, the sheltered workshops deny that they are 'day care' facilities, since they offer 'work and a wage'. Yet it seemed important to include them since they represent an extension of the activities of other agencies. While other day units offer a work programme to physically handicapped people and pay them money, they do not claim to pay a wage but rather to supplement income. But the sheltered workshops offered on average £40 per week, ranging between £24 and £60.[2] Of the sheltered workshops in the study, one was viewed as a 'mixed centre' and is described in Chapter 3.8. Another workshop catered only for the mentally handicapped and is dealt with in Chapter 3.2. Of the twelve workshops remaining, five were sponsored by the government-aided Remploy, four were run by social services departments and three by local voluntary agencies. Of the sheltered workshops, three catered in particular for blind people.

Six out of ten sheltered workers were middle-aged, aged from 40 to just under 60. Most of the rest were over 60 – there were very few young people in sheltered workshops. Eight out of ten sheltered workers were men.

The most distinctive point about the programme of sheltered workshops is its concentration on work. In ten of the fourteen units with sheltered work the work programme was the only activity offered to users. It may be helpful to reiterate that several different types of work seem to be available to users of day units. The first type might, as we have seen already, be called *simple work*. Simple work involves the sort of jobs accomplished without machinery, especially things which are done by hand and without tools or done with non-powered handtools; especially staplers, hammers and screwdrivers. The second kind of work is *machine work*: work with powered machines or powered handtools, the woodwork and metalwork machines or the electric drill. Then apart from simple work and machine work, some units offer *service work* – perhaps domestic work within the day unit, laundry work within the day unit, gardening or other out-of-doors work.

More sheltered workshops offered more machine work to more users than other types of units for the physically handicapped. The meaning and context of work within the sheltered work context is explored in Chapter 12. Half of the social services and voluntary units offered simple work and a rather smaller percentage offer service work. Half of the units for the physically handicapped – in both voluntary and social services units – offer both simple work *and* arts and crafts. But in these units there is a definite overbalance of work over arts and crafts, in terms of the number of users involved. In the social services and voluntary units overall, most users spent most time at work and second most time at arts and crafts according to staff.

Arts and crafts were never used in sheltered work. In the other units for the physically handicapped, where it was used it was never defined as 'work'. For a start, users were not paid for producing arts and crafts, in fact they were required to pay for the purchase of the materials used. Second, although sheltered *work* activities were usually supervised by a skilled tradesman, art and craft activities were rarely taught by either a skilled craftsman or a trained art/craft teacher. So arts and crafts were not treated as work, nor were they taught as a skill. This lends some support to the idea that arts and crafts are used often as 'fillers' – convenient ways of supplementing the programme. This different status makes the idea of comparing arts and crafts with work activities difficult and a more detailed discussion of this is contained in Chapter 17.

HEADS AND STAFF

As almost half the staff working with the physically handicapped were aged 50 or more, they are the oldest group of paid staff in day services.

(Heads and staff looking after the elderly were, overall, slightly older, but there were more volunteers amongst this group.)

Along with the staff of mixed centres and those caring for the elderly, the staff looking after the physically handicapped over-represent the unqualified staff of day services. At the same time there were marginally more former tradesmen represented in amongst the staff for the physically handicapped than other user groups. Apart from being older, heads and staffs were long servers. Four out of ten heads had been in the post for eight years or more, while this applied to a quarter of the staff.

In general, heads and staff could be characterised as relatively unqualified, unserved by in-service training of any type and not particularly interested in achieving qualifications. Heads were more interested in further training than staff and expressed a cautious interest in learning more about the CSS (Certificate in Social Service).

Why do people work with the physically handicapped? The most frequent reason put forward by heads and staff was a general interest in the area and field of physical handicap. The second predominating reason was the fact that the head or staff member needed a job – any job. Behind this requirement was a group of people composed of unskilled or blue collar workers, who found themselves out of work, or unable to continue for physical or health reasons with the hard manual work of their former occupation.

DISCUSSION

From information provided by users about their conditions it is impossible to estimate how many need medical rehabilitation, but it would be equally foolhardy to conclude that because users are in voluntary and social services day centres, none do. A similar point has been made about the many surveys conducted by local authorities on the needs of the chronically sick and disabled: no adequate figures are available about the users' potential for physical rehabilitation (Warren, 1977).

When the complaints of those in units for the physically handicapped are considered (regardless of their service provider), we find that the particular physical disorders mentioned most frequently are as follows: first, diseases of bones and joints, such as rheumatoid arthritis or osteo-arthritis (14 per cent), second, blindness (12 per cent), and equal third are unspecified cerebral vascular accidents (or strokes) and deafness (each 9 per cent). These figures are similar to the results of the national sample survey carried out by the Government Social Survey (Harris, 1971).

The point has been made that the trend is for each day service sector to operate in a self-contained way, without reference to other services. Experience suggests that if it is left to individual professionals or their departments to decide whether or not to co-ordinate together, most decide that it is not worth the expensive time and effort.

For practical purposes, co-ordination may be thought of as integration:

the gathering together of services on behalf of a common problem at several levels. One model analysing co-ordination between service agencies describes three different levels of co-ordination (Reid, 1964). At the lowest level is 'ad hoc case co-ordination' where activities are generated by individual practitioners who work together to meet the users' need. The next level involves systematic case co-ordination, where in the interests of an individual case the services of two agencies are meshed together, as in the case conference. The third level, programme co-ordination, implies the development of joint programmes between agencies, the loaning of specialist skills to each other and a mutual modification of policies and approaches, so it consumes inevitably a larger part of the resources of each agency.

At present, there is little indication that any kind of co-ordination *between* services is practised systematically on behalf of the physically handicapped. The present problem of co-ordination between potential rehabilitation services is not so much that of duplication of effort as discontinuity and incoherence. Discontinuity points to the fact that services related to each other and needed by the users at different points in time fail to follow on consecutively. Incoherence is the failure of relatively independent and specialised services to relate to each other (Rein, 1970).

Two potential strategies to overcome the problems of discontinuity and incoherence could be suggested. To overcome the problem of discontinuity in the care of the handicapped person who needs to steer through a maze of agencies, one idea is to appoint a named person, a professional whose personal responsibility it becomes to overcome discontinuity. This idea has been suggested by the Warnock Committee in connection with the handicapped school leaver (Warnock, 1978). He needs help to enlist services on his behalf at various points in time. Whilst some professionals, for example, a general practitioner or a social worker, see this as their role, others, preferring a functional definition of their job, do not.

On the other hand, to overcome the problem of incoherence, the difficulty of specialised agencies failing to overlap a new co-ordinating structure may be needed. A relevant model is the difficulty in co-ordinating the management of child abuse cases (Carter, 1976). Central government advocated setting up local area review committees: a new structure in each area with particular tasks which both monitors the performance of various agencies and acts as an interdisciplinary group to which the accountability of each service is expressed. There is some evidence to suggest that these have led the participating health and social services to over-invest in maintaining routines and bureaucratic procedures, but at the same time, each contributing organisation and each discipline has to surrender some autonomy in the interests of achieving a common goal and there is a legal and professional framework to support this. Such a model could be inspected and even tried on a pilot basis for rehabilitating the physically handicapped.

At present it will be noted that there is very little duplication of day services for the physically handicapped, although this may not be the case if health authorities increase their day services for the younger chronic sick. The danger implicit in duplication of services for similar groups will be discussed in the next section about services for the mentally ill. It may, in the long run, be better to ask local authorities to provide the day services and for health authorities to 'loan out' the requisite specialist skills.

Co-ordination of day services for the physically handicapped will become even more important as those presently in centres become older and join the ranks of the chronic disabled elderly and as increased numbers of handicapped children, who survived because of improved medical technology, take their place.

ROUTES

Other material dealing with day services for the physically handicapped can be found in Chapters 11 and 12. Chapter 8 discusses clinical assessment and treatment for an analogous group, the elderly in geriatric day hospitals, and Chapter 12 discusses rehabilitation, but mainly from a psychiatric point of view.

NOTES

1 But three heads of social services units were occupational therapists.
2 This is aside from one workshop where users were paid 97p per hour.

REFERENCES

Blaxter, M. (1975) *The Meaning of Disability* (Heinemann).
Carter, J. (1976) 'Coordination and child abuse', *Social Work Service*, No. 9, pp. 22–8.
Harris, A. (1971) *Handicapped and Impaired in Great Britain*, Part I (HMSO).
Mair, A. (1972) *Medical Rehabilitation: the Pattern for the Future*, report of the Subcommittee of the Standing Medical Advisory Committee, Scottish Health Services Council on Medical Rehabilitation (HMSO).
Mattingley, S. (ed.) (1977) *Rehabilitation Today* (Update Books).
Ministry of Health (1968) *Care of Younger Chronic Sick Patients in Hospital*, HM (68) 41.
Reid, W. (1964) 'Interagency coordination in delinquency and control', *Social Service Review*, XXXVIII, 4 (December), p. 418.
Rein, M. (1970) *Social Policy* (Random House).
Tunbridge, R. (1972) *Report of Subcommittee of Standing Medical Advisory Committee*, Central Health Services Council (HMSO).
Warnock, H. M. (1978) *Committee of Inquiry into Handicapped Children and Young People: Special Educational Needs*, Department of Education and Science, Cmnd 7212 (HMSO).
Warren, M. D. (1977) 'The need for rehabilitation', in Mattingley, op. cit.

CHAPTER 3.4

———◆———

THE MENTALLY ILL

INTRODUCTION

Now we turn to day units for the mentally ill. Our estimates indicate that there are 385 such units in England and Wales with 1,500 places for users. The day hospitals, sponsored by area health authorities, have the longest tradition of any form of day service. The first day hospital in the UK, and one of the first in the world, the 'Social Psychotherapy Centre', now the Marlborough Day Hospital, opened in London in 1946. The number of day hospitals opened in the 1950s trebled in the 1960s and then doubled in the first half of the 1970s.

Social services department day centres are more recent. Local authority social services departments were established in 1971 and have had less time to 'catch up'. Much of the section which follows will compare and contrast these two main sectors, the health and the social services, although the voluntary sector will be acknowledged. The section introduces three heads of day units for the mentally ill in one London borough. They explain why they took their jobs and what they get out of it. They comment on their users and say whether or not they would come to their day unit, should they find themselves suffering from mental illness. The verbatim comments have been edited, meaning that superfluous phrases have been removed and some passages consolidated.

EXAMPLES

Sister, St James' Day Hospital

I've worked in this day hospital for eight years now. Before that I had worked as a staff nurse in a mental hospital for sixteen years. This post was going as a staff nurse. I didn't want to travel and I didn't want the unsocial hours of hospital nursing. I was also a qualified and experienced mental nurse.

I'm 52 now. What I find satisfying about working here in the day hospital is that it's the job I've always wanted to do. When a very sick patient recovers it's a marvellous job satisfaction. It's the best day hospital in the area because it's small so that patients and staff are able to mix easily. It's a jolly good team here.

The patients are inadequates and need extra attention to bolster their egos. Would I come here if I were in the same position as the patients? I would love to – it would be heaven to be pampered and made a fuss of and looked after.

Manager, Parkville Centre

I've worked in this social services day centre for five years, before that I was a staff nurse in a nursing home. I'm 43 and I came to work here because I felt I needed something to occupy my time, utilising my training. I didn't want to continue nursing as such because I had a hearing difficulty. I wanted to work with people. My job is very satisfying, just looking after people and looking at their problems. My feeling of success is seeing their enjoyment at coming here. They really look forward to it and it gives the relatives a break and that is success. The ideal user is the person who is lacking in initiative and stimulation and we can bring them out. We like them to be responsible and bright and encourage them to be independent which is a great help. Co-operative types are ideal.

Would I come here if I found myself in a similar situation to the members? I wouldn't. We [the staff] don't wish to feel we are handicapped. I can't enlarge on this, this is just a personal feeling.

Organiser, Southborough Club

I've been here for four and a half years, I hadn't ever worked before although I'm 60. I had brought up a family and was asked if I would be secretary of the voluntary association for mental health. I'd done a social science degree at London University so I was also interested. That's how I came here. It's satisfying to see club members gaining confidence and to see their general health and well-being improve – to see them blossoming. Success is that the club is full of vitality – it's alive! We see lots of benefits to the members and the helpers themselves benefit a lot from the work they do. Our ideal members are those that take some responsibility for the club, to join in things and care for other members.

Would I come here if I were in a similar situation to the members? I would. There is always a warm welcome and a pleasant atmosphere. It's a pleasant place to be in.

Southborough: Example of Mental Health Day Services

Southborough is an outer London Borough. It is unusual because of its high number of day units: it has six units for the mentally ill sponsored by health, social services and voluntary agencies. Only two of the thirteen areas in the project had day facilities sponsored by all these three service providers. Moreover, Southborough is unique because it is the only area which attempts to co-ordinate pathways between the four day hospitals of the area, the one social services day centre and the voluntary day club. St James' is one of the four day hospitals in the area. It was progressive twenty years ago because it was located in a building in a residential street, rather than in the grounds of a hospital. Now a quarter of all health service day hospitals for the mentally ill are located outside the grounds of hospitals. The social services centre, Parkville, is found in recently constructed premises at a different end of the borough, while the voluntary day club, the Southborough, is in an old house in the middle of the shopping centre. Southborough acts as a drop-in centre to which people can refer themselves and their friends. This is unlike both St James' and Parkville which accept only professional referrals: St James' requires a medical referral and Parkville a social work referee, which is the pattern expected by most day units for the mentally ill.

The services in Southborough are a paradigm of national provision of day services for the mentally ill. Area health authorities provide most – three-quarters – of day units for the mentally ill. The social services departments offer only one-fifth. The voluntary organisations such as MIND concentrate more on offering clubs than day centres. The voluntary organisations at present provide a mere 5 per cent of the total day services for the mentally ill. In the thirteen areas of the project there were thirty-one day hospitals in the health sector, eight day centres in social services departments and two voluntary centres.

FUNCTION OF DAY SERVICES

Day places for those people labelled as mentally ill represent the fourth largest group of all those user groups catered for by day services. Other day services have clear relevance to services for the mentally ill: for instance, day services for the confused elderly are sometimes run in conjunction with services for the mentally ill. Family day centres are also related, for the same proportion of parents said they felt depressed as those users who used conventional mental illness day units. Services for offenders relate to mental illness, because a third of offenders claimed to have spent time in the past in psychiatric or mental hospitals. Finally, of the day units which provided for a 'mix' of user groups, two specifically incorporated some 'mentally ill' people. All these aspects are discussed later in Chapter 3.

Recent government policy has proposed different functions for the day services offered by the health and the social services sector. The White Paper of 1975, *Better Services for the Mentally Ill*, acknowledged that it was difficult to draw a clear-cut boundary between the two services but, in essence, 'the day hospitals should have facilities for treatment ... for group and individual therapy'. They should also provide a wide range

Checklist: Vital Statistics
Mental Illness

Number of units in national census			42[a]
Number of units sponsored by area health authorities (AHA)			32[a]
Number of units sponsored by social services departments (SSD)			8
Number of units sponsored by voluntary agencies (Vol.)			2[a]

	AHA	SSD	Vol.
Number of heads and staff interviewed	83	24	8
Number of users interviewed	126	39	13
Average size of unit (user places)	40	33	75
Range of size of units (user places)	6–100	20–50	75
Average ratio of staff to users	1 : 4	1 : 9	1 : 6

[a] Information is based on returns from forty units overall; thirty AHA units and one voluntary unit.

of occupational and rehabilitation activities. Thus the bias of the health-sponsored day hospitals was to be towards the treatment aspects of care while the social aspects of care should be undertaken by social services day centres. Day centres were to 'help with difficulties in forming or maintaining of personal relationships . . . adjusting or readjusting to the demands of work [and to] . . . encourage the realisation of the individual's potential'. As well, such centres were to meet clients' 'immediate needs for shelter, occupation and social activity' (DHSS, 1975).

Both the heads of St James' day hospital and the Parkville social services centre claim that their primary aim is to keep people out of hospital. At St James' the Sister amplifies this as follows: 'We keep people in the community and prevent further hospitalisation.' The head at Parkville expressed it this way: 'Our job is to keep a patient within the community and to slow down the rate of admission to hospital and to old people's homes.' Keeping people out of hospital was the most common aim mentioned by workers with the mentally ill in both health and social services centres. Whereas Parkville day centre claims to provide 'occupation and stimulation for people', St James' day hospital, in the view of its head, 'treats people: primarily most treatments given to inpatients could be given to day patients except when their phases become acute. When they are a danger to themselves they have to go to hospital.'

At the Southborough Club, the voluntary drop-in club, the head seems to place more emphasis on the club as a focus for human relationships than the heads of the other units.

> It's here to provide friendship, support and encouragement to people recovering from mental illness. People recovering from mental illness are socially isolated and the club is a place where members can meet people informally. We set out to be unstructured and non-directive – a place where members can be themselves and do what they feel like.

The heads in Southborough were middle-aged women: at the day hospital and the day centre the heads were nurse trained. Two-thirds of the heads of day units for mental illness units are women and three-quarters have a nursing qualification. Apart from a small group of heads with trades qualifications, practically none have 'other' academic or professional training such as social work, psychology or occupational therapy.

Administration occupies the heads at Southborough more than direct work with users. Paper work of all kinds, answering the telephone, arranging meetings, organising domestic and transport activities took each head on average fifteen hours per week. Personal and social contacts with users took each on average ten hours per week. This bias in the use of time on the job held for the heads of mental illness units in general. Three-quarters of the heads and staff in day hospitals and two-thirds in social services centres came to work in day units because the conditions suited them: the hours were good and there was no shift work. Half this number proposed more idealistic reasons: such as a commitment to work in the community, rather than a hospital; a concern for mental health work. Along with the heads of St James' and Parkville, many heads and staff had been associated with the day unit for a long time. A fifth had been in post for five years or more and the average length of service was well over two years.

One important difference between the heads and staff of day hospitals in health authority and social services day centres was that proportionately more workers are employed by the day hospitals than the social services centres. Another difference is that proportionately more of the health authority heads and staff have a qualification and training for the work they do than the heads and staff of the social services day centres. A more detailed outline of this matter is given in Edwards and Carter (1979).

All the doctors working with the mentally ill (including consultants and senior registrars) were employed to work in the health authority day hospitals. No doctors were seconded to or otherwise employed in the social services day centres, but in one day centre a psychiatrist did visit at least once a month. The role of psychiatrists in day services appeared controversial and is discussed in Chapters 7 and 17.

Nine out of ten paid staff work in the day hospitals. Yet if there were a rational distribution of staff between the two sectors, one might expect on grounds of size alone that seven out of ten of the workers would be in the day hospitals and two out of ten in the social services centres. What can be said about the users which might illuminate the issue of how staff should be distributed?

WHO USES DAY SERVICES FOR THE MENTALLY ILL?

Close resemblances were found in the users of the two main sectors of day services for the mentally ill. Their views of their mental health were similar. Their perceptions of their physical health had a great deal in common. They were remarkably uniform in their age, their sex, marital status and living circumstances. But they did differ in the amount of use they said they had made of psychiatric hospitals in the past. Half the social services users might be classified as chronic, on the basis of the length of time they had lived in psychiatric hospitals. Their health counterparts had spent less time, on average, in psychiatric hospitals which suggests there might be more chronic psychiatric disablement amongst the users of social services centres. But this is not to imply that social services users are simply 'chronics' and the health users are the 'acutes'. For when we looked for the users who had *not* been in hospital, or in hospital for less than a year, as an attempt to guide us to those whose conditions might be said to be 'acute', it appeared that almost half the social services users were 'acute' while almost four-fifths of the health users were 'acute'.

The traditional assumption is that an 'acute' workload needs a higher ratio of staff to users and more intensive staff skills. This may need to be re-examined. There is a possible alternative assumption, that 'chronic' users may need more, rather than less, intensive attention to progress. This issue is discussed at greater length elsewhere (Edwards and Carter, 1979) and in Chapter 9.

Most users attending both types of units considered that they had a mental or emotional disorder: but while the users of day centres were more likely to name psychotic-type conditions (like schizophrenia or manic-depressive psychoses), more of the day hospital users called their complaint 'depression'. However, both these groups were outnumbered by users who labelled themselves with their own view of their condition: phrases like 'bad nerves' or 'mental strain' or 'unable to cope with pressure'.

If a user *labelled* his or her condition as depression, he or she without exception *felt* depressed, too. But more users felt depressed than those who labelled their malady as depression. In fact two-thirds of the 178 users said they had been depressed in the previous month: four out of five of these said they had felt like doing away with themselves.

The severity of the depression was assessed from information about how often users said they felt depressed and how long the depression lasted. More users of day hospitals than social services centres had been depressed in the past month, on their own admission – and more of their descriptions of depression were assessed as 'considerable' or 'moderate' depression than users in the social services centres. (These assessments were rated by a research psychiatrist and a social researcher, independently of the study team.)

Although many of the users of day services for mental illness pass 'in and out' of the units quite rapidly, it also appears that there is a build up of long-stay users in day services. This is particularly true for the social services and voluntary sector where the average annual discharge figures are lower than in the health service. For instance, the social services day centres, on average, discharged twenty-eight users a year, while the day hospitals each discharged eighty-six users a year on average.[2] Not many of the day hospital users – only 2 per cent – went on to day centres after leaving day hospitals. The largest group of users leaving day hospitals and day centres (30–33 per cent) took jobs in open employment after leaving. Only a very few went to sheltered work (3–7 per cent) but many more just stayed at home: 34 per cent of discharges in day hospitals and 14 per cent in day centres. We cannot be certain whether this stay-at-home group represents successful discharges or failures. More work needs to be done on what constitutes a successful discharge from a day unit.

ACTIVITIES IN MENTAL ILLNESS DAY UNITS

The overlap between the health and social services sectors is reflected in the similarities by which heads in the two sectors outlined their programmes. Most units offered a number of different programmes each week – sometimes each day – which could represent a variety of activities. In the listing which follows, the programmes are presented in order of frequency. Then the three most frequently offered activities in both health and social services units follow the programme heading. When there is a difference between the two services, this is indicated.

(1) *Social programme:*   record sessions, table tennis, card games.

(2) *Physical treatments:*   by a doctor, nurse or therapist. Relaxation classes, special nursing care (injections or dressings, for example), medication dispensed by staff (day hospitals) or keep fit classes (day centres).

(3) *Arts and crafts:*   sewing, painting, toymaking.

(4) *Education classes:*   cookery, shopping activities, hairdressing or make-up classes (day hospitals) or drama classes (day centres).

(5) *Meetings:*   therapy groups with a trained leader to dis-

(6) *Work: industrial or domestic:*

cuss personal problems, discussion groups to discuss other matters related to the users, community meetings open to all to discuss the business of the day unit.

work without tools (for example, packing, sorting, labelling), work with non-powered handtools (for example, staplers, hammers, needles), domestic work (for example, cleaning, sweeping).

The users were also asked to say what they did during the week before. Their replies expanded the information: for example, the activity mentioned most often by users was spending some time chatting to each other. The second most frequently mentioned activity among social services users was doing arts and crafts. Amongst the users of health authority day hospitals the second most frequently mentioned activity was going to meetings or groups.

DISCUSSION

While it is true that social services centres seem to have more 'chronic' users than day hospitals, there are more similarities between users of the two sectors than differences. A number of factors may relate to this apparent overlap. The first is the method of the national survey itself. A national survey aggregates the views and characteristics of people in a wide cross-section of day units, and thus disguises a great deal of variation between individual units and areas. A national pattern of staffing or user views cannot predict the way individual day centres and day hospitals will operate. For example, how closely day centres and day hospitals are situated to each other might influence their operation and help determine the extent of overlap. In fact, only six of the thirteen areas surveyed had *both* health and social services units. Only two, including Southborough, sponsored health, social services *and* voluntary units. But the day hospitals in these areas where there was also a day centre, did not seem particularly specialised: they could not be distinguished in function from the rest. That is, overall, their aims were similar to those day hospitals in areas *without* day centres; the proportion of long-term users attending them was similar and at the same time they did not discharge significantly more users. Nor when discharged did it appear that any more of their users transferred to the social services day centre. So the general implication is that day hospitals and day centres run quite independently even when they are in the same area.

The exception to this was our outer London area, Southborough, with both day hospitals and day centres and a carefully planned administrative pathway of care between the two sectors. The day hospitals in Southborough discharged twice the national average number of users and three times the national average went on to the social services centres. But this kind of individual difference was rare enough not to influence the national averages.

In addition, the apparent overlap between the health and social services sectors may be related to certain recent social and organisational developments. Over the past decade, the health sector has shown an increasing interest in extending the hospital into the community. The day hospitals themselves illustrate this, but there are other extensions being developed – not without controversy. For instance, who is best to follow up users after leaving day hospitals – social workers or the new community psychiatric nurses? There were very few community psychiatric nurses working from a day hospital base. However, four out of five day hospitals in the survey referred some patients to a community psychiatric nurse for follow-up. Their presence points to a possible health sector trend towards maintaining a self-contained follow-up service which obviates the need for referral to social services. Alongside this, recently, some psychiatrists have become more active in extending their work to deal with the challenging field of the secondary handicaps of chronic patients, thus complicating the precept that it is the health service which provides acute treatment, while the social services deal with chronic care.

One or two of the day hospitals were interested in dealing with mental illness outside the medical context of the clinical model, and Chapter 13 describes one which had some features of the 'therapeutic community'. However, this day hospital remained under medical direction. In a few social services day centres there was an explicit trend towards the view that mental illness can be helped best outside a medical context altogether. This was the view of two day centres for the mentally ill in an inner London social services department. A number of day units for other user groups outside the health service, such as units for ex-offenders and young families, deal with people who have features of mental illness. In fact as many of the young parents in the national survey attending family day centres were rated as depressed as those users in units for the mentally ill, as we have noted already.

The fact that health and social services provided services with many similarities in a largely independent way was reinforced by the fact that the majority of referrals were being made along congruent paths – social services social workers referred most users to social services day centres, and hospital doctors referred most users to health day hospitals. On the other hand, the voluntary centres accepted self-referrals, uncommon in both the other sectors. However, a number of new centres in London, jointly funded by voluntary and statutory agencies, have adopted the 'drop in' system and will extend the idea of users helping each other with their difficulties.

Achieving a path for users out of day units is a goal shared by some staff in both the health and social services sectors. On discharge figures alone, this goal appears to be achieved more frequently in day hospitals but discharge is not the same as resettlement in the community. Only about a third of the users of both social services and health sectors considered that any staff member in the unit had discussed their future with them. So although day hospitals discharge more quickly, the majority of users appear not to be prepared systematically for this change. This is discussed in more detail in Chapter 9.

Clearly, providing for the range of requirements of those suffering varying degrees of mental illness at all stages is an enormous task. Whether the present differences between the services of day hospitals and day centres are distinct enough to offer real options to users and those trying to assist them is debatable, and needs further investigation. On the other hand, it is also important to consider how desirable it would be to perfect the distinctions between the health and social services and what repercussions this would have on staff and users. Past experience has shown that creating a venue for chronic care alone may depress staff and undermine user progress.

ROUTES

Further information about day services for the mentally ill can be found in:

Chapter 7   'Preventing Institutionalism': Keeping Users out of Hospital

Chapter 13   'We All Help Each Other': Aiming at Therapeutic Settings.

NOTES

1 Much of the analysis in this section and part of the text was written by Carol Edwards. A more detailed account of day services for the mentally ill is found in Edwards and Carter (1979).

2 This data does not reveal whether the day hospital users were perhaps readmitted again later in the year.

REFERENCES

Department of Health and Social Security (1975) *Better Services for the Mentally Ill*, Cmnd 6233 (HMSO).

Edwards, C. and Carter, J. (1979) 'Day services and the mentally ill', in J. K. Wing and R. Olsen, *Community Care for the Mentally Disabled* (Oxford University Press).

CHAPTER 3.5

---◆---

THE ELDERLY CONFUSED

INTRODUCTION

By the middle of the 1980s, 20 per cent of the population of Great Britain will be old enough to apply for a pension and the over 75 age group is expected to reach 3 million (Age Concern Research Unit, 1977). Although seven out of every ten units for the elderly confused have opened since 1970, there is little evidence that even if day units continue to grow at the present rate, they will be available to offer a service to more than a minute proportion of the expected number of confused elderly persons of 1985.

Defining the confused elderly or psychogeriatric population is a problem. One study suggests that there is a prevalence rate of 6.2 per cent of 'chronic brain syndrome' in the community amongst those aged 65 or more. This increases to 22 per cent at age 80 and over (Kay *et al.*, 1964, 1970). On the other hand, the incidence of mental disorders amongst elderly people aged between 65 and 74, based on diagnoses made by general practitioners, is much higher (291 per 1,000) (Age Concern Research Unit, 1977).

This chapter will adopt the term 'confused' to refer to users who would be considered as sufferers from 'chronic brain syndrome', 'senile dementia', 'arteriosclerotic dementia' or chronic brain failure, when these terms are used interchangeably (Levin, 1979). Whether or not day units for the confused deal with a wider group than this is one of the issues discussed in this section.

'The study of the senile and presenile dementias has been neglected to an extraordinary degree with little research either on fundamental or applied problems. Not only is there profound ignorance about causation but very little can be done by way of specific therapy. And so far empirical discoveries have failed to produce means of intervening in the disease processes' (Medical Research Council, 1977). This ignorance about the causes of confusion and the fact that it is said that very little can be done by way of therapy makes work with the elderly confused a difficult matter. To introduce the job of a staff member working with the confused, an occupational therapist speaks of what she does, and then about her rewards and frustrations.

Example: Marion, aged 45

I've only ever been a hospital therapist. I was given no choice about this day unit. I was sent down here on loan from the main hospital because they needed OT here with the dementia groups. As a trained OT, I now want to opt out because I realise since working with the dementias the hopelessness of the situation. I feel my skills could be used with better results with acute and hopeful cases.

I greet them each day, give them coffee and build up their security in a gentle way. I observe them and report anything untoward to the doctors. We see they go to the toilet and we see they wash their hands, we have a chiropodist, hairdresser and beautician. Socialising is done in all the activities we do: we have a very varied activity programme.

The important thing as far as I'm concerned is that I'm doing something worthwhile for patients. In some small way I make the end part of their life a little more bearable. I feel that benefit is gained from them coming here. I like people. I can't envisage doing any job where I wasn't in contact with people. But the patients we are having here are grossly deteriorated dementias and the work we are able to do with them is limited because of this. I feel that the community as a whole should be more involved with the elderly infirm to a far greater extent, especially as it may be the ultimate for all of us!

Checklist: Vital Statistics
The Elderly Confused

Number of units in national census	11[a]
Number where interviewing took place	11[a]
Number of heads and staff interviewed	44
Number of users approached for interview	66
Number of users interviewed	55[a]
Average size of unit (user places)	28
Range of size of units (user places)	16–50
Average ratio of staff to users	1 : 5

[a] Nine were sponsored by the AHA and two by local authority social services departments.

To assess the degree of confusion of those in units for the confused elderly is something of a problem. No independent view exists as to the *degree* of confusion of the old people other than that reported by themselves and noted by the interviewer. Of the fifty-five users who were interviewed eventually,[1] four-fifths understood all, or nearly all, of the questions put to them. They answered 'open-ended' questions in sentences and the interviewer rarely used the code 'question not understood'. At the other extreme one-tenth of the interviews had to be abandoned at some point in the discussion. For the rest (13 per cent) most questions appeared to be comprehended by the users but were answered in single words or phrases rather than full sentences.

These figures raise immediate questions about the composition of the 'confused' group of the elderly confused people interviewed. Significantly more (52 per cent) reported 'feeling muddled and unable to remember things' than other user groups aside from the mentally ill. Nearly two-thirds admitted having a physical or mental disability, the most common of which was a non-specific emotional or mental complaint. Four out of ten thought their health was only 'fair': and there tended to be fewer elderly confused users than other users who thought their health was 'good'.

The extent to which these old people may represent long-standing sufferers from chronic psychiatric conditions rather than newly discovered psychiatric problems relating to the dementias of old age is unknown. But one-third of the users said they had spent a minimum of three months in mental hospitals in the past. Of this group, nearly half reported spending over two years in the hospital. If this reporting is reliable (and there is no way to check it), the implication is that the elderly confused in day units may be composed of two socially and clinically distinct groups. First, there is the smaller group of those with a long-standing history of mental illness who may be part of what has been termed the 'new chronic' population. These are elderly people with long-standing conditions who have been discharged from mental hospitals with mental illnesses incurred *before* they became old. They are a separate group from those afflicted recently with the mental disorders of old age. The other possible explanation of the one-third who reported mental hospital admissions is that it is composed of old people who had been admitted to hospital for short periods of treatment for dementia. However, admissions of the elderly to mental hospital have decreased since 1970 (Schulman and Arie, 1978) and other evidence suggests that once admitted to mental hospital, patients with diagnoses of dementia rarely come out.

Users came to day units on three days each week, on average. Two of every three users were women and the average age was 72 years. Just over half the users lived alone. Although this was a similar proportion to the numbers of old people in general attending day units who lived alone, it exceeds the proportion of elderly persons in the general population who live on their own, since only 26 per cent of those of pensionable age live on their own (Age Concern Research Unit, 1977). This is a point of some importance which will be discussed later.

Aside from the group who lived alone, 40 per cent of the users in units for the elderly confused said they lived with relatives. Of these 17 per cent lived with a spouse, 12 per cent with adult children and 10 per cent with other relatives such as a brother. But of those users aged 70 or more there was a marked increase – nearly threefold – in those who lived alone. This implies that the death of a spouse may uncover cases of mental disorder which would otherwise perhaps remain contained within the family for longer periods. In fact, of those users *least* able to cope with the interview, four out of five still lived with relatives.

THE STAFF AND THE TASK

'Heads' of units were usually married women aged between 40 and 60 and over half were psychiatrically trained nurses. The largest group of staff were also trained nurses. A quarter of staff interviewed had no training at all but this figure compared favourably with other user groups. Consultant medical staff (who of course worked only to the health-sponsored units) were psychiatrists.

Half the heads and staff nominated the actual conditions of services of the day unit (particularly the daytime shift) as the prominent reason for coming to work in a day unit. This was followed by an expressed commitment to work in what was seen to be a 'community' rather than a hospital-based service. (The day hospital is seen by some as the interstice between institution and community, as discussed in Chapter 10.)

As the staff member who introduced this topic indicated, the elderly confused are the least favoured potential users of day services. More staff working with other user groups wanted to exclude an elderly confused person ahead of other users from their unit. However, such repudiations were not common amongst those who worked with the elderly confused. Three-quarters of staff were women; their ages ranged from 18 to 63 years old and most were clear-sighted about a certain basic lack of glamour inherent in their occupation. They acknowledged unpleasantness consequent on dealing with old people whose most common self-perceived disability was mental muddle. According to the heads, one in every six users needed considerable help from the staff to go to the lavatory effectively and one in twenty were incontinent. In discussing this one said: 'You have to be game for anything here, including diarrhoea down your leg.' Work with the elderly confused was sometimes seen as part of the 'dirty work' of day services. An occupational therapist declared: 'You have to be a humanitarian and never forget that. You have to like other people and have the personality to be able to make allowances for the bad behaviour we encounter – physical violence and erratic mood swings.'

Those who work with the elderly confused considered that the personal attributes required with such elderly people were kindness, patience and understanding ahead of practical, academic or organising skills. At the same time staff were unequivocal about the rewards of working with the elderly confused. Fewer staff complained about the nature of their users (their characteristics, their suitability for day care or their responsiveness) than other staff groups in day services. As rewards, the following items were listed: first, pleasure at seeing the development of 'happiness' in the users. This meant knowing that confused people were happy, comfortable and glad to attend the unit: this gratified nearly three-quarters of the staff. Comments such as 'I'm so happy watching them come out of themselves' or 'It's such a reward to see the old people happy' were common. 'Sometimes when they first come, they can't even smile. Satisfaction is in the help I give in little things – like having a bath – and the happiness it gives that old person.' The second reward was in relating to the users: in talking to them and getting on with them (although the numbers reporting this were fewer than those working with other groups). The third reward lay in observing distinct improvements in the phsyical status of the patient. Although the elderly confused were described as being 'at the end of the road', or as 'hopeless cases', significantly more staff than those working with any other user group except the elderly counted successes in the physical improvement of users as part of their satisfactions. What might be regarded as quite minor advances by other staff groups were viewed as dignified human gains. One young male nurse said he liked to be able to show the relatives that the patient 'had done just one thing more than they did before they came in'. A fourth reward for staff lay in feeling that they 'gave a break' to the families of the elderly confused. This is discussed in more detail in Chapter 10.

Complaints from staff concerned their working conditions more than the patients. The poor state of the buildings and the lack of space is discussed in more detail in Chapter 17. In fact relatively few day units for the elderly confused were purpose built (only a quarter) and almost every head declared the premises of the unit to be 'partly suitable' or 'unsuitable'. All but one of the health authority units were found in the grounds or on the premises of a hospital, usually a psychiatric hospital. Half the heads felt this was 'unsuitable' or only 'partly suitable'. So day services for the elderly confused appear to lag behind other user groups in how suitable heads and staff evaluate their premises and surroundings.

Staff also were frustrated by inadequate transport services. Four out of five users came to the unit by special transport which all units provided: but nearly all the heads reported problems. These were very similar to the difficulties of the geriatric day hospitals detailed in Chapter 3.1. The most common complaint hinged on difficulties of timing the ambulance services to accord with the 'day'[2] of the day unit. A second problem related to the supply of transport: some heads could take in more users but had to keep the use of the ambulance service down to an agreed minimum. And the problems of long distances to be travelled by some users was a concern. Transport problems are summarised in Chapter 17.

DAY UNITS AND THEIR ACTIVITIES

Nine of the eleven day units for the elderly confused in the sample were

sponsored by area health authorities.[3] The two units in the sample provided by social services departments were the oldest and opened before
the reorganisation of the social services in 1971. Nearly half the units
were situated in semi-rural or rural surroundings. The high proportion of
day hospitals situated in the grounds of outlying psychiatric hospitals
obviously contributed to this. A quarter of the units were in suburban
areas of private housing, and another quarter were in highly urban
surroundings. Three-quarters of the units were to be found within the
boundaries of county councils, as opposed to the metropolitan districts or
London boroughs.

Day units for elderly confused people offer their users eclectic programmes. The variety of the programmes were summed up by the
occupational therapist introduced earlier who explained:

> We have a very varied activity programme. A session of gentle exercise
> and group activities which involve physical contact with other people.
> Conversation is vitally important. Simple craft activities satisfy the
> desire for pretty things. Music and poetry refresh the spirit. Gentle
> gardening and bird-watching help make life a little more bearable. We
> always bear in mind that we can never cure these people.

Nearly all the heads of units said the following activities were offered to
users in the week before the survey: *arts and crafts* (particularly knitting,
sewing and painting), *physical treatments* (mainly drugs and nursing care)
and a *social programme* (mainly record sessions, bingo and outings).
Further, nearly three-quarters of the units had held meetings for users,
the most common meeting being a discussion group; normally a topic-
centred discussion about news of the day or activities related to patients.
Perhaps even more surprisingly, just under half the units offered contract
work and/or 'educational' classes to their users. The contract work
centred on simple work like packing plastic car parts or on domestic work
around the day units, such as setting the lunch table and washing up.
Gardening, baking, jam-making and preserving were on the domestic
'work' agenda of the more rurally located units. The 'educational' classes
mostly included shopping trips and self-care classes.

COMMENT

What does all this activity mean? The impression is that those working in
the day units seem to be well aware of the potential of their task in staying
the deterioration of their patients. 'Put plainly', said one charge nurse,
'we want to get involved with the preventative aspect of psychogeriatric
care. We realise we are not one of the sophisticated day hospitals now to
be found in the psychiatric field. If we are limited in our day-to-day
aspirations, it is because our patients are limited.'

Day services for the elderly confused have entered the field of 'moral
management'.

The comfort of a warm bath ... often occasions expressions of remarkable satisfaction. The refreshed patient is taken out of the bath, carefully dried and has clean and comfortable clothing put on; he is then led out of the day room and offered good and well prepared food ... Wherever patients go they meet kind people, and hear kind words; they are never passed without some recognition and the face of every officer is the face of a friend. (Conolly, 1856).

Although this description does not come from a late twentieth-century day unit, but from the early nineteenth-century advocate of 'moral management', Dr John Conolly, his comment could have been made by members of staff in a psychogeriatric day unit. The rural surroundings, the site within mental hospitals, the multiform activities and the stress staff place on kindliness and patience are reminders of the days of 'moral management' in nineteenth-century psychiatry. The judicious regime of a lack of physical restraint, a philosophy of kindness, good food, varied occupation and personal contact between staff and patient, characterised the treatment of the mentally ill before the growth of large institutions and the population explosion of the mid to late nineteenth century (Jones, 1972). The belief that 'lunatics' were suffering human beings inspired the 'moral management' programmes of the era. Similarly, the belief that 'dements' are sad old people informs the activities for the elderly confused in the day units of today. In this light it is important to note that half the staff are nurses who have come out of long-term hospitals to the day hospitals. Some interpret this as a highly progressive step which makes them feel optimistic about their patients. (The problems of maintaining the morale of staff working with psychogeriatric patients in long-stay hospitals have been described (Arie, 1977). There was slight evidence to suggest that if a staff member's training had been geared to achieving clinical 'progress' (as in the cases of four doctors and three occupational therapists), the stronger were the reservations expressed about working with elderly confused people because the full range of 'skills' were thought to be under-utilised.

At present the morale of staff seems relatively high. First, there is the motivation of staff, which appears to come from combining personal convenience with a sense of mission. Second, there is a relatively high staff–user ratio. Third, there is a varied programme (which may be as important for the staff as users). Fourth, there is an acceptance on the part of staff of the erratic behaviour of the elderly confused person along with an ability to be satisfied with achieving minimal personal and physical gains for users. This replaces a desire to 'cure'. All these factors seem to contribute to what might be termed staff morale.

A second matter relates to the question of which users in particular might best be helped by psychogeriatric day units. A high proportion of elderly confused persons enter hospital or residential care from the day units. Four out of ten of those discharged from day units for the elderly confused in the previous twelve months were admitted straight into long-term permanent care. At the same time we know that the highest proportion of elderly confused persons in day units live alone. The policy of offering day places to those who live alone has recently been questioned (Bergmann *et al.*, 1978). It may be important for the future to consider offering day services for the elderly confused to those who have family support – particularly the support of their children. Those with relatives to care for them may be helped to stay in the community longer if they are given the support of a day service, as the elderly patient living alone with dementia presents a very poor short-term prospect for survival and patients living with spouses were more likely to be admitted to hospital than patients living with their children (Bergmann *et al.*, 1978). There is therefore an argument in favour of using scarce day unit resources to bolster the care of those elderly persons who are most likely to remain in the community – those living with family support.

ROUTES

Chapter 10 discusses other aspects of the care of the elderly confused.

NOTES

1 This figure does not include patients from the eleventh day hospital where the district Division of Psychiatry refused us permission to interview patients.
2 This was usually a five-day week although one day hospital was open six days and another social services centre was open seven days a week.
3 Four health authorities were unaware of the existence of units for the confused in their areas until the survey 'discovered' them!

REFERENCES

Age Concern Research Unit (1977) *Profiles of the Elderly,* Volume 1 (1), 'Who are they?' and Volume 2 (4), 'Their health and the health services' (Age Concern).
Arie, T. (1977) 'Issues in the psychiatric care of the elderly', in A. Exton Smith and J. Evans (eds), *Care of the Elderly* (Academic Press).
Bergmann, K., Foster, E. M., Justice, A. W. and Matthews, V. (1978) 'Management of the demented elderly person in the community', *British Journal of Psychiatry,* 132, pp. 441–9.
Conolly, J. (1856) with an introduction by R. Hunter and I. McAlpine (1964) *The Treatment of the Insane without Mechanical Restraints* (Dawsons of Pall Mall).
Jones, K. (1972) *A History of the Mental Health Services* (Routledge & Kegan Paul).
Kay, D. W. K., Bergmann, K. *et al.* (1970) 'Mental illness and hospital usage in the elderly: a random sample follow-up, *Comprehensive Psychiatry,* II, 1, pp. 26–35.
Kay, D. W. K., Beamish, P. and Roth, M. (1964) 'Old age mental disorders in

Newcastle upon Tyne', pt 1, *British Journal of Psychiatry*, 110, 465, pp. 146–58.

Levin, E. (1979) *Personal communication*.

Medical Research Council (1977) *Senile and Presenile Dementias: A Report of the MRC Subcommittee* (Medical Research Council).

Schulman, K. and Arie, T. (1978) 'Fall in admission rate of old people to psychiatric units', *British Medical Journal*, 6106 (21 January 1978), pp. 156–8.

CHAPTER 3.6

———◆———

THE FAMILY DAY CENTRE

INTRODUCTION

Family day centres are a minute fraction of day care for pre-school children. Our estimates indicate that by 1976 no more than 100 such centres could have existed in England and Wales. Family day centres are neither day nurseries nor nursery schools nor playgroups. They are 'different' to the bulk of day care for under 5s because parents either help to run the centre or receive a service themselves from it. Of seven family day care centres the average ratio of staff members to adult users was 1 : 1.5, although of course this ratio omits the children in the centres.

Of the six family centres in the study four were found in an inner London borough (Innerborough). Voluntary agencies were responsible for four of the six. The section which follows, however, omits one of the Innerborough centres, a day care programme for child minders held in a double-decker bus. In a number of ways this 'unit' fell outside the terms of reference of the study, hence its omission from the discussion which follows. Another unit omitted is a day centre for parents who hurt or batter their children which opened in Midshire just as the survey finished.

In the 1970s, increased research attention has been paid to the stresses encumbent on the parents of young children. Although it was John Donne who said 'poore mothers cry that their children come not right or orderly', this was echoed by the twentieth-century mothers in family centres. One of their themes was their loss of control. They find it hard to control their children, their own tempers and their surroundings. Here is one mother who introduces the problems faced by some users of family day centres:

Example
Mary is 27 and lives with her 7-year-old daughter and a kitten in a council flat in inner London. Unmarried, she has no relatives apart from a brother in Nottingham. She left school at 15, took live-in jobs as a maid in a hospital, became pregnant, came to London and had her baby. She has been coming to the centre for fourteen months, having found out about the centre from her health visitor. 'I was depressed about the electricity bill and it had been cut off – I told the health visitor and she sent me up here.'

Most times she feels depressed.

My kid makes me depressed. I worry about money [she is on statutory benefits] and getting things for the kid. This place is a talking centre, to help give you friends and somewhere to go to work out your problems. It's like a club – someone to talk to – it brightens you up – it's very friendly.

Mo [the leader] solves problems for me – you can talk to her and she knows who to contact. I don't get so many problems now because of the centre. I can talk about them before they get too big, the problems.

Who runs the centre is important. The most important point is staff need to be friendly, that makes a hell of a difference. They need to get on with people. You couldn't take a problem to someone you couldn't talk to. You need to be able to talk and joke. They need to be passed by the welfare so education is important: you need to be educated to solve problems. You have to be able to talk to important people and you have the backing of the unit behind you if you're educated. They have to be careful with you if you're educated.

Checklist: Vital Statistics
Family Day Centres

Number of units in national census	6[a]
Number where interviewing took place	6[a]
Number of heads and staff interviewed	19
Number of users interviewed	29
Average size of unit (user places)	4–9
Range of size of units (user places)	6
Average ratio of staff to adult users[b]	1 : 3

[a] Only five of these units are reported in the section which follows.
[b] The ratio is calculated on the number of parents attending the centre and should be at least doubled to take account of the children attending the unit.

THE PARENTS

Twenty-nine young parents in six family day care centres were interviewed.[1] Their losses of control were over their children, themselves and their surroundings. Over a third mentioned that it was difficult to manage their children. 'My children are always fighting, they never sit nicely', complains a 30-year-old mother from Cyprus. 'I just could not control my little boy', states a 22-year old mother of two, separated from her husband.

He had been back to and fro from his dad and I just did not know if I was coming or going. I could not understand why he was taking it out on me. I can understand better since I've been coming here why children do things now. Before they were aggressive and they'd tear the wallpaper down [at home]. Here they tell you how to understand it and they suggest ways to get them to do certain things. Since coming here I can cope with life better, before I just wanted to get out of it [she had taken an overdose] – now I can cope.

Further, these parents – the average age was 29 – confess to difficulties in controlling themselves. More users in family day centres than other forms of day care admit to feeling upset and irritable with those around them – and have trouble controlling their temper. ('Every day I start quarrelling with my husband and then I hit my children.')

Nearly two-thirds mentioned they were depressed: and one-quarter of these were assessed as being 'considerably' depressed. (In fact more users of family day care were rated as suffering from considerable depression than users in day units for the mentally ill.) Although not asked directly about causes of depression, the two most frequent spontaneous explanations related to lack of money and feelings of being lonely, or both. Lack of money was mentioned by over half the parents. All but two of the families with a depressed head of family existed on state supplementary benefits, thus below the poverty level. In the twenty-nine families two-thirds of the families relied on supplementary benefits.

Twenty-five-year-old Cathy, mother of two living in local authority temporary 'part three' accommodation and existing on benefits, commented: 'Well, if there's one thing that gets me down its not having enough money. On days I don't have enough money I feel rotten about everything.'

Two-thirds mentioned feeling lonely and lacking friends: over half the families were headed by a single, separated, divorced or widowed parent (one was a single parent grandparent). For example, a 25-year-old former machine operator, now the single mother of two, commented: 'I've been very depressed in the last month especially at night when the kids are asleep. I always have to do something during the day to keep me occupied, I do the housework all over again, I'm so lonely.'

Further, parents in family day centres indicated that they have problems in controlling their locality. More problems arose than with other user groups: a third considered that they had difficulties about which their local community could be more helpful. Predominant amongst these were requests for full-time day care facilities. Six of every ten parents came to the unit on only one or two days per week. Better housing, especially housing which offered adequate play facilities for the children, was also considered a need. A few also complained about the restrictions on movement imposed by the neighbourhood. 'There is so much traffic where we live: I can't leave the children to play out or cross the road to go to the park: the traffic is so heavy', said a single 23-year-old mother of two.

Perhaps because of these material and practical problems, parents used the services of general practitioners, health visitors and local authority social workers more frequently than other user groups, including the elderly and the mentally ill.

FAMILY DAY CENTRE 'STAFF'

Three of the five centres were run by staff and the other two by a parent management committee. However, as the centres run by staff promoted a high degree of parent participation, we shall call them the 'parent-involved' centres. The other two centres will be known as the 'parent-controlled' centres.

Staff members in family day centres were younger than staff members in other branches of day care except offenders. The average age of both the heads and staff was 34 years: all the heads of units (apart from one of the two 'parent-controlled' centres) were tertiary educated in either social work, social science or teaching. However, half the staff were unqualified (more than most other user groups). This implies that the leadership of family day care is more qualified than the average while the staff are slightly less qualified than the average.[2] Three-quarters of heads and staff were female, but one of the 'parent-involved' centres had a man as a leader.

Heads claimed to have sought their job because of their commitment to improving the quality of family life. In contrast to all other user groups, none of the heads mentioned 'conditions of service' or 'promotion reasons' as reasons for taking the job. Over half the staff in family day centres acknowledged that they had sought their jobs for reasons similar to the heads but the same number related their choice of job to the convenient hours and proximity to their home.

PARENT-CONTROLLED CENTRES

In the parent-controlled centres, five playleaders were employed and thirty-one parents worked on the rota. Of the two 'parent-controlled' centres in London, the first (partially grant aided by Innerborough) was set up to offer community day care for pre-school children as part of a neighbourhood project which would eventually cater for other groups such as the elderly. Opened in 1975, it occupied an old house and was open five days a week. Parents constituted the managment 'collective', hired the staff and also worked themselves on the nursery rota (with nominal pay) to support the three full-time paid play leaders. A weekly meeting of all parents set policies. According to one of the parents, it was set up 'to enable people to take more responsibility for their lives and to challenge the assumption that the mass of people do not want to have active involvement in their children's day care. People work together and make a large commitment to a project that comes from their own needs.'

On the other hand the precarious and interim funding of the centre led to problems for parents. One mother explained:

> We have to spend too much time on political issues like fund-raising and campaigning for premises at the expense of the day-to-day running of the nursery. This means we don't give the children what they need: the right kind of atmosphere and play facilities. There's not the rhythm and peace that children need to develop individual and social capacities. The lack of structure is potentially damaging to children.

The second 'parent-controlled' project, funded by the EEC, was more financially secure. It was set up by the branch of a self-help organisation for single parents in Outerborough. As well as providing care during the day for pre-school children, it offered after school care to school age children because most of the single parents using the centre went to work. 'This centre is to help single parents who want to work and otherwise wouldn't be able to because of insufficient care facilities. It provides a forum for play for children that's not too loose and does not involve leaving them to their own devices.' The project was managed by the branch committee who hired staff who were usually, but not always, single parents. About one in six parents also helped on the roster as volunteers.

In the 'parent-controlled' centre the functions of the staff and the parents are indistinct because parents are users and sometimes staff.[3] There was also a tendency for users in 'parent-controlled' centres to hold higher educational qualifications than those interviewed in the 'parent-involved' centres.

PARENT-INVOLVED CENTRES

Fifteen heads and staff worked in the 'parent-involved' centres, in other words, those centres which were staff controlled. Two of the three centres were sponsored by voluntary family agencies in Innerborough and the Midshire county social services department. Two of the three centres were headed by qualified social workers and the third by a former teacher. Each offered discussion groups in which all parents took part and a limited range of arts and crafts programme, mainly sewing or knitting.

The Midshire unit, sited in a new town, was led by a male social worker. There were two groups of users, each representing six to seven families who had been defined as problem families: each came two days per week for about six months. In contrast to the other two 'parent-involved' units, relationships between parents and their children were discussed very closely in this unit. The aims were described by a 25-year-old father like this: 'I think the aim is to help parents unwind. To unwind here so they don't unwind on the children at home. To sort out their problems here and not at home. To stop worrying so they don't take it out on the children. You tell them any problems, they do their best to help you.'

The second 'parent-involved' centre run by a social worker was in Innerborough. Basically a parents' group which ran as an adjunct to a voluntary day nursery, the care of the children was separate from the group for parents. While the social worker worked with the parents, nursery nurses ran the nursery. 'It's for isolated and depressed mothers', explained one. 'It's here if you want to talk or be with other adults.'

The third project, also sponsored by a voluntary family agency, operated as a 'parent-involved' centre for three days a week in a community hall. It offered a club for local mothers and was the only unit where children were not deliberately involved in activities (a fact complained about by several parents). It was described by a mother as 'a place to give you somewhere to go to work out your problems but it's more a talking centre to give you friends'.

IMPACT ON USERS

What parents got most out of the day centre was, first, the contact it provided with other parents, second, the practical services it offered and third, the way they felt it modified their children's behaviour.

First, two-thirds of the parents delineated the benefits of meeting with others. Sharing common experiences appeared to lighten the burden.

It's helped me to make friends which I can't do on my own.

It's given us a family life.

Working with other people in a group has given my life a focus.

When I started coming here it was the high spot of my week. My marriage had broken up. It was so important to me – I've made a lot of friends.

Second, half the parents alluded to the help of the centre either in improving their children's behaviour or in contributing to their own confidence in feeling that they could cope with the children.

Now he eats his meals which he didn't before.

It helps me to cope with the children better.

It's helped me with Thomas and his potty training: if you have a problem with the children they help you out. Everything they have spoken to me about has worked out all right.

Third, more parents than those in other user groups, except offenders, said that the day centre had provided or arranged special help for them. Of this 17 per cent, one 25-year-old father declared:

> I've had a lot of help with family problems. When my son was in hospital they arranged for us to be taken and brought back. They helped me to sort my bills out and with information, how to get extra time. For me it couldn't have done more as it has helped me to adapt and talk my problems out and see how others are in the same way.

The particular climate in most of the family centres was often based on the rationale of a therapeutic setting, an aim discussed in more detail in Chapter 13. As we have seen there was more opportunity for parents to be involved in family day centres than in other kinds of day units. In practical terms over half the parents (slightly more than in other groups) considered they helped to run the centre. They spoke about serving a committee, helping to contribute to the daily maintenance of the unit by doing chores like cooking or shopping.

There was a tendency for more parents to claim to have talked to staff about their personal problems than users of other forms of day centres.[4] This may relate to the parents' assessments of the staff's ability 'to handle anyone and to deal with their problems' and also to frequent comments that the staff were 'good with children'. The approachability of the staff is also discussed in Chapter 13 but was a point of agreement by almost all parents. One said: 'They're not stuck up here, they don't class themselves better than the likes of me.' Others said:

> The thing is, they're not snobs. They have to talk proper and work with people. They are polite and when you come in they always give you their attention. They have to understand people and not lose their temper.

> They have to be approachable.

> They have to get people involved: training gives confidence.

The facility of staff in getting on with children in a family day centre is consistently visible to parents. Half the parents noted this, and 'relating to the little ones' added to the credibility of the staff. These comments come from parents in the Midshire family day centre:

> The staff need to be loving and affectionate to all the kids and that's what they are down here all the time. Some of the children are really wild and need a lot of patience.

> Tommy was very crabby but the social workers didn't mind that. Everything they have tried to help me with has worked out all right.

They are good with children . . . they help you with anything you can't
do and find a way around it for you. They have to know what to expect
from children.

They have to cope with children without getting depressed.

Parents in day care tend to talk to each other more about their worries
and problems than other users. More said they were able to discuss
personal problems with the parents' group and an equal number were
able to talk with at least one other parent. One mother commented: 'We
begin to depend on each other: that's what friends are for.'
One centre which combines the 'parent controlled' and 'parent
involved' approaches is the London Borough of Camden Langtry Young
Family Care Centre (Brill, 1976). This social services family day centre
has aimed to employ mothers of children as paid workers in the centre
along with other staff, as a prelude to seconding them to professional
training courses. This scheme is similar to the 'New Careers' movement,
but unfortunately was cut back in local authority expenditure trims
during the financial crisis of 1976. In the long term, however, involving
parents or other close relatives in the day unit may be a sound investment.
Consider the moral of the tale told by Eric Midwinter about young
Timothy Shy:

'A Cautionary Tale'
(with sincere apologies to Hilaire Belloc)

The Tender Years of Timothy Shy
Were slightly incommoded by
His marked reluctance on request
To recognise with Vocal Zest
The simplest shapes and colours bright,
Or pile his tumblers up aright.
In every field he Fell Behind
The others of his Age and Kind,
All of whom could gaily prattle
Ere Timothy could grasp his rattle;
Nor did he greet with Deep Elation
His fellows in close conversation,
Refusing all their hopes of play.
His parents soon felt quite distrait . . .
. . . Thus, after Laboured Negotiation
Of a nature which defies narration,
Timothy Shy, it came to pass,
Joined a brand-new Nursery Class,
With vivid hues from wall to wall
And a Tropical Fish-tank in the hall.

Hopefully, his mother took him
To the school, but then foresook him,
Because, emblazoned on the gate,
She found a notice which did state
For every's mother's steadfast guide:
'Parents are Welcome to Wait Outside'.
Tim was therefore flatly landed
In spheres well-watered and well-sanded,
With climbing-frame and all the frills
Equipped to nurture Timothy's Skills,
Under the eye and at the knee
Of a Nursery Nurse (NNEB)
Who offered him from Head to Toe,
An ample chance to learn and grow
And free himself into the bargain,
And, 'socialise' (Excuse the jargon).
But Mrs Shy, a homely dearie,
Knew naught of modern Childhood Theory,
With access to the place denied
Wherein she might, at teacher's side,
Learn by what Method to what Goal,
The modern pre-school child's made whole.
So cudgelling her unsharpened wit,
His mother did the opposite
Of all the school contrived for Tim.
It was a Trifle Blurred for him.
Now school time very fast expires
Compared with hours before home fires,
And mother's influence though perverse,
Was more pronounced than that of nurse;
Where they did 'number' she did 'sums';
'Free' art for teacher; the 'lines' were mum's;
They laid off letters: she went 'phonic',
Leaving Tim a confused and chronic
Case of academic schizophrenia,
In which his mother played the senior
And more crucial role, so that the cost
Was a Nursery Schooling largely lost.
Pre-schoolers should remark the thought:
'Hearth is Long: Cloisters Short'.
To give each child a Valid Start
Both Home and School must Play its Part:
And they must take a combined grip
To share in fruitful partnership.

(Midwinter, 1977)

COMMENT

Family day care centres can be distinguished by the type of involvement of parents in running the centre. In the 'parent-involved' centres, those where parents have less control in running the centre, the centres also varied in the integration of the service for the parents and that offered to the children. At one end of the scale, in the Midshire centre the programmes and activities of parents and children were organised together, whereas in an Innerborough unit the children's service and the parent programmes were organised quite separately, since a separate staff cared for the children. In the third 'parent-involved' centre children came to the centre only occasionally. In contrast to this, the 'parent-controlled' centres did not have a separate staff caring for parents and children. This fostered closer contact between parents and children in the unit.

One possible speculation for the appreciation of parents for their centres could relate to their perceptions of involvement in the day centre. We have pointed out that these parents feel 'out of control' in everyday life. Some have drawn attention to the lack of power perceived by parents beset by social and emotional problems, particularly by those considered to be 'at risk' for possible child-battering (Carter, 1974). If family day care can provide an experience for these parents which contradicts their assumption that they cannot control themselves, their children or their everyday life, it suggests that this type of day care should be explored more for its potential.

Tim Shy's mother illustrates two related situations which will come up again in this book. The first situation is the low degree of involvement of users themselves in the centre. The second is the low degree of contact that families of users have with the units. By regarding parents as co-users of the centre, family day centres have overcome many of the conflicts that other day units describe as 'normal' in dealing with the families of users.

If the degree of control of the *centre* by parents is a critical factor, further work is needed to determine the way this might relate to the parents' perceptions of being in control of *themselves*. For example, the amount of depression reported by parents in the 'parent-controlled' centres was less than that expressed by parents in the 'parent-involved' centres. Five times as many parents in the 'parent-involved' centres were depressed as those in the 'parent-controlled' centres. However, more parents in the 'parent-involved' centres were on supplementary benefits, on average they had a lower level of education, and the parents in the two types of centres are probably recruited rather differently.

Despite these qualifications, parents in family day care can be regarded as a highly vulnerable group. Half are single parent families, two-thirds are on supplementary benefits and two-thirds are depressed. This profile accords with the picture obtained from recent population studies about the burdens of mothers of young children. Working-class mothers of pre-school children who are at home and who lack someone to confide in are at high risk of psychiatric disturbance (Brown and Harris, 1978) and their children also appear to be at greater risk of developing behaviour disorders (Richman, 1977). Although more parents than users in other groups mentioned spontaneously that the centre had benefited their home life, more exploratory work needs to be done in this area.

ROUTES

Other aspects of family day centres are mentioned in Chapter 13.

NOTES

1 Twenty-six of the twenty-nine users interviewed (90 per cent) were mothers.
2 But no information is available about the qualifications of twenty-one of the thirty-one parents who work on the rotas of the 'parent-controlled' centres.
3 Parents were randomly assigned to be interviewed as either parents or staff.
4 Family day care users were very unlikely to say that they did not have personal problems compared to other user groups.

REFERENCES

Brill, J. (1976) 'Langtry young family centre – a method of intervention', in M. R. Olsen (ed.), *Differential Approaches in Social Work with the Mentally Disordered,* BASW Occasional Paper No. 2 (BASW).
Brown, G. and Harris, T. (1978) *Social Origins of Depression* (Tavistock).
Carter, J. (1974) *The Maltreated Child* (Priory Press).
Midwinter, E. (1977) 'The Tender Years of Timothy Shy', in *Education for Sale* (Allen & Unwin).
Richman, N. (1977) 'Behaviour problems in pre-school children: family and social factors'. *British Journal of Psychiatry,* 131, November, pp. 433–47.

CHAPTER 3.7

———◆———

OFFENDERS

INTRODUCTION

Day services for offenders are new. The first day unit to be opened in this sample started in 1973 and by 1976 it can be estimated that fifty units operated in England and Wales primarily for offenders.

The four accounts which follow introduce the activities of each centre, then a member of staff and a user, selected at random. The staff members discuss the aims of their job, and say what they get out of it. The users say what they interpret as the function of the centre and report what it has done for them.

EXAMPLES

(1) *Centre 112*, a day training centre, is sponsored by a probation service in a northern city. The Criminal Justice Act of 1972, which aimed at halting or at least slowing down the continuing increase in the prison population, provided courts with sentencing powers that could be used as alternatives to prisons. One alternative, the day training centre, required an offender as a condition of a probation order to attend a day training centre for a period 'not exceeding sixty days' – in practice, three months.

Centre 112 opened in 1973 as one of four experimental day training centres. Every three months an intake of about fifteen 'clients' arrives (the number depends on the interest and commitment of sentencing judges and magistrates). The centre occupies part of an old building in the inner city. Staffed by trained probation officers, arts and crafts specialists and educationalists, the programme is comprehensive: arts and crafts, meetings and discussion groups, a work programme and social activities (especially outdoor games), education classes (especially literacy and numeracy). A great deal of use is made of video equipment as a technique to communicate many of the activities, to impart simple social skills in a relaxed way: how to talk politely to a stranger in the street, how to deal with a job interview, and so on.

As an example of a staff member at the centre, meet Marie, a 28-year-old probation officer with a BA in Swedish. She, along with all probation officers in this centre, is trained. After four years' conventional case work in probation, she took this job because she wanted the opportunity to do 'more intensive work and more time to work with individuals in different settings'. She felt she was successful at her job 'when an offender didn't return to court, when he gained greater communication skills, when he had a better idea of himself and his problems, and had been helped to find new ways of resolving them'.

Peter is one of Marie's clients. Aged 26, he had been at the centre for three weeks when he was interviewed. Single, he lived with his parents and two brothers and had worked as a labourer in the building industry although he had been unemployed for the past eight months. He had spent fourteen months in prison, for an earlier conviction. He saw the centre as 'aiming to get to know a person, why he gets into trouble, to see if they can do something about it'. So far, apart from getting rather fed up filling in all the forms, he said the place had opened him up a bit. 'I was very shy – it has helped me to be able to talk to people.'

(2) *Northend Centre* was the only centre in purpose-built premises. Opened in 1976 by the same probation service as Centre 112, it has thirty places each day. Although its overall aim is the same – 'to prevent people from re-offending' – its *modus operandi* is very different to that of Centre 112.

For a start, attendance at Northend is voluntary and up to the users. Paradoxically, however, its front door is kept locked. Nearly all its users are ex-prisoners, although users do not have to be on probation. Attendance at the Northend Centre has no defined time limits, whereas the amount of time a user spends at Centre 112 is carefully defined. The staff at Northend are, in probation terms, untrained. The head of the centre is an ex-policeman, a matter which he says hinders his work ('people just think of you as an ex-copper'). Northend Centre offers no activities to its users apart from offering them a warm place with an informal atmosphere, a cheap lunch, and some restricted social activities such as card games or irregular outings to museums. There are also showers and washing machines for people to do their personal washing. This is considered important, as few of the attenders live independently: most go to hostels or a night shelter, or sleep rough.

Mary has worked in the day centre for four months. She used to do residential work with children. She saw the centre's role in these terms:

> We provide a comfortable, non-threatening environment to try to stabilise many of the wandering population, by encouraging them to use the day centre, thus alleviating persistent callers on the town's probation officer. Also self-help and self-esteem with the aid of showers and clean clothes is important: when they come in they are dirty and horrible, and when they go out they feel a bit cleaner and have more self-esteem.

She defines the most crucial bit of her job as listening to people. She enjoys doing something for a member and having him feel grateful for it, but also finds her job frustrating, feeling that she is not always able to get to the help that a member needs.

Peter is a member of the centre. Now he lives in a bedsitter, although most of the other members live in hostels or the night shelter. He spent three years as a child in an orphanage, and has had two recent prison sentences. Now aged 34, he recently lost a job as warden of a hostel for homeless men. He said: 'All of the lads here are potential thieves. Without this place 79 per cent would be in prison.' This sentiment was expressed by other users, who saw the main function of the centre as keeping them 'out of the nick' in a time of high unemployment. 'I like coming here', said Peter. 'I've made friends and it gives me somewhere to go. It's filled my day.' He explained further: 'Like the OAPs have a club, well, here this is a homeless club. They've all got something in common: unemployment or offending. Only thing is, though, it closes too early – at 3 p.m. 3 p.m. to 10.30 p.m. is a long time for a homeless bloke.'

(3) *The John Smith Project* offers employment and housing to single homeless people in an inner London borough. Not all the users had been in prison, although all have been in mental hospitals in the past. Basically it offers a hostel plus workshops for homeless people on social security benefits. It is hoped this will develop into full-time employment for a few. At present, soft furnishings are made for the houses in which the users live and for sale in a shop. An attempt is being made to develop a printing project, to produce notepaper and cards.

The staff interviewed were former degree students who were working with the project, hoping that it would provide an entrance to college training for a social work qualification. Although the staff agreed to be interviewed about their job, they decided not to complete the postal questionnaire. Its questions offended, it was said.

> By implying that the participants of the workshop were divided into two very separate categories: the helpers – who might be professional or unprofessional – and the helped – be they alcoholic, elderly, or physically handicapped . . . The helpers are defined in terms of their abilities, and the helped are defined in terms of their disabilities. Instead, the workshop must present itself as a vital opportunity for people to discard their labels and to be seen primarily as workers in a work situation where they will survive well or badly according to their skills and more importantly, their ability to work with others. If the workshop can provide this opportunity, then it can play a vital part in breaking down the barriers between the so-called able and disabled.

The current staff leader was a former sociology student. When interviewed about the project, John, aged 23, defined his main use of time in the working week as 'supervising the users'. This included 'watching users at work, supervising their movements, giving instructions, reprimanding users, and so on'.

The users were paid 40p an hour for their work, an amount which kept their earnings inside the social security disregard limit. Gail, a 59-year-old user, lived at the hostel next door. She gave an account of a varied institutional career: first a children's home, then a TB hospital. Seven admissions to mental hospital were interspersed with six admissions to prison. In between these she had worked as a waitress in hotels and bed-and-breakfast places across England and Wales. She saw the purpose of the centre as this: 'to control people, to keep them sane, and to make them able-bodied'. (Her claim that she had been awarded six Victoria Crosses, and that her past bills in the children's home were paid by King Gustav of Sweden, are unlikely.) But she did say: 'This house has made me feel better than the hospital and the gaol. They got my dole through. They've made me feel normal. I've had a bath every day. I watch TV.'

(4) *Peterborough House* is a centre in a northern city which is run by a voluntary agency with help from a probation and after-care committee. Opened in 1974, it provides 'unlimited' day places, although the average daily attendance is four to six. The head says: 'The centre tries to give persons who come – voluntarily – a place of identity, a place to feel relaxed, and we try to put some therapy into action.' There is a programme of arts and crafts, a meeting-cum-discussion group each week, and a social programme along with cricket and football. As well as this, the attenders are expected to help in the cooking and in cleaning and decorating the day room which is attached to the hostel.

Doreen, aged 26, is the deputy head, married to the head of the project. Without formal qualifications, she is a former cadet nurse. She describes her job thus:

I start off with the basic needs of the lads by making sure the house is clean and tidy. Food and cleanliness: if you substitute 'mother', that is it. Their emotional needs too, remembering them as a person by being here and talking to them: letting them think they have made decisions when really I have manipulated them into it. Making sure that they are secure is the most important thing.

Three of the five offenders interviewed in this centre had been in a training centre, two in prison, and three had spent time in children's homes. This might have been unexceptional if their average age was not 17. All except one lived in the hostel and all were currently unemployed: two of the five had never held a job. Martin, aged 17, living at present in a Salvation Army hostel, claims that he felt like doing away with himself often. 'I don't feel a part of those around me. Everywhere I go, I feel in a trap.' His other theme was wanting to do a job, or get on a course – 'a woodwork course, I'm full of ideas'. He had spent seven years in a boarding school for maladjusted children, and then three months in a 'training centre'. He had held a factory job for three months but now unemployed, he can see little hope in the future. 'I can't see any improvement in me. But I know they are trying their hardest to help me here.'

Checklist: Vital Statistics
Offenders

Number of units in national census[a]	4
Number where interviewing took place	4
Number of heads and staff interviewed	12
Number of units interviewed	24
Average size of unit (number of user day places)[a]	23
Range of size of units (user places)[a]	15–30
Average ratio of staff to users[a]	1 : 5

[a] Three units returned postal questionnaire.

Centres for offenders, of which there were these four in the study, opened between 1973 and 1976.[1] An active debate ensued immediately about the principles on which such centres should run. These dilemmas will be mentioned because they apply in greater or less force to issues which will arise with other user groups. First, should these centres work with offenders on a voluntary or a compulsory basis? In other words, should it be up to the users to decide whether or not they want to come, or should they be legally compelled to attend the centre? In three of the four centres in the study, users came of their own volition; in the fourth, the court had the power to order a potential user to attend a day training centre for a period of 'not exceeding sixty days' as part of a probation order. This change came about after the Criminal Justice Act of 1972 which aimed at slowing down the continuing increase in the prison population by providing courts with sentencing powers that could be used as alternatives to prison (Pearce, 1974).

A second dilemma is whether centres for offenders should aim to rehabilitate offenders to 'normal' life outside in the community or whether to allow users to stay in the centre long term – if necessary on a life-long basis. There is a related issue here: how long should users be allowed to spend in the centre? At least one London day centre was recently closed down by the management because the users were not 'rehabilitated'. By contrast, the staff saw the idea of 'rehabilitating' their clientele of 'old lags' (mostly with inadequate personalities and a lifetime of convictions and imprisonment behind them) as essentially unrealistic. They considered that offering a day centre as a warm, secure place to which chronic offenders could be encouraged to retreat from the temptations of the outside world was a valuable contribution to reducing the crime rate. If the men were at the centre they could not be pinching toiletries at Woolworths or throwing bricks through bathroom windows.

A third dilemma is the degree to which centres for offenders actually gear themselves to work on the offender's *offence*, or alternatively concentrate on the background social problems which seem to accompany the offence. One of the four centres was, strictly speaking, a centre for homeless people who also happened to be offenders (or many of them were). The other three centres dealt with homeless people but secondarily to their offence. This is not an academic point, as another important fact which emerged in day centres for offenders, as we shall now see, is the high proportion of mental illness amongst the users of centres for offenders. In fact a higher proportion of users attending centres for offenders had spent longer periods in psychiatric or mental hospital than in prison.

OFFENDERS AND INSTITUTIONS

Who uses day centres for offenders? For a start, as already implied, offenders were a group who had passed many years of their life living in an institution. Over a third (nine of the twenty-four interviewed) had spent two years or more in children's homes (proportionately more than any other user group). This institutional beginning extended into the adult life of the users: nearly two-thirds had spent a year or more in one kind of adult institution or another. For half, ten years or more had been spent in institutions. The bulk of this time was not spent, as one might think, languishing in prison, but in a mental or psychiatric hospital. In other words, as already mentioned, more of those in centres for offenders spent longer in hospital than they did in prison.

Two-thirds of the offenders were under the age of 40: on average their age was 34 years. Men predominated. Over a quarter lived in hostels, more than other user groups. Offenders were also the least 'married' group in day services, aside from the mentally handicapped: only 8 per cent were married. But unlike the mentally handicapped they were comparatively the most physically robust group in day care: all could walk a quarter of a mile alone or climb stairs alone.

As far as qualifications went, the users in centres for offenders were no worse off than any other group. There were marginally more with a trade qualification, but set against this it must be remembered that two out of three had no qualifications at all. The context in which this needs to be interpreted is that the offenders represent the youngest group of people in day care apart from those in family day centres.

More offenders, almost three out of every four (more than those in any

---

other user group), planned to leave the centre at some stage. Half of these thought that some attempt had been made by the staff to discuss rehabilitation and their future with them. This is double the proportion of mentally ill users who thought that rehabilitation had been discussed with them.

STAFF

Twelve staff members of centres for offenders were interviewed. Unlike the imbalance of men over women amongst the users, there were equal numbers of men and women staff in the centre. One-third were trained probation officers.

One distinctive feature of centres for offenders was that the staff and users interviewed both reported that regular discussions about rehabilitation and training took place in the centre. Of the twelve staff, half agreed that regular discussion took place with their users, and the same proportion of users considered that someone on the staff had discussed their rehabilitation or their future with them. As a comparison, consider the mentally ill units where nearly two-thirds of the staff thought they discussed these matters with their users, but only a fifth of the users thought this had happened while they had been in the unit.

DISCUSSION

Users in centres for offenders make a point which has wider application than this one user group. What happens to users after they leave the centre is beyond the scope of this study, but it is an important question often discussed in the field of dealing with offenders. In many ways those staff working with offenders appear to be under much more community and agency pressure to justify their results than those working in other fields of day care. This could be partly related to an increasing scepticism about the role of rehabilitation and treatment in penal policy, illustrating that the community has a different attitude to those deviants who offend against the law, than to other kinds of 'deviants'. For example, the community cares less, perhaps, whether a mentally ill person has another breakdown or a physically handicapped person a relapse, than whether an offender commits another crime.

It is not very meaningful to compare the outcomes between these four centres because the assumptions on which these centres were set up were so very different. Certainly the number of users who went back to prison from Centre 112, where attendance was compulsory, was rather less than the number who went back to prison from the Northend Centre. Only six out of 120 users went back to prison from Centre 112 in one year: but twelve out of forty attenders at Northend went back to prison in the same time span.

Yet return to prison is not the same as reconviction rate and even if it were, it would not say much about the effectiveness of the two types of centres, largely because they have a different kind of intake and also because the users in each centre are exposed to potential criminal risks for different lengths of time because of the different discharge policies of each centre. A rather different point is that examining the effectiveness of day units only in terms of reconviction rates ignores the implicit success of those who do *not* re-offend. For this group – as well as those who re-offend, we need to ask whether their specific abilities to cope in the community have improved. One centre discusses this question by asking whether a user's 'survival kit' has strengthened. Has the centre improved his skills in coping with life outside?

Day centres for offenders deal with a very damaged group of people, just by virtue of their extensive institutional background. On the one hand it seems unreasonable to expect that staff should be expected to unravel the multiple social deprivations and psychic insults experienced by the graduates of mental institutions and children's homes, all in a three-month period. On the other hand, given time, it appears that day centres for offenders – perhaps more than most organisations which offer a service to the offender, or the community – have a chance to persuade offenders to look at issues of personal responsibility more systematically than either prison or probation. Day centres introduce the opportunity for users to take practical and visible responsibility for their own lives. Two centres which have been particularly articulate about the strength of this are the Barbican Centre at Gloucester and the London Day Training Centre (MIND, 1978; Inner London Probation and After-Care Service, 1978).

Both centres work within very different constraints about, for example, whether attendance should be voluntary or compulsory. But the impact of past institutional confinement on the users and the constraints of their current social disadvantages are fundamental issues tackled by each centre. Underlying every aspect of the programme is an attempt to involve the user in the running of the centre. There is less control by users at the day training centre where users stay a shorter period. But at the Barbican, for instance, the guiding principles are those of self-help. Meetings during the week give an opportunity to discuss progress and problems, and the essential direction of how the day centre and its resources are to be used comes from the members themselves. Participation comes during twice-weekly community meetings. A realistic appraisal about the lack of conventional work likely to be available to members has led the members to take on a community service project in a local residential village. Members not only participate in running their own activities and deciding on their own personal programmes but they run activities for others: for example, some members run a club at weekends for some homeless dossers in the area. Some 'graduate' members go on to become staff members in the centre; one ex-offender is the present careers counsellor. Others get jobs: some don't and become community service volunteers.

At a personal level the relationship between the offender and staff member is recognised to be crucial in users' taking personal responsibility. The centre forms a contract with those who after visiting the centre for an initial period decide to join it. The contract is an agreed set of social, personal and work objectives which a member wants to achieve in his time there. The activities in the centre are planned in relation to the contract: a record system (the Kardex) is used regularly by staff and member to record the member's progress, or lack of it. Renegotiation of the contract is possible.

One important aspect of the Barbarian Centre is that it holds out a possibility for a user of eventually becoming a staff member. This penetration of the staff side by the user has, as we have seen, been used in a rather different format by some of the family day centres. In a highly professionalised society, this must be an extremely powerful potential reward for users. As an incentive to persuade users of the value of taking more responsibility for their lives, it suggests an interesting theme for a potential research project. This could look at the comparative outcomes of users with parallel past experiences in centres which allow the user the potential of moving on to the staff with those that do not.

Finally, there is the issue of the amount of time needed to 'rehabilitate' an offender. This matter is discussed in a slightly different context in Chapter 8. But this aside, if it is agreed that short-term day centres for offenders are a viable sentencing alternative to prisons, this does not deal with the issue of reconstituting damaged users within a time scale pertinent to the needs of an individual. So it is important to consider making a pathway from the short-term to the long-term facility. This is due less to the assumption that short term equals acute while long term equals chronic than to the fact that human problems cannot be discretely fitted into predetermined time slots.

ROUTES

For other chapters pertinent to the problems of offenders please turn to:
Chapter 9:   'A Normal Life': Aiming at Rehabilitation
Chapter 13: 'We All Help Each Other': Aiming at Therapeutic Settings
Chapter 14: Listening to Users': Aiming at Relationships

NOTE

1 A fifth opened just as fieldwork concluded.

REFERENCES

Inner London Probation and After-Care Service (1978) *Day Training Centre:*

The Third Progress Report (Inner London Probation and After-Care Service, London).

MIND (1978) *A Study of Day Centres* (MIND, London).

Pearce, W. H. (1974) 'Community-based treatment of offenders in England and Wales', *Federal Probation,* 38 (1) (March), pp. 47–51.

CHAPTER 3.8

◆

MIXED CENTRES

INTRODUCTION

Centres which mix groups of users together by combining two or more disabilities or two or more age groups are something new in day services. All the six units in this study were the product of the first half of the 1970s. The section which follows will explore some aspects of this new development.

This section begins by introducing a user from a centre which mixes the physically handicapped and mentally ill. She comments on what the centre has done for her and how she views mixing together.

Marjorie, aged 57

I'm fifty-seven and I've come here for sixteen months, just two days a week. I wear a caliper due to a gangrene operation in 1972 and my knee is not co-ordinated. I also have psoriasis. I'm a bit confused and have a slight loss of memory.

I think the main aim of this centre is to get us out of our homes and meet other people and compare notes. This place mixes physically handicapped people with the mentally ill. Mixing mentally ill people with normal patients helps them. It helps them to be jollied up and cheered up. For people in my position it does you good to get you out of your homes where you are on your own and mix with people in a worse situation.

Orders here are more or less from upstairs, where the mentally ill users are. We [the physically handicapped] more or less obey them. As long as the mentally ill are cared for here, the head doesn't really bother about us. The rules are that we're not supposed to leave before 4 p.m. and behave ourselves. No rules otherwise. Anything serious and a patient would be dismissed.

Coming here was to get me out of my flat two days a week. I suppose it has helped me mentally, otherwise I would have moped. Seven days a week, honestly you can't be on your own *that* long.

In one sense, most day units are mixed. The official label on the door of

Checklist: Vital Statistics
Mixed Units

Number of units in national census	6
Number where interviewing took place	6
Number of heads and staff interviewed	23
Number of users interviewed	36
Average size of units (user places)	45[a]
Range of size of units (user places)	13–65[a]
Average ratio of staff to users[a]	1 : 15[a]

[a] Based on postal returns from three day units.

the unit ('mental handicap', 'elderly' or 'offenders') is not the last word about the people inside. Most units have groups of people under the roof who the planners and architects had not envisaged as regular users of the place. For example, heads of units for the elderly confused considered that technically only 69 per cent of their users were *both* elderly *and* confused; 12 per cent were just plain elderly, 7 per cent were elderly and physically handicapped and 5 per cent were handicapped physically, not confused. One user in twenty in social services centres for the mentally ill was mentally handicapped in the head's view while one in ten was said to be physically handicapped rather than mentally ill.

But these unofficial amalgamations of users which are part of everyday life in most units are different to those units which mix users by official purpose. This section will consider these units which arrange deliberate mixes of their users. For the purposes of this project, to qualify as 'mixed', a day unit needed to have at least a proportion of 75 per cent of one type of user group against a minimum balance of 25 per cent of another. An additional part of the definition was that both of the user groups comprising the 'mix' would use the same building and facilities. However, in practice, as we shall see, there were a number of ways of organising the use of the building and the facilities which did not necessarily assume – or require – much coming together of the users.

There are two kinds of mixes found in the six units which mix their users. First, there are those mixes which bring together people of differing disabilities. For example, physically handicapped people may mix with the mentally ill, or the mentally handicapped, or both together. Second, there are the kinds of mixes which bring together different age groups, for example, the elderly and children under 5. These kinds of mixes will be now considered in detail.

MIXED DISABILITIES

Physical handicap was the one disability which was common to all four units which fell into this part of the study. It will be simplest to describe these units in turn.

(1) *County Lodge*. This centre, sponsored by a county social services department, has sixty-five places, of which 75 per cent were 'reserved' for the mentally handicapped. The aim of the unit (in the words of the head) is 'to teach trainees work habits, to eventually get them into open or sheltered employment. To give them a fuller life and to train them to be more independent – not to rely on their families.' Contract work (packing sterile supplies for the local hospital, packing kites and stapling together cards) occupied most time for most users. For this work, payment of amounts between 85p and £2.00 per week are offered to supplement supplementary benefits. At County Lodge mixing is a secondary consideration. What this means is that users are allocated primarily to a job rather than segregated according to their particular disability. So mixing the user groups is not the primary principle of organising the centre and the mixing which takes place does so on an *ad hoc* basis.

(2) *Borough Lodge* is a 150-place unit under the aegis of a London borough social services department in a built up area of mixed industry, business and housing. On the day of census 116 users were present. Thirty-one per cent were mentally ill, 29 per cent were mentally handicapped and 22 per cent were physically handicapped. The 'factory' at Borough Lodge is divided into two sections: a sheltered workshop and an 'assessment and rehabilitation' section – all new users stay here for a year before being placed either in the sheltered workshop part, or transferred to open employment. The head sees the aim of the unit as that of 'providing a sheltered workshop for those who would otherwise be unemployable . . . and to give opportunities for outside employment by training and encouraging them in their work so they can resume a more normal life'. Most time is spent by users at industrial work, mostly packing and assembling work. However, there is some straightforward work done by machine which occupies a few users and some limited domestic and gardening tasks for others. Payment ranges from £4.00 per week for the assessment group to about £30 per week, a union-negotiated rate paid to those in the sheltered workshop. Once again, the organising of mixing is *ad hoc*. A mentally ill user may find himself alongside a mentally handicapped person or someone with a physical handicap, depending on the job.

(3) *St Gordon's* has forty official day places, but is usually oversubscribed. Two-thirds of the users are mentally ill, the rest are physically handicapped. The head said that the aim of the centre is 'to act as a stepping stone from psychiatric hospital into the community and to avoid admission into psychiatric hospital. Also we maintain the chronically ill in the community.' There is not the same emphasis on industrial

work at St Gordon's. Users do arts and crafts, and some simple packing and assembly work. They also spend some time at unit meetings and go on outings, particularly in the summer. St Gordon's is located in a two-storey house in particularly attractive gardens. The mentally ill users inhabit the top floor and the physically handicapped occupy ground floor space. Tea and lunch are taken separately. So in this centre the label on the user is the principle by which the users are organised.

(4) *St Mark's* is described at greater length in Chapter 15. Sponsored by a voluntary charity, of thirteen places each day, *all* places on two days each week are taken by persons who suffer from a chronic physical handicap, such as disseminated sclerosis. On the other three days the users are those in the advanced stages of suffering from malignant disease: the terminally ill with limited prognoses. This day unit is attached to a hospice for the dying and its aim is 'to give patients an environment where they realise they are being cared for . . . to give them a social day . . . to relieve their families, they need a day off too'. The users' activities focus on making simple crafts, such as small pottery animals. Many of these objects are sold at fund-raising ventures for the hospice. Mixing between these two groups of users, the terminally ill and physically handicapped, is rare, for each group uses the centre on different days.

STAFF AND USER VIEWS OF MIXED UNITS

Each head, in the four centres described already, was happy about the given mix of users within the centre and wanted to leave the mixture as it was. Not so the staff, whose opinions were more equivocal. Staff at St Mark's and St Gordon's, where users of differing disabilities were separated either by a day of the week or a floor of the building, were happy to leave their units be. In other words, in these two units the random sample of three staff interviewed in each centre approved of the mixed policy. But at County Lodge and Borough Lodge, where mixing between groups was *ad hoc* and unplanned, the staff interviewed in both units wanted the 'minority' group, in each case the physically handicapped, to be excluded from contact with the majority group, the mentally handicapped.

> I would exclude the physically handicapped unless they were mentally handicapped. They need different training to what we can give them. (61-year-old instructor, at Borough Lodge for seven years)

> I think the physically handicapped would be better off somewhere else. I have overcome a severe disability myself and I would try to do it again. (55-year-old instructor, at Borough Lodge for seven years)

> Exclude the physically handicapped. We haven't got the proper facilities. (47-year-old ex-fitter, at County Lodge for seven months)

Exclude the physically handicapped people. Spastics and wheelchair
people are often intelligent and resent being with the mentally handicapped. (39-year-old former sales assistant, also at County Lodge for
seven months)

What about the users? The users at St Gordon's and St Mark's[1] do not
want to exclude anyone. St Gordon's, of course, is the centre where users
of different disability are separated effectively by using different floors of
the building. But at County Lodge and Borough Lodge some physically
handicapped people disagreed. A minority (two out of eight) would
exclude not themselves, the physically handicapped, but the mentally
handicapped. Here are some of their comments:

I dislike the working together of the physically and mentally handicapped [said an 18-year-old lad at County Lodge with a spastic condi-
tion]. I just don't think it's right to mix handicapped people who are
very bad. It makes you think you are the same as them and you're not.

I do think there are too many mentally handicapped and the staff treat
you as if you are mentally handicapped. You can't have an intelligent
conversation [said a 56-year-old spastic man at Borough Lodge]. The
work's not interesting and the people, being mental, are not stimulating at all. The mentally handicapped should be in a special place for
backward people.

On the other hand, those who did not feel strongly *against* mixing with
other disability groups did not discuss their reasons for this. It is not
possible to say whether it is the actual presence of mentally handicapped
people or the actual type of mixing together that the physically handicapped users objected to. For example, in two other centres, not strictly
speaking mixed because the units were divided into two separate wings,
one each for mentally and physically handicapped users, the implication
was that there were fewer complaints about mixing. (It is right to be
cautious about this, though, as the evidence is not strictly speaking
directly comparable with that of mixed centres.)

MIXED AGE GROUPS

Two centres offered a service to those aged over 60 and to children aged
under 5.

(1) *Centre Point*, operated by a local community association and grant
aided by the local council, is in a deteriorated part of inner London. In a
reconstructed building there is a day centre for the elderly, with lunch
facilities for about eighty each day, and a playgroup for under 5s – this can
cope with about ten children each day. Both age groups have their own

'space' and there are no planned activities which combine the two groups. Three old people (but no parents) are on the management committee for the centre. The main activities for the elderly, aside from lunch, are some limited crafts (mostly knitting), cards and bingo. The aim of the unit, as the organiser sees it, is to try to meet the needs of the elderly living nearby. 'It's one part of an integrated project to provide in the one building a mixing of different ages in the one setting, not isolating of one age group.' The degree to which both age groups actually *mix* rather than just use the same building is restricted.

(2) *Petra St Centre*. This started as a centre for the elderly, the main emphasis being a lunch offered by the WRVS. This gives a meal to an unrestricted number of old people – in practice about fifty each day and some stay into the afternoon to join in with bingo or perhaps an outing. There is a clear division of responsibility, as far as the volunteers are concerned, between the long-established service for the elderly and the newer pre-school playgroup which uses a spare room on the premises. For the elderly people, the 73-year-old leader (formerly a clerical officer in the Ministry of Food) had these unambiguous aims: 'It's feeding the old people, mainly giving them somewhere to go.' The 34-year-old leader of the playgroup, who described herself as a former depressed mother, said of her work:

> It's to help the mums to mix with each other. The children as well. If we weren't here they would have nowhere to go. We have started a sewing circle which some have never done. We have jumble sales to help buy toys and fix them ourselves. That's the only help we get. It's nice to see the children enjoying themselves.

In both these centres heads, staff and most users were clear that the centre supported two distinctive age groups. Heads, staff and users were also clear that they wanted the centre left as it was. They neither wanted the other age group removed nor did they want any other group included.

DISCUSSION

It should be said, to start with, that the evidence on which to discuss the 'mix' of mixed centres is based is tenuous. The size of the sample of units – just six – is small. Also, if the survey had been geared towards examining mixed centres only, a more intelligent method of selecting the users to be interviewed than the random sample might have been adopted. For example, we might have found a method which stratified the sample either by disability or age group. This might have been more enlightening for as it is, there are two few representatives of each disability group who have been interviewed to do much more than indicate initial trends.

Given these limitations, some matters do, however, raise themselves for further exploration. The first matter is the way that mixed centres organise themselves to use their space, the building in which the centre lives. Basically two different formats emerge. The first format offers separate space to each user group. Within this separate space a separate programme is run for each. For examples, take Centre Point and Petra Street; St Mark's and St Gordon's. The second format offers common space to both sets of users and amalgamates them by a common programme to both. Examples here are County Lodge and Borough Lodge.

The provisional outcome is that while heads of mixed units are committed to whatever format the centre has already, more staff and users appear to be happier with the first format (that of separate space and separate programmes). The degree of complaint increased in those units in the second format (that which utilised common space and programmes). It is also worth observing that staff in the second format were required to work with both user groups whilst staff working within the context of the first format specialised by working with a particular user group at a particular time: the elderly or the under 5s.[2]

The second matter for discussion is the ratio of staff members to users. Mixed centres employ fewer staff members to each user than any other user group. While one staff member, on average, works to eleven users in a physically handicapped unit, or to nine in a mentally handicapped centre, or to five in a mentally ill unit, there is only one staff member, on average, to work with every fifteen users of mixed centres. As if to confirm this, no mixed centre offered its users an individual timetable developed around their individual needs and capacities – or lack thereof. Thus one question is the extent to which the rationale of mixing users, which is sometimes described by policy makers and administrators as a policy of 'genericism', is, in actual fact, little more than a cover for a convenient strategy for economising.

A third matter is the question about which group of users might be predicted to get on comfortably with another group of users with a different disability or age span. This information implies that in those circumstances which do not demand an actual sharing of activities and facilities, the elderly and the very young can coexist under the one roof. It should also be added that this appears to be the case when the elderly are the larger group numerically. On the other hand, some physically handicapped persons are offended by the reality of merging with the mentally handicapped, when the latter are the group in the majority.

At Borough and County Lodge it appeared that the culture – if it can be termed that – of the day unit was aimed at the mentally handicapped majority. For instance, both heads were trained to work with the mentally handicapped rather than the physically handicapped; the aims of the two centres were similar to those aims which as we will see predominated in units for the mentally handicapped. These concerned the 'training' of 'trainees' – as evidenced in Chapter 6. The rules and the sanctions of the two units paralleled those of units for the mentally handicapped, also described in Chapter 6.

One piece of information missing from this discussion is the question of how the mixing was arranged in the first place and how it was conceived initially by the staff and the users. This could be a most important matter as the following example illustrates. A centre designated an adult training centre for the mentally handicapped – Brightways centre, described already in Chapter 3.2 – decided to introduce a small number of middle-aged physically handicapped users, initially about a dozen. When they first arrived at the centre, for a few months the physically handicapped people used a room of their own. But later the manager decided to 'integrate' the small group of physically handicapped people with the larger group of the mentally handicapped and to situate the physically handicapped within the same workshops as the mentally handicapped – even though their tasks were different. The mentally handicapped users were employed on contract work and were paid for this. The physically handicapped worked at arts and crafts – and were expected to buy their own materials out of their supplementary benefits; no payments were made. This led to a revolt by the people with physical handicap and half of them left the centre immediately. Those who were left complained that they felt that asking them to integrate with the mentally handicapped indicated that the management regarded *them* as mentally handicapped too.

One moral of this story could be that a minority group in a day unit will interpret mixing as a loss of status, unless the majority group is already perceived to have a higher status than the minority group. The principle seems to be that the more vulnerable you consider your status to be the more you will feel you have to lose by mixing. The other moral seems to be that mixing which involves sharing space and facilities is more problematic than mixing which involves separate space and separate facilities. Further support for this is indicated by the two other centres already referred to and neither classified as 'mixed', which provided separate wings for the mentally and physically handicapped within the one building. No complaints from staff or users of either group were received about the other, largely because each wing was interpreted as a separate centre.

In general, it seems then that mixing which involves separating the space and activities between two user groups seems agreeable to heads, staff and users. Mixing which involves sharing space and facilities is more problematic, particularly for the minority group. More detailed work needs to be done on the specific sources of dissatisfaction and on situations under which mixing different user groups is acceptable. For example, is officially organised mixing more distasteful to users than that which just 'happens' in centres in an unplanned way?

What can be said at least is that establishing mixed centres as a rationale for amalgamating facilities ('building two for the price of one') appears to have a lot of question marks. To be blunt: it appears that for some users the experience of mixing with another user group represents a late twentieth-century parallel reminiscent of the nineteenth-century workhouse. In treating unequal disability equally, the result, for some user groups, may be not so much an increase in status but an unwitting maintenance of equal deprivation.

ROUTES

No other chapter in this book deals with mixed centres. A more detailed discussion of this matter is in J. Carter (1980) *To Mix or not to Mix* (A report for the Department of Health and Social Security: in preparation).

NOTES

1 No physically handicapped people were interviewed at St Mark's because interviewing took place on a 'terminally ill' day.
2 The exception was St Mark's, where staff worked with both the physically handicapped and the terminally ill but on separate days.

PART TWO

Chapter 4

———◆———

AIMS OF THE STAFF

Very little is known about the aims of day units. As Chapter 2 points out, sometimes official statements such as government White Papers describe their intentions in phrases like 'the provision of community care' or 'rehabilitation', but there has been very little probing beyond official statements to see how people in day services think about them.

The views that have been held to date of the aims of day services might be dealt with in two main groups. First, the aims of day services could be seen as the same thing as statements about the objectives of the organisation made by top people. These might include the example of the government White Paper on services for the mentally ill which sets out a list of aims for day units for the mentally ill (DHSS, 1975). These statements imply either that the aims of day hospitals and day centres for the mentally ill are standards for the day unit to achieve, or that the aims of day units should be applied as a kind of prescription. In this latter sense, the aims of the top people are applied as a measuring stick of orthodoxy, to assess the right thinking of those in the day unit. Writers about geriatric day hospitals sometimes have taken this line: prescribed aims are 'diagnosis and treatment . . . and these functions are performed concurrently with rehabilitation, maintenance and monitoring of functional ability' (Keet, 1979).

A second approach might be to think of the aims of a day unit as the same thing as its needs. Researchers who subscribe to this approach try to identify those needs critical to the survival of the day unit by measuring what they call the input–output process, in other words, what goes in across the boundary and what goes out of the day unit. From this they infer what the aims are. But a recent study of adult training centres demonstrated that the researchers' views of the 'input' and 'output' process were a very long way from the practical shopping list of the aims as seen by the heads or managers of adult training centres (Whelan and Speake, 1977).

These views of the aims of day units leave numerous problems about adequate definitions. Some of these problems have been summarised succintly by Perrow who makes many points, rediscovered whilst exploring views about the aims of day services (Perrow, 1970).

(1) It can be argued that, strictly speaking, day units do not have goals, only individuals do.

(2) Goals are hard to observe and measure. For example: should we focus on the behaviour of all members of a day unit, or only on the powerful ones? Should we take at face value the statements of the top administrators, or even the heads? Or, should we ignore these and examine only what they actually do?

(3) How do we distinguish between a goal and a means? What one observer calls a goal, another may equally well designate as a means towards some higher or more general goal. Production in a day unit, for example, may be viewed as a goal, or as a means of keeping users occupied or giving staff a job. These and several other problems have made the concept of goals, or aims, one of the most ambiguous in the social science literature.

APPROACHING THE AIMS

We decided to look at the aims of day units by asking individuals about the aims. A randomly selected sample of staff and users was a wider group than the 'top people'.[1] When we reviewed the information, we discovered that one man's aim was another man's means and that it was difficult to distinguish between the aims and the means.

A person's view of the aims of his unit seemed to represent his own point of involvement in the unit. A member of the domestic staff might hold a different view of the unit to that of the consultant or sister-in-charge. We would not want to assume that the domestic's account was less adequate; in everyday life we accept that the vantage-point of observers affects their view. For example, commentators at a Test cricket match or a royal procession each tell a story slightly differently according to their own vantage-point, but each is clearly describing the same event. In the same way respondents usually appear to be describing the same event even if their reactions are not identical.

CONTENT OF AIMS

In the discussion which follows, the themes found in heads', staff and users' accounts of the aims will be discussed. These are presented in a numerical order from largest to smallest and then the frequency by which they refer to particular user groups discussed. Table 4.1 outlines the themes of the aims. The rest of Part Two consists of chapters which discuss the way in which aims related to other information provided by the staff.

(1) *Aiming to provide practical services for users*
Offering company, food and occupation was an end in itself for some. For example, one user attending a voluntary day centre for the elderly said: 'It's to get people together and to see that they have a meal each day.

Table 4.1 *What are the aims in days units?*
(in rank order)

As seen by heads and staff (N = 500)		As seen by users[a] (N = 535)	
1 Practical services	143 (29%)	1 Practical services	225 (48%)
2 Training	105 (21%)	2 Practical services for therapeutic improvement	66 (12%)
3 Keeping users out of hospital	95 (19%)	3 Rehabilitation	64 (12%)
4 Clinical assessment or treatment	83 (17%)	4 Training	54 (10%)
5 Rehabilitation	71 (14%)	5 Clinical assessment or treatment	51 (10%)
6 Relieving relatives	68 (14%)	6 Other aims, e.g. to occupy time	32 (6%)
7 Practical services for therapeutic improvement	63 (13%)	7 Industrial production	26 (5%)
8 Industrial production	59 (12%)	8 Relationships with users	15 (3%)
9 Establishing a therapeutic setting	36 (7%)	9 Establishing a therapeutic setting	5 (1%)
10 Relationships with users	12 (2%)		
11 Preparing users for institutions	8 (2%)		
12 Other aims, e.g. liaison with other agencies, practical services outside the unit	11 (2%)		

Note: Numbers are expressed as a percentage of those whose replies were coded, that is, 500 staff and 535 users. More than one aim may be coded per person.
[a] User data was not coded for the aim of relieving relatives.

They come and mix with people and they enter into games and other indoor activities.'

Although this was the most common aim attributed to the day unit by heads, staff and users, it was one of the two aims where the views of heads and staff diverged. A few more staff (44 per cent) than heads (32 per cent) saw offering practical services as an aim of their day unit. On the other hand, more heads than staff discussed their aims in the light of certain values. For instance, a straightforward service like serving a hot lunch is redefined by some heads in the light of a value like the maintenance or improvement of users' nutritional state. Chapter 5 deals with these issues in more detail.

(2) *Aiming to train or to socialise users.*
Training users up to a desired standard was often called 'developing full potential', 'developing social acceptability' or 'making users independent'. These appear to be values which were strongly held but were not always fully explained, as the following example from a head of an adult training centre for the mentally handicapped shows: 'Our aims are to provide on-going training and further education in social training and work training to enable as many of the mentally handicapped as possible to maximise their potential and to lead as full and happy a life as possible.' Users thought more concretely and less often mentioned such values. For example, a mentally handicapped user in an adult training centre said, 'They're trying to teach you grown up things, something like work and writing and sums. Things you don't do at school.'

Chapter 6 will discuss this theme at its most common amongst staff in units for the mentally handicapped. It went almost unmentioned by staff working with other groups. Those users who were mentally handicapped mentioned this aim when they answered the question.

(3) *Aiming at keeping people out of hospital*
In this view the aim of the unit was to prevent the admission of users to institutional or inpatient care. This was either phrased as the need to 'keep users in the community', or as the object of saving beds in hospitals or institutions. No reference to the needs of individual users was made; nor were specific means or activities to achieve this aim important, although some reference to the need to 'occupy' users was common. One head of a local authority day unit for the mentally ill put it like this: 'It seems the aims of this unit are to keep them out of hospital and in the community.' This subject is expanded in Chapter 7.

(4) *Aiming at clinical assessment of treatment*
The clinical theme stressed assessment and treatment of physical dysfunction. It is close to what has been called the 'medical model', the main approach of which is to search for a cause so that the relevant treatment can be given and the prognosis determined. Thus the object was physical or mental dysfunction and the accompanying assessment and treatment modalities were physiotherapy, occupational therapy, nursing care, speech therapy, and so on. The means included the whole range of techniques available to the various therapies, from drugs to specialist nursing procedures. The following response from a sister-in-charge of an AHA day hospital for the elderly indicated that 'the aims are the

rehabilitation of elderly people. It's to mobilise them and to continue medical care, occupational therapy, physiotherapy and the maintenance of supportive therapy.'

Not surprisingly, this theme came up almost exclusively among staff and users working in health service day units rather than social services or voluntary agencies. Half the health staff and a quarter of health users mentioned it. The consequence was that clinical perspectives were usually adopted for user groups in day hospitals for the elderly (32 per cent of staff), the elderly confused (26 per cent of staff) and the mentally ill (26 per cent of staff). However, clinical approaches are almost ignored in units for the mentally handicapped and the physically handicapped (2 and 7 per cent of staff respectively), since their services, almost without exception, were provided by local authority social services departments or voluntary agencies. An extended discussion of clinical assessment and treatment is given in Chapter 8.

(5) *Aiming to rehabilitate users*

This was the only theme which was congruent with getting the user out of the day unit, into life in the community. The assumption was that users were to pick up the threads of a former life outside the day unit in the community so this was rather different to the training theme which aimed to teach users skills for the first time without necessarily associating these skills with a previous life outside the unit.

Of a wide range of activities the most common were work, meetings or groups, and clinical treatment. A user attending a SSD centre for the mentally ill commented that the aim was 'To get you out into the community and get a job. They help you to mix with other people, go to clubs and generally lead a more active life.' The conception of rehabilitation in the day unit is discussed in greater detail in Chapter 9.

(6) *Aiming to give relief to relatives*

Some people saw the day unit as a place to which users came by the day so that a break could be given to their tired and over-extended families. 'Relieving pressures in the home is what we're here for', explained the head of a day centre for the elderly confused. There was a recognition that admission to an institution could be halted or, at times, deferred indefinitely, if the day unit was prepared to help relatives to support their frail and confused users. This is outlined in greater detail in Chapter 10.

(7) *Aiming to give practical services to achieve therapeutic improvement*

Sometimes values like well-being or self-esteem were mentioned as possible outcomes of providing practical services to users. The head of a day centre for the physically handicapped told us, 'Well, it's to occupy people, really to give them a sense of belonging and to be useful. To continue rehabilitation and to help them mix socially.' A 70-year-old lady attending another day centre for the physically handicapped put it in different words when she averred: 'Well, it's to make life worth living for a lot of us. People find they have friends they never realised.' The staff and users most often adopting this view were in units for the physically handicapped. See Chapter 11 for more information about this aim.

(8) *Aiming at industrial production*
The theme of industrial production values work as an end in itself so that the result is profit. To achieve this, users doing contract or industrial type work were closely supervised by staff to control their output and the quality of the product. The main focus was therefore the product or the work process. There was also a recognition that industrial production provided employment for incapacitated or disabled people. The manager of a sheltered workshop said: 'We aim to employ severely disabled people of all categories and train them to make them capable of producing at an economical rate.' Chapter 12 investigates this aim in more detail.

(9) *Aiming to establish a therapeutic setting*
Here the emphasis shifted from the individual user to the user's relationships as a member of a group in the day unit. Many values often associated with the so called therapeutic community such as mutual support, sharing of feelings and democratisation by group decision-making were strongly expressed. Group (therapy) meetings were of crucial importance and activities such as arts and crafts enhanced the communal amosphere. According to a staff member of a day hospital for the mentally ill the aims were 'The treatment of various sorts of mental illness. The methods and the treatment is supportive and relies on social forms of group therapy rather than on intensive psychological and physical methods.'

However, few staff and even fewer users thought that the aim of the unit was to provide a social milieu. Users were extremely conscious of the influence of other users, but in the more limited sense of providing company for each other rather than as a specialised therapeutic setting. Chapter 13 is a further discussion of this.

(10) *Aiming at relationships*
This was one of the least frequently mentioned themes, even in units for the mentally ill. Its object was the development of a relationship between a user and a staff member usually developed during 'one to one' sessions. Usually the values associated with this approach included the users' personal development, particularly the encouragement of self-esteem, self-confidence, personal responsibility and psychological growth in users. As the head of a voluntary unit for ex-offenders said, 'We try to give the persons who come – voluntarily – a place to identify with, to feel relaxed and just some therapy. We act as a counsellor for them and get them back into the community.' More discussion on this is included in Chapter 14.

(11) *Aiming to train for institutional living*
A few held to the view that day units prepare users for eventual hospital
or residential living. This was never mentioned by users, but heads and
staff believed that providing services such as food or company today
could assist users to make a good adjustment when they were admitted to
institutional or hospital care tomorrow. A head in charge of a day centre
for the elderly, attached to a residential home, described the aim of her
unit in these terms: 'It's a sort of stepping stone before permanent
residential care. So we give them an insight into what will ultimately
become their permanent home.' Although a very few heads and staff
mentioned this – and no users, the theme of training for institutional
living was most prominent in those day units attached to residential
homes, where a third of those interviewed talked about it, as Chapter 15
illustrates.

(12) *Other aims*
There are other aims which do not fit into any of the themes already
discussed. The first of these was the notion of dealing with users'
problems *outside* the day unit. Examples were 'to encourage users to
learn the types of grants etc. they can obtain from the government' or 'to
help, advise and encourage users with regard to domestic financial
problems'. The second was promoting a link with outside social and
health agencies concerned with day care users. This included things like
'co-ordinating agencies to give advice to the handicapped persons and
their families' or the idea of the day unit 'acting as an intermediary
between, for example, local authority social services, hostels, group
homes, and the Salvation Army and the parent hospital'.

FREQUENCY OF AIMS

The information set out below refers to the frequency in which heads,
staff and users spoke of the aims.

(1) *Elderly*
As we have already seen, there are three providers of day services for the
elderly: social services departments, the various voluntary agencies and
the area health authorities. In the health authority day hospitals most
agreed on the aim: clinical assessment and treatment was paramount.
Amongst the heads and staff keeping people out of hospital was considered important. The users of day hospitals also thought that an aim was
to provide them with practical services, although staff did not. But in
social services units for the elderly, as well as in day centres run by
voluntary organisations, most users, heads and staff said that the provision of practical services, such as food, and the company of others was
pre-eminent. A different slant was given by users (but not the volunteers)

in the voluntary centres who stressed that users' well-being improved greatly by providing practical services; paid staff and users of the social services centres also considered this important.

(2) *Mental Handicap*
We have seen that most day units for the mentally handicapped are adult training centres provided by local authority social services departments.

More than half the users in centres for the mentally handicapped (and more than users in any other group) were omitted because they did not understand the question about the aims of the centre. (This included all users in two special care units.)

Leaving the exceptions aside, the view of five out of six heads and staff and half the users who could answer the question was that the aim of their unit was to train the users. Providing practical services for users such as company and food came second among both staff and users but more users than staff stressed this. A couple of users mentioned industrial production as an aim of the unit but more staff thought it was important enough to mention.

(3) *Mental Illness*
Most of the users in the twenty-one day hospitals sponsored by health authorities thought that the aim of their unit was to get them back to life in the outside community. The second group thought that the aim was to provide clinical assessment and treatment. But turning to the staff, most in day hospitals thought their aim was to keep people out of institutions. A second group put trying to rehabilitate users on a par with providing clinical assessment and treatment.

What about the views of those in the social services day centre? Most heads and staff in such day centres agreed with health authority staff that keeping users out of hospital was their main aim. The provision of practical services came a close second. Rehabilitating the user to life outside the centre came third. But for users in social services day centres for the mentally ill, most thought that provision of practical services was more important than rehabilitation.

In two units sponsored by voluntary agencies, most staff and users considered that provision of practical services like food and company was the main aim.

(4) *Physical Handicap*
Most staff and users in the day units for the physically handicapped within the social services departments nominated the provision of practical services as their important aim. A smaller group of staff stressed the link between practical services and the therapeutic improvements – the psychological well-being of users. Even fewer emphasised the importance of getting users back to the community to be rehabilitated. But the

priority of some users was to acquire new skills by training – particularly by craft skills.

In the voluntary sector, units for the physically handicapped were either work units or sheltered workshops. Most users saw the purpose of these as providing them with straight practical services which included company and money. In comparison most staff saw the aim of sheltered work as industrial production. This was considered important by far fewer users, just as to see the unit as a way of providing practical services to users rated lower with the staff.

(5) Confused Elderly
There were no differences between the aims of the two providers, health and social services units. In the main, both groups wanted to keep users out of hospitals and give them practical help. Of those users who understood the question (four in five of those interviewed), just over half thought the aim of the unit was to provide them with practical assistance, the main one being the company of others. Half the heads and staff agreed, though a main preoccupation from their point of view was the aim of giving relief to families of users and almost as many staff were conscious of the need to keep users out of institutions. Amongst users, a small group thought the unit's aim ran along the lines of improving their health whilst another small group even spoke of the unit aiming to help them develop new skills. As one old lady attending one of the SSD centres said: 'It teaches us things that perhaps you wouldn't have done, so they teach us to knit and crochet.' However, heads and staff did not express an optimism that psychogeriatric users might be retrained.

(6) Units for Families
One of the most obvious clashes of perspective between heads, staff and users came in these units. Whilst most users thought the aim of the centre was in offering practical services such as company, material aid and social activities, amongst staff and heads the provision of an appropriate therapeutic setting for parents came first. Actually four times more users than staff named the matter of providing practical help. With the staff, returning parents to the community came next while providing practical services came in third.

(7) Offenders
It will be remembered that attendance in one day unit was legally compulsory, while attendance in the other three units was voluntary. Despite this heads, staff and most users concurred that the aim of day services was to try to return users to the community: in other words, to rehabilitate them. Next aim for all was thought to be training – helping the users acquire new skills – for example, being able to read competently. Where more staff were inclined to opt for psychological help to users, fewer users

saw this as important as providing practical services for more concrete needs.

(8) *Mixed Units*

Mixed units were a difficult group to discuss in this context. It will be clear that it is illogical to lump together units which encompass the elderly and children, the mentally handicapped and physically handicapped. Mixed units are 'one off' ventures and it would be difficult to draw conclusions from the fact that both users and staff and heads opted for practical services as the major aim.

DISCUSSION

What this chapter suggests is that the aims of day units are complex sequences of means and ends. Each staff member and user can be located at varying points according to his or her perspective or vantage-point. The aims provide people in day services with a theme – or themes – which are really shared understandings. These can provide either a springboard for joint action between the staff members – as in the case of those working with the mentally handicapped – or a springboard for potential misunderstandings or conflicts, particularly if the holders of one aim do not comprehend or reinforce the aims of others. An example of potentially conflicting sets of aims between users and staff, where nevertheless one group gives the other room to operate their own views of the aims without apparent conflict, is family day care centres. More heads and staff in family day centres want to run therapeutic settings: more users want practical services. Yet other information indicates that staff are seen by users to deal with their material and concrete needs substantially. If staff ignored the practical needs of the users there might be more dispute.

How do understandings about the aims affect day services for a particular group? One example is day services for the physically handicapped. The main aims mentioned in units for the physically handicapped emphasised giving and receiving practical tangible services by staff to users. There was also a less dominant view that giving practical services in themselves achieved psychological well-being for the users. Further, there was an accent by some staff on industrial production. Thus it could be argued that assumptions about the aims imply the following things about the physically handicapped. First, physically handicapped people need day services and staff to give them welfare services. Second, such services improve the way the physically handicapped feel about themselves. Third, physically handicapped people are useful in the profit-making of the unit.

However, equally logical but alternative understandings could be constructed from those aims which are *not* found in the views of those in day units for the physically handicapped. To extrapolate from the other given aims, these might include some emphasis on developing relationships with users, or training the skill potential of the physically handicapped. Another possibility is aiming to return them to independent life within the community (the aim of rehabilitation). Even aiming to improve the physical status of the users by the techniques of the clinical approach might be considered logically possible. So the point is that omissions of aims are as significant as those which are given, because the omissions indicate that there has been a selection in the aims attempted for a user group.

Take another example, that of services for the elderly, where overall the staff and users in all services for the elderly considered that the main aim was the provision of practical services, but where a more specific picture is provided once one looks more closely at the staff and users of geriatric day hospitals where the provision of clinical services to users was the main aim. For a second group of users in geriatric day hospitals the provision of practical services like food and company was important. Aside from clinical services staff wanted to keep users out of hospital, provide for their practical needs and affect their clinical status. These aims do not acknowledge that day services for the elderly might attempt to reintegrate old people into their communities (rehabilitation), support their everyday roles aside from that of the patient (such as father, grandfather, neighbour, gardener). So the question is this: is the understanding about day services for the elderly a reflection of certain social attitudes to ageing in our society; an acknowledgement that the roles and psychological hopes of the aged lie in their past? If this is so, to what extent do understandings in day units collude with the dislocation of the old from their social fabric? This matter is pursued in Chapter 5.

So far in the examples discussed there has been agreement between the staff and users' views of the themes of day units. This was not always the case and those in units for the mentally ill provide an example. The major theme of the staff was to keep users out of hospital. But the users saw the main aim as that of trying to return them to everyday life in the community. This lack of agreement between staff and users in units for the mentally ill contrasts with the substantial agreement about the aims between staff and users in units for offenders. In the latter it was staff and users who saw the day unit as a forum for helping users to resettle in the wider community or to rehabilitate. One important difference between these two groups is the employment background of the staff. Staff working with offenders in day care have never worked in institutions, whilst almost half of those in day units for the mentally ill have spent the longest part of their working life in institutions such as mental hospitals. Given this, Chapter 7 will ask if their preoccupation becomes protecting users from further institutional damage, rather than exploring the possibilities of returning them to normal roles in the community.

This discussion implies that many of the understandings which inform aims for different user groups, far from being rational and logical can be arbitrary in their influence. At the same time, a particular understanding may alter over a period of time. For example, it seems likely that the aims in units for the mentally handicapped may have altered over time: fifteen years ago centres for the mentally handicapped were more orientated to industrial production than training users.

In summary, the aims of day units as they apply to a particular user group may be far from logical or rational, they are the social constructions or understandings of the people in day units, and it is very difficult to separate ends and means: both may be regarded as part of the aims.

With these matters in mind we will now explore the aims of day services through the perceptions of the heads and staff. We will begin with the aim detailed by the largest group – practical services – and finish with the aims mentioned by the smallest group. Each aim will be discussed as it applies to a user group where more heads and staff nominated a particular aim. So we discuss practical services, particularly from the point of view of heads and staff in voluntary units for the elderly and social services centres, as these were the two groups which nominated practical services as their aims most frequently. This gives the opportunity of linking the themes behind the aims of the units to other information about them, of providing case studies about certain user groups and offering a way into thinking about day units in a critical way.

NOTE

1 The Appendix at the end of this chapter describes the method employed to do this.

REFERENCES

Department of Health and Social Security (1975) *Better Services for the Mentally Ill*, Cmnd 6233 (HMSO).

Keet, J. (1979) 'L'hôpital de jour gériatrique en Grande-Bretagne', *Gérontologie et Société*, 9 June, pp. 89–100.

Perrow, C. (1970) *Organisational Analysis* (Tavistock).

Whelan, E. and Speake, B. (1977) *Adult Training Centres in England and Wales: Report of the First National Survey* (National Association of Teachers for the Mentally Handicapped).

APPENDIX TO CHAPTER 4

We collected information about the aims of day units from 559 heads and staff members and 888 users in day units. Information about the aims of day units was sought by an 'open' question in a semi-structured questionnaire. Interviewers asked *'What are the aims of (name of unit)?'* and then recorded the respondent's answer until he or she had no more to say on the subject. Extensions to each aim were sought by asking 'Anything else?' on the subject. Information about other possible aims were sought by using the standardised probe 'What else?'

The next job was to classify the answers whilst preserving their meaning and the context in which they were offered. One frequent difficulty in trying to preserve a certain line of thinking in an answer was that often one statement made by a person connected with the next. Or perhaps three or four points linked together in the respondent's mind. We wanted to avoid reducing complex answers to lists of items which would have wrenched the information from its context, thus cancelling the achievement of the interview in collecting as full as possible a version of the person's views. Another practical difficulty was in dealing with material at very different levels of abstraction. For example, a statement like 'Developing the full potential of users' is obviously of a different order to a statement which might be checked empirically, like 'giving the users a good hot lunch'.

From a random sample of all the answers, outlines of the themes appearing in the answer to the question about the aims were drawn up. All responses were rated independently by two researchers and disagreements were discussed in an attempt to achieve agreement about how an answer should be rated.

We grouped the common elements of answers into themes. We found that the views of an individual might contain all or any of the following four components.

(a) statements about the main *values* connected to the aims;
(b) details about the aim's *object* of attention;
(c) reference to the most appropriate programme of *activities* accompanying the aims;
(d) comment on the means employed to achieve the aims.

Occasionally all of the components of a theme were found in one person's response but more often one or more parts was omitted. For example, heads of units were more likely to report the *values* connected with an aim. As pointed out already, we took this to be a reflection of the vantage-point of the head, rather than an indication of the truth or falsity of the response. Users most often described the *activity* as the aim (for example, 'to provide us with a dinner and we do crafts in the afternoon') which again emphasised that the vantage-point of the respondent was an important factor in the way the aims were perceived.

A further issue was the way respondents interpreted the question. Most respondents saw the question as applying to the 'here and now' but a few contrasted the 'here and now' with the aim they thought the day unit *should* achieve. We coded only the 'here and now' responses, that is, the 'is' rather than the 'ought' aims.

Then again we discovered that whereas some respondents nominated one aim for their unit, others nominated multiple aims for the unit. For example, to take the heads of units, six out of every ten nominated simple aims (that is, only one aim) for their unit. Relatively few heads (6 per cent) nominated 'multiple' aims, that is, three or more for the unit. It was also found of multiple aims, that some were more associated with each other than others. For example, the clinical aim and the aim to keep users out of hospital often went together.

The fact that some heads and staff see the aims of their day unit as multiple and interlocking will not be obvious from the way the aims are treated in this book but it is an important additional point to remember. In discussing the themes explicit in the aims, we are of course ignoring many other things which might be said about the aims, for example, the degree to which aims might conflict or support one another. An important limitation of the information is that we are able to talk about the aims of individual respondents, but not of day units, unless, as Chapter 3.1 indicates, we are clear that we have interviewed a substantial proportion of staff and users within any particular unit.

The information in this chapter is based on the replies eventually coded: that is, 500 of the 559 heads and staff and 535 of the 888 users. Some responses could not be classified because the answers were too vague or non-specific (9 per cent of staff and 13 per cent of users). Others were left on one side because a large number of users, particularly the mentally handicapped, did not understand the question (17 per cent). A further group of users said that they did not know what the aims were (9 per cent).

Chapter 5

'MEETING OTHER PEOPLE, HAVING CUPS OF TEA': GIVING PRACTICAL SERVICES

> We offer somewhere for old people to meet and for them to come with their queries. It's something the town does for them. They get their deaf aid batteries and food. It's a social thing. We [the volunteers] don't do anything. They can sit here all day if they want to, meeting other people, having cups of tea. (Volunteer aged 78)

Some day unit heads and staff offer their users services which are practical and straightforward. The medium itself is the message, unbuttressed by theoretical or philosophical beliefs. In the eyes of those who work there, serving meals, providing company, offering information and organising entertainment are aims. These matters are not viewed as means to more abstract ends: for example, it is not said that serving meals is done to improve a user's nutritional health nor is company offered to reduce depression or to combat loneliness. Intrinsic ends in themselves, providing these down-to-earth practical services is, as Chapter 4 points out, considered by more to be an aim of the unit than any other single aim. For many it was an aim which overlapped with others, for offering practical services was not the be-all-and-end-all of the aims of the unit. But this was not so in voluntary units for the elderly. Of the forty-eight heads and staff interviewed in voluntary units for the elderly nearly all – 96 per cent in fact – reported that the aim of the centre was offering services defined as practical. Of these 83 per cent viewed the practical services as the sole aim of the unit.

Chapter 3.1 has pointed out that nearly all 'staff' in voluntary centres for the elderly are, in fact, volunteers. In this chapter the word 'volunteers' refers to the head and staff of those voluntary centres for the elderly. Aside from the voluntary centres for the elderly, heads and staff in the centres for the elderly sponsored by community-based local authority social services departments were the next largest group advocating the aim of presenting practical services. But fewer staff than volunteers thought the aim of the centre was to provide practical services to users, and those who did were confined to particular centres; as were the staff who thought the aim of the centre was to provide the aim discussed in Chapter 11, practical services for therapeutic improvement of the users.

What this means is that in certain centres people tended to talk the same way about aims. Heads and staff who saw the aim as providing practical services tended to work together, while those who provided practical services for more therapeutic reasons (see Chapter 11) were also found under the one roof. In three out of the thirteen areas where there were community-based social services centres for the elderly as well as voluntary centres, the differences in aims between those in social services and voluntary centres could be explained in part by an attitude on the part of the social services of providing a service for a more selective and problematic group of old people, for example, the socially isolated who lived alone. This point will become clear later in the chapter.

But to illustrate the use of practical services as an aim in day services, this chapter will compare staff and users in two kinds of centres: those day centres for the elderly run by voluntary groups and staffed by volunteers on the one hand; community-based day centres for the elderly run by social services departments with paid staff on the other.[1] A comparison between people in the two versions of day care seems important, since the elderly users of the two kinds of centres are very close in age and in their ability to get about.[2] The users differ in the respect that almost three-quarters of the users of the social services centres live alone, whereas less than half of the users of the voluntary centres are on their own.

What are the most common services issued by those in the centres? The four services offered most often were these: first, the company of others; second, food, usually a hot lunch; third, some social activities, usually entertainment; and fourth, information and advice about welfare matters. These aims will now be considered in turn.

COMPANY

This means offering a place where old people can be with others. It does not imply any personal exchange between the elderly users, although this does happen at times. Nor does it imply that the volunteers see themselves as part of the 'company', although the largest group of volunteers, in their 70s, were past retirement age themselves.[3] These comments made by volunteers in voluntary centres about the aims of the centre indicate their views on the social side of the centre:

> Basically the centre supplies social contacts and companionship for the elderly.

> It gives a meeting-point for our elderly where they can socialise and meet contemporaries.

'Company' was also critical for the elderly users of both voluntary and social services day centres. The most often reported benefit of coming to the centre for the elderly users was the company: around two-thirds in both kinds of centres pointed this out.

The company here gives me a sense of belonging to our own age [asserted a man of 85 in a voluntary centre]. We are out of the rat race and we're forgotten people but we're not forgotten here. When together we are able to help other people to get to know their needs and make their last days happy.

There are so many nice people here and it's such a happy place [said a 77-year-old widow, living alone]. I think I'd be dead without it. It gave me something to live for when my husband died three years ago. You meet all sorts of people, some you've known for years. It gives you friends to talk to. You introduce others who are alone. There are some awfully nice men here, they're jovial and happy. I'm trying to persuade a lady friend of mine who is 60 years old and alone to come and join us.

However, other information helps us qualify what company means to users. What is does *not* mean (for the users of the voluntary centres, at any rate) is being able to talk over personal difficulties with the volunteers. Very few old people (only 6 per cent) considered that they had talked over their problems with the volunteers. But talking to the staff in the social services centres about whatever the user defined as a 'personal problem' was more frequent, since a quarter of the users confessed that they had opened up and discussed their personal worries with staff.

Nor does 'company' imply that users can talk to their fellows about personal problems. Six out of ten users in the voluntary centres had spoken to other users about personal problems in the previous month or in the recent past, but in social services centres eight out of ten had talked about matters classified as 'personal' with other users. Nevertheless, most users in both types of centres had spent some time chatting to other users in the previous week.

So the impression is that the significance of 'company' in day care for the elderly relates more to sociability than to intimacy. A comparison can be made with family day centres where the company of other parents seemed to relate to the development of emotional intimacy. Four out of ten of the parents asserted spontaneously the personal value of talking openly to other parents: and three-quarters spoke of involvement and open communication with staff. As one parent said: 'Before I came here I couldn't speak with people. Speaking to one another has helped me more than anything. Cracked the shell a bit.'

FOOD

After company, the second component of practical services related by volunteers is the food, since over half considered that serving a meal was part of offering practical services. Eating dominated the thinking of the social services staff rather less, for less than a third nominated a meal as an aim of the centre.

Preoccupation with food was important to volunteers and users in a number of ways. To take the volunteers first, actual descriptions of the lunch were central to retailing the aims for some.[4]

'The centre aims at providing a good midday meal, piping hot', stated a volunteer, aged 73. 'They need a cheap meal, reasonably priced', argued another, herself aged 71. 'Balanced eating' asserted a 61-year-old volunteer organiser, predictably, an ex-dietician. Over a quarter of the volunteers in the voluntary centres were formerly employed in industries associated with food, which represented the largest recruitment pool for volunteers.[5] Some volunteers considered their culinary experience a qualification for voluntary work. For instance one elderly volunteer maintained: 'I worked at Eton College doing 100 dinners a day and I think that was plenty of training. I did train under a French chef too, but that was a long time ago.'

The significance of food to the elderly related to other aspects of the centre such as the rules. A third of the volunteers considered that their centres had no rules at all, but some of the remainder indicated that what rules there were related to eating.

Lunch must finish at 1.30.

Sign in for your meals the day before.

Eat at set times.

Members are not allowed to bring in their own sandwiches.

No smoking while the meal is served.

Sherry only for members' birthday parties.

Most voluntary centres had a kitchen on the premises where lunch was prepared and served.[6] Users never helped to buy, prepare or serve food. In only one centre did users and volunteers work together. A choice of menu was rare and the logistics were such that volunteers ate their meals separately from the users, either afterwards or in a separate room.

Turning to the users, it was clear that those in voluntary centres found the meal as integral a part of their day as the volunteers. It was the major consumer of time at the centre after chatting to other users. Twice as many of the voluntary centre users (23 per cent) as those in social service centres praised 'the dinner' as one of the benefits of the centre, and in both kinds of centres the relative cheapness of the meal (a charge was made in all centres) was a big consideration for some.

Our meals are much cheaper than we could cater for ourselves.

You wouldn't get the dinner outside for the same price. I'm healthier now from the fresh vegetables I get. Being a man on my own I wouldn't like to cook cabbage and carrots for myself.

Complaints about food were rare. 'Macaroni-cheese or peas isn't good enough even if it's cheap', said one lone complainer. 'They don't tell you the day before what you are going to eat so you don't have the chance of buying and eating somewhere else if you don't like it.' The degree to which complaints were inhibited by gratitude to the centre is not known.

Four or more 'dinners' per week were eaten at the centre by four out of ten users of both types of centres.[7] Very few users used domiciliary meals services aside from the centre, such as meals-on-wheels. Eating at the centre represents a considerable nutritional and temporal investment for users, so it was not surprising to find that routines and rules about eating were built into the thinking of elderly users as much as for the volunteers. Those users who did consider that the centre had rules related them to food. One-fifth reported their perceptions of rules as prescribing when meals would be served (or when they would not), where food could be eaten (or where it could not), or how one should conduct oneself at the meal table (or how one should not).

Pay for your dinner.

Order your dinner a week in advance.

They are stricter here now – we can't eat anything of our own like we used to.

She likes everyone to be in on time. Lunch is served at 12.30 and she likes everyone sitting at the table at that time. There are no other rules.

PROGRAMME

The main metaphor used by volunteers to describe voluntary centres for the elderly is the 'rest centre'. It is seen as a place for the elderly to put their feet up, a retreat for retired people from the burdens of life.[8]

It's mainly a rest centre for the elderly: it gives them somewhere to go.

It really is to give elderly people somewhere they can relax and get together, they can come here anytime during the day . . . they can come in for a cup of coffee – it's basically a rest centre.

Social services staff, however, stressed a more active than passive conception of the purpose of the centre. Although in practice social services centres offered little more than voluntary centres by way of actual activities, the attitude to doing things seemed different. 'Stimulation', 'keeping active minds', 'introducing new activities' were more common metaphors and, in keeping with this, over half of the staff of the social services centres stressed the practical service of offering social activities to the users. This was mentioned by only a third of the volunteers. This difference in perspective was illustrated by the head of a social service centre who said:

> It's first and foremost the meals, the companionship, new interests and new hobbies. All sorts of things open up when you start with certain aims and become enthusiastic. One thing leads to something else: for example, we found a new member recently turned out to be a choir master. Because someone else had an interest we decided to form a choir and within a week this was founded.

Whether or not the day centre acts as a rest centre or a stimulant for the old people themselves, it is clear that the centre is crucial in helping to structure a virtually timeless landscape for elderly users. About a half of the voluntary users detailed the benefits of the centre by the way it 'occupied time', rather than by the effects of the activities, and these comments are culled from the assessment made of the impact of the voluntary centres by the users.

> It gives me a break from the house [said an old man].

> I've come to an age where I'm satisfied with anything. When you're 84 you can't pick and choose.

> Now I've got somewhere to come it takes me out of myself a lot. If I didn't come here I'd sit at home and get morbid.

This last comment came from an anxious, almost blind and hard of hearing old lady who was seeking a transfer from her flat to be nearer the centre. 'Well, the main thing is it took me out of the house and relieved me thinking about myself', said a 64-year-old woman, whose fractured pelvis had limited her ability to look after herself.

However, a few old people tentatively asked for a more active programme in voluntary centres. This is amplified in Chapter 17 but some requests were as follows:

> I think they could do more in the evening, getting games, dominoes and bingo going.

> I'd like to do a little job: doing labels like we did in hospital – anything at all really, just to do something.

They could not do more for us here except that I have been hoping for occupational therapy; it's useful for all.

In the social services centres, the users indicated that they were more active in structuring their time. Less thought that the centre had merely 'occupied time', and more users than in the voluntary centres related what the centre had done for them by recounting their part in specific activities: the chiropody had benefited them, or perhaps the contract work or the craft activities. A skill learned since coming to the centre was attributed to the centre's activities by a third of social services centre users, compared with 4 per cent of voluntary centre users. Examples of specific opportunities for learning were as follows:

[On the craft work:] Well, I've got something for me, ten days I've come. I know I'm coming. If I was at home I'd be going to the toilet. Well I've just learned to do things, knitting. I feel more settled in myself and not so depressed.

[On contract work:] It's kept me going, kept my health. If I hadn't got this job to go to I'd lose interest, and it gives me interest to live.

A few also recounted specific skills learned since coming to the centre: 'Well, it's made me speak. It taught me how to play dominoes and cooking and make jam and marmalade. Oh, I've had to be patient. It's helped me a lot.'

As well as being more involved in the programme of the centre, more social services users considered that they helped to run the centre than the voluntary users. By contrast, more users of voluntary centres were inclined to say they didn't want to, or to feel that they lacked the skills or capacity, or to define running the centre as the business of volunteers, not users.

More social services users took part in leisure activities away from the centre and outside their homes than the voluntary users. For example, twice as many social services users as voluntary users had been out to church, or to bingo, in the previous four weeks. A few more had used the local library, or gone to the cinema. This paradox needs to be explored, because as we shall see, technically the social services users are a more isolated group: more lived on their own and were thought to be 'lonely' by the staff.

INFORMATION AND ADVICE

The supply of welfare information and advice was a practical service offered at some centres, and was seen as an aim of the centre by 17 per cent of the volunteers. Very few staff of the social services centres mentioned this as an aim, but as we shall see, more social services staff saw the centre as aiming to deal with information and advice – not so much as an aim in itself, but as part of a context which viewed the old person as a person in need;[9] for most of the social services staff (85 per cent) saw their users as people with 'special needs'. Primarily, these special needs were personal needs, of which the most crucial problem was loneliness. But rather less than half the volunteers saw users as having special 'needs' in the same way as the staff of the social services centres.

How did users view themselves? Those in social services centres – three-quarters, in fact – concluded either that they had no outstanding needs or that their needs had been met. But rather fewer in voluntary centres considered that their needs had been met, and many more talked about needs to which they hoped their community might pay more attention. Practical needs were mentioned a lot, the most frequently mentioned examples being:

> There should be someone in authority to repair windows, as I'm disabled and have no income and the windows are falling apart and the house will collapse [said a man aged 60].

> We should have a telephone for emergencies [said an 83-year-old married woman]. Also I need a rail to help me walk from my door up to the path.

> I should like to help with the garden. I can't weed it as I used to [said a woman over 80].

The paradox was that more social services staff saw their users as problematic, while, in turn, more social services users considered that their needs were met. But the volunteers saw their users as problem free, while more users of voluntary centres were conscious of their difficulties. How can these apparent contradictions be explained? Do the differences reside in unknown differences between the two groups of users themselves, or do they reside in the perceptions of the volunteers and staff and the mental constructions they make about their groups of users? For example, how does the process of entry to the two types of centre differ and contribute to these differences?

For a start, users of social services centres say they first came to the centre after an official referral from a professional such as a social worker rather than by the informal advice of a friend or relative. So perhaps more social services users arrive in the centre with a 'dossier' about their background and an established definition of their problems than the users in voluntary centres who refer themselves, or are sent by friends. If staff of social services centres have more information about users upon which to base their perceptions of the user as a 'needy' individual at the time of his or her entry to the centre, this may formulate the view of the elderly person as someone in need, since they do not spend long periods talking to users. Neither group, volunteers or staff, spent a lot of time talking to users. In the social services centres more staff devoted time to talking to users about personal problems than the volunteers, but in the main this work was done by the heads in voluntary centres. From the users' point of view, it has already been noted that those who use voluntary centres say they are disinclined to discuss personal problems with the volunteers and that more users in social services centres had discussed problems or difficulties defined as personal with staff. Further, a few more social services users (56 per cent) spontaneously mentioned the personal help they were given by the centre than the voluntary users (42 per cent). If voluntary users have more unmet needs than their social services counterparts, where do they go for help? Voluntary users do not have higher rates of attendance on GPs or more visits from the home help, and fewer voluntary users are in touch with a local authority social worker than the social services users. Three-quarters of voluntary users say they *never* see a local authority social worker, whereas only half of social services users never do so. Less than one in ten voluntary users see a local authority social worker less than monthly, but three in ten social services users have some contact, even if intermittent, with a local authority social worker.

When explaining their notion of an 'ideal' user in the day centre, more volunteers described the ideal user as a person with an 'extroverted' personality. Nearly all volunteers reported that the ideal user was the friendly outgoing mixer, who was always ready with a joke and prepared to make light of any difficulties or complaints.[10] Certainly, the extrovert was a favourite 'type' for the social services staff, but more in these centres nominated the virtues of the 'dependent' user: the user who relied on the staff for support, and who was grateful for whatever succour the centre offered. Perhaps these different views convey themselves to users and affect the extent to which they approach staff or volunteers for help?

DISCUSSION

There are many differences, practical and symbolic, in the services that people in the two types of centres offer the users. On the one hand there is the volunteer, usually elderly, rather practical and busying herself about the food for today's lunch rather than the social and personal context of the users' lives. She wants the elderly users to be able to relax and put their feet up. But she wants to maintain an active interest in the world herself. At the social services centres, the middle-aged staff member is concerned about the life of the user outside the centre and advocates interests and involvement for users. But can these staff facilitate these involvements for users, inside and outside the centre, and appreciate the delicate balance of supporting whatever independence the user had left in life without eroding it?

The chapter to date will have indicated that it is not entirely clear whether the users of voluntary day centres and social services centres differ considerably in their 'needs', or whether the real differences reside in the perceptions of the staff and volunteers. Assuming that 'real' differences in users exist, and that the social services users have special needs because they live alone and are lonelier, what process dictates their entry to a social services centre ahead of a voluntary one? In fact there is no real choice, because in no area was a choice between different kinds of centres available and at no point did a social services centre and a voluntary one serve the same local elderly population.

A different issue, but one which relates to the question of a choice between different types of services, is the degree to which both kinds of day centres offer services which reinforce what has been called 'disengagement' philosophies about the elderly.[11] Such theorists tend to imply that an elderly person, to make a 'good adjustment', should be happy to retire to a rocking chair by the hearth and they view old age as a period of growing detachment from the affairs and business of everyday life. It might be argued that some day provision for the elderly reflects this passive philosophy. Do volunteers in voluntary centres who assume that old people need 'rest centres', and the company of their own age group alone, reinforce a philosophy of 'disengagement'?

Of course, the history of voluntary centres for the elderly has a great deal to do with their current format and in particular their emphasis on food. This is a legacy from an earlier period. One of the larger voluntary organisations now involved with some day care for the elderly, the Women's Voluntary Service (now the WRVS), was established to deal with national emergencies. During the Second World War keeping the nation fed was high on its agenda (Walker, 1974). Meals were wheeled by pram and trolley through blitzed streets to elderly folk, food was served to the occupants of shelters, and pies were distributed on bicycles to argricultural workers. During the war, too, the WVS worked in communal feeding centres, renamed 'British Restaurants' by Churchill and established in major cities to offer a good cheap meal at a low cost to the civilian populace, with special reference to elderly people (Rowntree, 1947).[12] After the war, with the national emergency over, the WVS needed to find a new function and instead of dismantling, the WVS continued to serve meals to the nation's elderly by developing their services of meals-on-wheels, lunch clubs and day centres. So feeding the nation in national emergency has translated into feeding the elderly a good hot meal in day centres – and other places, like luncheon clubs, too, of course. Whether this should be the main focus for voluntary day centres, given the other needs of their users, needs re-examination.

Social services department day centres have a different focus. On the one hand there are the day centres in residential homes dealing with frail old people who require physical help. On the other hand, there are the community-based day centres discussed in this chapter, which do have some frail old people, but which on average deal with physically fitter old people, at risk for social and physical deterioration. Other research (Goldberg et al., 1978) has demonstrated that many old persons known to a social services department live alone. On the brink of admission to residential care, they take up an inordinate amount of social work time in terms of alert surveillance and practical support. Day care, directed strategically to this group, may, in the end, save considerable time and energy in field and residential services.[13]

When the users of the voluntary and social services centres are compared, it seems that those in community-based social services centres are more involved in activities, perhaps because paid staff have more time to organise them. This gives the social services centres, in potential at least, a role which could make them less 'disengaging'.

Three recent developments which concentrate on 'engaging' old people in day services might be mentioned. The first, a day centre sponsored by a county social services department, is used by the county education department for adult education classes held outside day centre hours. The low take-up of elderly people in conventional adult education classes has been noted and social services may aim to link old people with such services. Old people can 'learn' (Elder, 1977; Marcus, 1978): at the Charlie Ratchford Centre in north London, old people drawn from a working-class population take adult education classes. The French class holidays in France each year, and the screen-printing class holds an annual exhibition. Although 71 per cent of the elderly people attending day services left school at age 14 or earlier, indicating that formal learning is not a habit, this does not mean it cannot be tried.

One interesting idea is to wed the concept of day care with that of providing a social role. One new day centre is the 'workforce' for an amateur dramatic company of younger people. No ordinary day centre, the members make costumes, print tickets, distribute programmes, man the box office, paint scenery. The lighting man, aged 70, manages a 'team' who are still involved: the box office is manned by three-hour shifts of elderly volunteers, six days per week. In between, members play Scrabble, drink tea and talk (Pilch, 1978).

But extending roles for the elderly as a part of day care is very new. Perhaps more day centres for the elderly should be part of a children's home, close by a hospital for mentally handicapped children, so that 'having a purpose' can be continued by those who wish this. Foster-grandparenting has been introduced with great success in some parts of the United States (Hobman, 1978). Grandparents visit children in long-stay hospitals (Reynolds, 1978), help out in day centres for children, visit children of battered parents, give talks in schools about their jobs when young and their entertainment before the advent of television, and so on. These possibilities have not been thoroughly explored in day services for the elderly. If the primary task in day services were to work on a project, rather than to offer company, day care might appeal to a wider group. Other research indicates that many old people are not interested in clubs and that some would prefer to stay isolated than suffer an unstimulating atmosphere (Tunstall, 1966). Although users of voluntary centres did not, on the whole, want 'more say' in running their centres, one local authority grant-aids voluntary centres on condition that they develop self-management and elect their own committee.

But at present, the main group of elderly persons in day services to have their roles extended are the elderly volunteers. Most achieve considerable personal satisfaction and success from their work. Yet fewer of the volunteers 'identify' with the day centre than the staff of the social services. Over a third of the volunteers (more than the staff in any other user group) stated they would not attend the day centre 'if in the same position as the users'. The inactivity, their views of the users as 'different' and self-sufficiency were the main reasons for the volunteers' reservations. 'I hope to God I never have to come to one of these places – as most of them probably said in the past', said one. 'To be sitting here all day long would drive me round the bend', said another. 'I'm too active.' The organiser of a centre said: 'To be candid, no, I wouldn't like to come here. I don't mind working for them, but I wouldn't want to be one of them. I don't like the pettifogging chatting and jealousy.'

Very little is known about the actual quality, as opposed to the quantity, of social relationships in late life. Some claim that successful 'disengagement' presupposes a loss of the intensity of relationships which characterise younger people. Certainly the expression of relationships between old people in day care lacks the vigour and concentration of the expressed attitudes of, say, the parents in family day care, or the offenders. But then, as old people are offered much less *opportunity* to develop intensity in their relationships in day care than these groups, this may be a lack of exposure or lack of encouragement as much as due to the innate characteristics of ageing. The elderly volunteers, after all, seemed highly 'attached' to what they were doing.

More understanding of the quality of attachments of elderly people might provide a basis for determining the range of needs which services like day care might fulfil.[14] If younger women need an intimate confiding relationship in their everyday lives to protect them against psychiatric breakdown after severe adversity, is this the case for the elderly too? (Brown *et al.*, 1975) The degree to which the companionship offered at the elderly day centre is any substitute for an intimate confiding relationship needs to be explored, as well as the potential place of day centres in facilitating roles for the elderly – whether volunteers or users.

This chapter has begged the question about the social position of the elderly in our society in general and in day centres in particular. Day centres for the elderly might be said to reflect wider social values which emphasise the peripheral and essentially passive role of old age. When a person's economic vitality ceases, our current society shows little further interest in him, apart from arranging services to prevent his financial and physical decline. The attitude of marginal maintenance of the elderly has been caught by W. H. Auden's interpretation of old age in an old people's home:

All are limitory, but each has her own
nuance of damage. The elite can dress and decent themselves, are ambulant with a
single stick, adroit
to read a book all through, or play the slow movements of
easy sonatas. (Yet perhaps their very
carnal freedom is their spirit's bane: intelligent
of what has happened and why, they are obnoxious
to a glum beyond tears.) Then come those on wheels, the
average
majority who endure TV and, led by
lenient therapists, do community singing, then
the loners, muttering in limbo, and last
the terminally incompetent, as improvident
unspeakable, impeccable as the plants
they parody . . .
one tie, though unites them: all
appeared when the world, though much was awry there, was more
spacious, more comely to look at, its Old Ones
with an audience and secular station. Then a child
in dismay with Mama, could refuge with Gran
to be revalued and told a story. As of now, we all know what to expect, but their
generation
is the first to fade like this, not at home but assigned
to a numbered frequent ward, stowed out of conscience
as unpopular baggage . . .

(Auden, 1972)

That attitudes to ageing are conditioned by the type of society we live in can be illustrated by a different outlook, that of the German Democratic Republic (Groupe Gamma, 1978). The *official* position of the elderly (which may of course be quite different in practice) is that 'the foundation of the involvement of the elderly in social life rests, in the GDR, on the right to work and to do a job, irrespective of age, sex and religion'. Presumably because of the drive to involve as many people as possible in production, old people are guaranteed jobs and work well beyond what we would consider the 'normal' age of retirement. As productivity diminishes, elderly people are said to transfer to sheltered work projects, to community work, or to work in clubs of the 'People's Solidarity'. We do not know, of course whether this policy involves compulsion or what old people themselves think of this; but the point is that a different economic structure leads to different thinking about the place of elderly people in a society.

There is also an official, recent move to help the aged in East Germany to take part in the intellectual and cultural life of the community. Unless the elderly join in with the intellectual and cultural life of the community, they are doomed to a life apart. For instance, there is particular emphasis on art as a source of intellectual and emotional stimulation in preserving and developing personal relationships between old people and the rest of the community. This does not imply imposing the cultural values of an elite on an elderly population which has grown up without these values. 'It is a fundamental tenet of the GDR's cultural policy that only those things which have found their way into the daily lives and habits of people count for anything in the realms of culture.' [15] Whether this works in practice is an open question, but it is a provocative contrast in theory, at least, to our concept of day care for the elderly.

NOTES

1 This chapter compares users' and staff opinion in thirteen voluntary day centres for the elderly with nine local authority social services day centres. Forty-eight volunteers were interviewed in the voluntary centres and twenty-seven staff were interviewed in the social services department centres. Among the users, seventy-nine were interviewed in voluntary centres and fifty-seven in social services centres. For definitions of 'voluntary' centres see Chapter 3. Day services attached to a residential home for the elderly as described in Chapter 3 have been omitted from this analysis.

2 For example, the average age of users is 73 years in voluntary centres and social services centres. While 63 per cent of the users in voluntary centres could walk alone outside their house for a quarter of a mile, so could 66 per cent of the users of the social services centres.

3 The average age of volunteers was 64 years. The largest group were in their 70s whereas the average age of social services staff was 47 and the largest group were in their 50s.

4 No information is available on how many of these voluntary day centres have grown out of luncheon clubs, which as Chapter 3.1 indicates have been omitted from this study.

5 More volunteers came from backgrounds in food industries than staff of social services centres, only 11 per cent of whom were formerly employed in the food industry for the longest period of their working lives.

6 The information in this paragraph alone comes from observations by the researchers in nine of the thirteen voluntary centres in the sample, not a random sample. In a tenth centre, there was no lunch because users attended for only a morning or an afternoon period.

7 About 50 per cent of users had three or more meals a week. According to Stanton (1971) five meals per week on meals-on-wheels service are of major nutritive importance, but meals provided for fewer than four days a week made no significant nutritional difference to the elderly.

8 To be over-literal about putting one's feet up, it was noted that 78 per cent of the voluntary centre users and 86 per cent of the social services users said they always – or almost always – sat in the same seat when they came to the centre.

9 Social services users were equally likely to visit others and have visits from friends and neighbours as voluntary users, and there was no difference in the rates at which they used GP and home help services. However, the social services centre users were more likely to have support, if intermittent, from a social worker than were voluntary centres' users.

10 Volunteers who did not mention extroversion as an ideal characteristic worked in a mobile day centre, sited in a caravan. Relentless extroversion may be more problematic in a confined space!

11 Disengagement theory, in essence, proposes that a gradual severing of ties takes place between an old person and his society. Roles are abandoned and there is a reduced intensity in relationships before the disengagement of death (Cumming and Henry, 1961).

12 In 1945 there were 1,600 British Restaurants in the country. By 1953 this number had dropped to 250 (Townsend, 1961).
13 A qualification to this view in the case of the elderly confused, those with progressive dementias, has already been expressed in Chapter 3.5.
14 And of course there may well be specific differences between the young-old (the under 75 group) and the old-old (aged 75 or more) on their need for attachments to others.
15 In 1972 7.5 million old people were said to take part in 10,599 cultural and political events in about 10,500 local branches and clubs run by the People's Solidarity (Groupe Gamma, 1978).

REFERENCES

Auden, W.H. (1972) 'Old people's home', in W.H. Auden, *Epistle to a Godson and Other Poems* (Faber).
Brown, G. W., Bhrolchain, M. and Harris, T. (1975) 'Social class and psychiatric disturbance amongst women in an urban population', *Sociology*, 9, pp. 225–54.
Cumming, E. and Henry, W. (1961) *Growing Old – The Process of Disengagement* (Basic Books).
Elder, G. (1977) *The Alienated – Growing Old Today* (Writers and Readers Publishing Co-operative).
Goldberg, E. M., Warburton, R. W., Lyons, L. J. and Wilmott, R. R. (1978) 'Towards accountability in social work: long-term social work in an area office', *British Journal of Social Work*, 8, 3, pp. 253–87.
Groupe Gamma: Comité Européen d'Action Gérontologique (1978) *Synthèse du travail effectué par le groupe restreint charge des responses données au questinnaire Gamma sur la politique nationale en matière de vieillessement* (forthcoming).
Hobman, D. (1978) *The Social Challenge of Ageing* (Croom Helm).
Marcus, L. (1978) 'Ageing and education', in Hobman, op. cit.
Pilch, M. (1978) 'Drama down at the day centre', *New Age*, Spring, pp. 25–8.
Reynolds, D. (1978) 'Getting better with a new granny', *Community Care*, 16 August, pp. 16–19.
Rowntree, B. S. (1947) *Old People: Report of a survey committee on the problems of ageing and the care of old people* (Oxford University Press for Nuffield Foundation).
Stanton, B. R. (1971) *Meals for the Elderly*. (King Edward's Hospital Fund for London).
Townsend, P. (1961) *The Development of Home and Welfare Services for Old People, 1946–1960*, Association of Directors of Welfare Services, unpublished.
Tunstall, J. (1966) *Old and Alone: A Sociological Study of Old People*, (Routledge & Kegan Paul).
Walker, S. (1974) 'Meals on wheels', *Health and Social Services Journal*, 25 May.

Chapter 6

'BRINGING PEOPLE FORWARD': AIMING AT TRAINING

> I suppose they come here because they have nowhere else to go like
> me and nowhere they can get a job. (Johnny, aged 23)

INTRODUCTION

Almost all mentally handicapped users in most adult training centres can
expect to stay for the rest of their lives, according to estimates made by
the managers of centres.[1] Training the users is the aim of three-quarters of
those staffing the centres for mentally handicapped adults.[2] What is
training aimed at?

It needs to be remembered that there have been recent shifts in the
interpretation and meaning of 'training' as it applies to the mentally
handicapped. In the mid 1960s, training seemed to mean two main things
(if the 'model of good practice' of the Ministry of Health in 1968 can be
taken as a guide). Training was about developing specific 'work habits'
and also about continuing formal schooling for mentally handicapped
teenagers who came to the training centres straight from school. But
when it came to a conflict, education was an adjunct of work rather than
central to the programme of the centre.

> The adult training centre should meet the needs of the mentally
> handicapped adult in a setting of adult social and working conditions.
> It should offer realistic work training so that some at least may in due
> course find a job in open or sheltered employment. Others who are
> unable to progress so far should be given opportunities to develop their
> abilities to the full and all trainees should be given further education
> and training. (Ministry of Health, 1968)

By 1977, the view that education was secondary to work appeared to
have been superseded. Far from being peripheral to the training centre,
education should be central to it:

> The first and most general need is for continuing education . . . there is
> a substantial body of evidence both from research and from practice
> which indicates that mentally handicapped people of all ages are able
> to improve their abilities and respond to skilled teaching. On the other

hand there is also considerable evidence that very little development takes place spontaneously or without a deliberate and systematic approach . . . (National Development Group, 1977, p. 7)

This chapter will try to explore, amongst other things, the extent to which the views of those working in training centres parallel the official policy. In other words, how far do they see the training they offer as 'deliberate and systematic' education? This raises, of course, the question of what is meant by the word 'training'. According to the Oxford Concise Dictionary, 'training' means bringing a person up to a desired state or standard, something close to that social science neologism – 'socialisation'. Although social scientists are not agreed on the meaning of socialisation, the end product is thought to be 'socialised man – the individual [who] has learned to think and feel in the ways that someone of his age, sex and placement is supposed to think and feel, given the necessary skills to perform accordingly' (Clausen, 1968, pp. 9–10).

But what is the standard or reference point for training a mentally handicapped person? If a mentally handicapped adult is fully 'socialised', does he think and feel like his instructor in the training centre, or his father, or a reasonable but mythical member of the public, the man on the Clapham (or Blackpool or Brighton) omnibus? Who is to judge when socialisation has been achieved in the training centre and how long does it take? These questions apply in most educational spheres: when applied to mentally handicapped people they become particularly difficult.

Recent public policy statements imply that a mentally handicapped person's problems are more a failure to learn whatever 'roles' are considered to be 'normal', rather than a result of innate deviant or unrespectable behaviour. The implication of this is that a mentally handicapped person is not so much *badly* socialised as *under*-socialised. The point of this distinction will become evident later.

AIMS AND THE PROBLEMS OF POLICIES

Chapter 4 indicates that those who expressed the intention of 'training' most frequently in day services were those working in centres for mentally handicapped adults. Perhaps this is hardly surprising when units are called training centres, but three-quarters of all instructors and managers took this line.[3] Every adult training centre had at least one person expressing training aims, but in well over half the units everybody stated that their unit trained users. All managers of social services department adult training centres regarded their units as training institutions.[4]

Although those working with the mentally handicapped were the largest group aiming to train users, a few working with other user groups (excluding the elderly and elderly confused) considered that their unit had a training function too. For example, all those working in the day training centre for offenders thought the unit 'trained' their users. A fifth of the staff members of family day centres commented on this too, as well as small numbers of those working with the mentally ill and the physically handicapped.

Alterations of policies for the mentally handicapped were reflected by instructors who commented on recent changes in the inventory of activities offered by units. For example, a 41-year-old woman who had worked for eight years in the same centre explained: 'The centre has changed a lot since I came. Then the workshop was more active but now it's not used as much and there's more training for them to be resourceful in their capabilities.' Another staff member had noted an interregnum: 'We're passing through a transition period: in the past eighteen months we've changed. When I first came it was just work, like a factory. Since then we've started development work in education and social training. (But they still do a lot of contract work and they get paid on Thursday.)'

In short, most people working with the mentally handicapped appreciate that training is vital. What dispute there is centres on how the syllabus should be constructed to achieve training ends. Two-thirds of the managers and instructors reported that most users spend most of the week doing simple factory work. Only 7 per cent considered that educational classes and programmes occupied most users for most of the week. And sharp disagreements about the syllabus were expressed by different people working under one roof. For example,one manager said: 'We have a training function – to cater for the assessed educational needs of the client and to provide a conducive environment for the training to be undertaken.' But one of his instructors questioned the relevance of unskilled factory work for 'training' users and said emphatically: 'This is not a training centre in my opinion. It's an occupation centre – we are supposed to cater for a balanced programme in providing social training and further education but what takes up most time? – The contract work.'

In a nutshell, some query the relevance of unskilled factory work as a means of achieving training ends. Others disagree: those who believe that factory work is 'training' have two specific images behind their view. The first image endorses the value of training a user to be a *worker* because the centre can then offer him a protected work environment, the next best thing to working outside the centre. Thus: 'The centre exists to be a permanent and stable environment for those likely to progress to open employment. By this I mean that it provides social and work training for those with possible work potential.'

The second image holds that work is valuable training for users because of its potential to transmogrify the user from working in the unit to working in outside employment: 'It's to get everyone to outside employment or sheltered employment. A lot won't ever leave here though.'

When these two groups are added together, about a third of the managers and instructors consider the centres train users to be working inside or outside the centre. But the rest want to train to rather different ends. The most frequent image was of training users to reach individual 'self-sufficiency' and 'independence'. The second image spoke of developing what was called 'full potential', while the third image addressed itself to the issue of the 'social acceptability' of the user in the outside society.[5] There was very little unity about these images. For instance, one person might endorse training a 'good worker' while colleagues (and very often the managers) might talk about the priority of developing each user to 'full potential'. A third might emphasise developing 'self-sufficiency' and 'independence'.[6]

These images are abstract and best described in the words of their advocates. 'Self-sufficiency' or 'independence', for example, is:

> Making our people independent within their own sphere, it's whether a person can keep himself clean and travel around in the community. Everything in the centre is channelled towards this independence: cooking, social insight, vocabulary, woodwork, number work, money, visits to the community to see how public places work, transport and crossing roads.

The development of 'full potential' is a more elusive idea:

> It can be achieved by creating an environment in which an individual can be extended in all aspects of personality and ability. We are as much interested in their mental and social ability as we are in the practical and physical side of life. We want to enrich the quality of their life so that they really become the adults that they are and have the respect and dignity that this can hold for them.

'Social acceptability', another key image, was explained by an untrained staff member close to retiring age: 'It's to try to get the kiddies suitable for society but in my opinion I would rather see society come to meet them halfway.' About half mentioned two or three different images at once. Developing 'full potential' coexisted with offering a sheltered work situation while trying to make the trainee 'socially acceptable'. Some of these combinations of images, in strictly logical terms, seem to be at odds with each other for sometimes the practical consequences of one image might result – at best – in a diminished status, or at worst no gains at all for the other. One 19-year-old mentally handicapped youth was an extremely talented artist, but he spent all his time at the centre in the workshop packing sterilised pads for the local hospital sterilising department. His paintings were done at home and kept in a cupboard in the manager's office, for the manager aimed to train 'good workers' as well as to develop 'full potential'. For this user the latter aim had no impact at all.

Images of training also relate to the way that people in training centres think about the world outside the centre. Some older, untrained women instructors likened the centre itself to the outside world, presumably because their starting assumption was the mentally handicapped person closeted in the family. On this basis, the centre did indeed represent the outside world. But most viewed the centre, and the family, as the 'inside' world and saw the comunity beyond as the 'outside' world.[7] Despite this, only a quarter of managers and instructors saw the aims of the centre as getting users into the 'outside' world, into employment. More – just under half in fact – considered that the training aims of the unit were confined to the development of the user *within* the orbit of the unit itself. A further quarter also seemed to consider that the users' future lay with the unit but saw their training as providing a notable spin-off for the mentally handicapped user in everyday life, perhaps by aiding him to catch the bus and do his shopping at weekends or enabling her to buy stamps and post a letter on her way home from the unit.

In short, the most common images underpinning the broad aim of training the mentally handicapped are about 'self-sufficiency' or 'independence', developing 'full potential', promoting 'social acceptability' and training for work: in the unit, or occasionally outside. A further question is the extent to which the activities in the training centres match these aspirations. Chapter 3.2 has already mentioned that users spend the majority of the week doing simple factory work. Seventy-five per cent of managers were aware of a gulf between aspirations and activities, and the comments of one reflect this gap:

> We need some clear indication of standards and criteria for activities. In many cases [standards and activities] are completely at the whim of social services administrators who fail to understand the true nature of the problems and tend to view them with some idea of pseudo-adventure into industrial/commercial fields without either resources or staff. They also equally expect staff to not only supervise and control outwork (necessary to pay the handicapped) but expect them to achieve educational miracles with an equally dire lack of material and manpower expertise.

Another manager, who tried to be committed to the development of 'full potential', complained: 'We also believe that each user should be treated as an individual and his/her needs catered for but it would be unreal to say that we achieve this at all times – lack of staff of suitable experience and qualifications prohibits us from doing all we should!'

USERS: HOPES AND DISAPPOINTMENTS

How does the debate about whether training should be achieved by education on work impinge on the users of training centres? Many users had perspicacious views on what coming to the training centre had achieved for them, and their beliefs contribute to an understanding of this complex issue.[8] Users views were classified into three divisions: those who felt they had improved (18 per cent); those who felt disgruntled and unhappy about what the centre had done for them (17 per cent); and the largest group, nearly two-thirds, those who felt the centre had maintained them or kept them going.

Take the group of users who were classified as improved. Common to them was the belief that education classes were responsible for the gains they had made at the centre: three out of four attributed their improvement to educational classes.[9] About half the 'improved' users also spoke of the development of a particular educational skill. And although the users of training centres emphasised strongly the importance of friendships with other users, more of the 'improved' users mentioned this.[10]

Jane was an example. Aged 21, she lived with her mother and her unemployed father. Staff said she was slow at grasping the meaning of questions and she took a long time to answer, but commented on the impact of the centre in two years of attendance: 'It's helped me a lot, because it's brought be more forward. I'm more intelligent now than I was before. That's what my Mum and Dad say . . . I can read more, I can spell more too. I couldn't go swimming before but I can now. I see what's happening in the world today and before I couldn't see what's happening.'

Twenty-three-year-old Paul would recommend his centre to others like himself, largely for its educational benefits: 'It's for people who are handicapped and backward at school. They could learn to do things here . . . it's brought me on quite a lot in the education part. With reading and arithmetic, I couldn't get on with it all before I came here.'

Seventeen-year-old Marcia was an aspiring waitress. She summarised her educational achievements and hopes by saying: 'I can enjoy my writing now. I could not even write my own address when I came but Mr Smith showed me how and now I can do it . . . I hope it can improve my reading too, I'm not very good at that, I can read a bit, but not hard books. At school I did not know what 1 + 1 was and I couldn't even write my own name but I can now.'

Developing social relationships with others was emphasised by more users who had 'improved' [11] than by users who were maintained or by those who were disgruntled because they thought that no change had taken place. Eighteen-year-old James would recommend his centre to people 'even more severely handicapped' than he because 'they help you to get confidence and find out about jobs'. The centre had helped solve problems just through talking to people: 'It keeps me interested in helping people, other people who come here.' He hoped to get his friend Kevin along to the centre too because: 'He needs encouragement and educational advice. I feel the people here help to educate you and give you a chance you wouldn't otherwise have.'

Gains in getting on with people were sometimes slow developments. Looking back on twelve years at the centre, Lucy, now aged 31, commented: 'It's certainly made me more friendly. When I first came here I couldn't speak to anyone. I like the staff, especially one. Oh! I thinks she's lovely.' Other ways in which the 'improved' mentally handicapped people considered that centres had helped them were in doing cooking, washing up, doing the garden, or even making a shirt on the machine ('I've never used a machine before'). Less tangible personality increments were noted too. The thought of coming to the centre brought David out of his common depressed moods: 'I look forward to coming because when I get up and get dressed I have somewhere to go.'

Susie confessed that she used to get into tempers, throw things and stand and cry. She was relieved to have overcome these problems with the help of the centre because, as she said: 'If I had thrown things in the road a policeman might have put me away.'

Gratitude and hopefulness permeated the attitudes of users who felt they were 'improving'. Almost none of the 'improvers' wanted better things from the centre (apart from Jill who felt the time had come to leave the centre and find a job 'in the fresh air – because I don't want to be here all my life'). Further, all but one of the 'improvers' were distinguished from the disappointed users by wanting to recommend the centre to others.[12] This enthusiasm related to the approachability of their instructors (about two-thirds of these users said they had discussed personal worries with them in the past fortnight), more than for the mentally handicapped users as a whole.[13]

The second group of users were those who said that coming along to the centre had done nothing at all for them personally. Most of them had detailed complaints about the centre, particularly about the tedium and lack of interest of the contract work.

Eighteen-year-old Tom, a recent school leaver, would rather be motorbike scrambling than coming to the centre. He felt that the centre might have given him something he *liked* doing: ' . . . like woodwork or something. Coming here hasn't done much for me: it's boring. I suppose it's made me some friends.' He would never recommend the centre to anyone else 'because they don't treat you right here, because you don't get much work to do. They don't run it right – they let people roam around and do nothing.'

Another recent school leaver, Mark, aged 16 years, who had been coming to the centre for five months, said: 'I thought it would be great here. I'd do work and get paid for it. It has given me some work but I want to do more work. I would like some help to find a job – I would like to be a joiner. I'm very good at woodwork.'

Michael, aged 21, usually 'screwed screws into little slots' but had spent the previous week chatting, as no work was available. Although he confessed that the centre at least kept him occupied he commented: 'Most of the work here doesn't really interest me. I wish they'd let me help with things more.' Personally he refused to say that he felt satisfied on the whole with the centre: 'One day I'm satisfied, one day I'm not.'

Another small group of disgruntled users were those who had been out working at a job before returning to the centre. Beryl, aged 25, admitted that the centre had 'learned' her some things particularly 'about what to do and what not to do'. But she had been employed for a short time in a cake shop and said: 'All the work we do here I can do straight off. I could do a lot more.'

Peter, a 30-year-old user who had worked outside for a time, reflected from a 'before and after' perspective: 'Well, I don't know, I used to enjoy my work down here at the centre. I used to be happy going to and from here. I should be doing a man's job really. A friend of mine got me a job at a sawmill, sawing logs up for a good wage. This meant me working up in the woods, but I wasn't good enough. I would like to have a chance in life.'

Some of the training centre's problem in translating users to the working world outside was caught by one user who complained: 'They should help me learn to do a job, but when I say I want to leave they seem to put me off working.'

Although too small a sample of users was interviewed to make confident statements about the centres, it is reasonable to note that only one of the units containing unhappy users had regular monthly visits from the disablement resettlement officer. This implies that the capabilities of these users for open employment had not been assessed, at the unit at least, recently. Further, none of these unhappy users spent most of their time at education classes in the centre.

As an aside it might be noted that most mentally handicapped users are young people who live at home with their parents. But more of the disgruntled users live in hostels or hospitals than their peers and unsolicited distress intruded into their comments. Peter, who felt he wasn't good enough to work in a sawmill, now lived in a hostel attached to the day centre where he said he was very unhappy. Beryl, who lived in a hospital, complained she was not allowed to do things she was good at, like cooking. Tom was in a hostel until his behaviour was said to have become too difficult a month before. He had been taken into the home of one of the staff on a temporary basis. He was 'wondering what was going to happen to him'.

Aside from the 'disgruntled' users and the 'improved', two-thirds of users were rated, on the statements that the centre had kept them going, as having been 'maintained'. Although these users almost never claimed to have learned a skill or to have benefited from educational classes, about half commented favourably on their work, about a third mentioned their friendships with other users and about a quarter on the way the centre had affected them personally. All these factors contributed to keeping them going. One example is George, aged 23: 'It keeps my mind occupied which I don't at home. Mr Valentine tried to get me work in the factory. I've been tried on several sections here. Coming here helps my mother as I was under her feet all the time when I was at home all day.'

Few users however, discussed the effects of the centre on their life outside the centre.[14] Apart from the rare comment, 'Well, it's made me kinder to my mother', nearly all users were silent on the way the centre affected the hours outside of it. It was mentioned earlier in the chapter that most staff confine their statements about aims to the centre itself. All the action takes place within the building too; very little activity takes place outside the four walls of the centre. For example, only one centre in five used the facilities of local adult education centres. Only half the units assisted users to use local libraries, and as the trips to the library were made by small groups, very few users per centre visited libraries regularly as part of the centre's activities. In the same way, although most of the units used local shops, on average twice a week, not many users from an average-sized centre could be taken on each trip.[15]

STAFF: EDUCATION AND WORK

So far we have discussed the debate about what training should equip the users to do; but there is also a parallel problem with the staff and their training. Should instructors be trained by formal courses or by practical experience in industry? This has been an issue for years, but it appears that formal education has made some headway, for four out of ten managers and instructors possessed the approved one-year qualification, the Diploma of the Teachers of the Mentally Handicapped.[16] Almost as many are unqualified although many of these have trades or industrial skills and some consider these to be relevant training. But this group will for the purposes of this chapter be regarded as unqualified. A third group (two out of ten) had qualified in an associated vocational occupation such as nursing or occupational therapy, but they will be omitted from the ensuing discussion.

Alterations in the structure of instructors in training centres over recent years are discernible, although whether these relate to planned shifts in recruitment policies or to alterations in the occupational structure of the workforce as a whole is a question discussed in Chapter 3.2. It was demonstrated that significantly more of those working with the mentally handicapped came from either a skilled manual background or a clerical occupation than those working in day services for the mentally ill, the elderly or the elderly confused. Further, there has been an increasing proportion of women entrants to the service, most of whom are recruited from skilled non-manual, mainly clerical occupations. There has also been a recent decrease in the number of men recruited from skilled manual occupations.

The background from which managers and instructors are recruited and their subsequent training is important in adult training centres discussed earlier in the chapter. There are specific differences in the way that qualified and unqualified people viewed the aims of centres. More qualified staff talk about images of 'full potential' or 'independence' as part of their view of training for users. On the other hand, more unqualified instructors see the aim of training in terms of developing 'social acceptability' in the trainee and trying to cultivate him into being a 'good enough' worker to get a job outside. The inference is that the aims of the centre – in the eyes of unqualified instructors at least – is less concerned with development of 'full potential' or 'independence' than in fostering the social adjustment of the user to the outside world.

When considering the tasks in the centre and the way these tasks are performed, there are not large differences between qualified and unqualified staff. Likewise, large differences in the strategies used by qualified compared to unqualified instructors did not exist, but some incompatibilities did. The task in the centre as seen by both the qualified and unqualified is a teaching task. Two particular notions amplify this. In the first, the instructor views himself as a transmitter or carrier of his own culture. One middle-aged man said, 'I try to educate them in the things of the world and impart all my knowledge.' Another stated: 'When a boy comes in here, it's to get a boy to grow up and get him into manhood.'

The second notion was that some instructors saw themselves as coaches, helping the users to practise the components of a particular identity. The most common identity was that of the worker. 'My aim is to teach one group of mentally handicapped people the basic skills of a workshop and to carry out jobs to date requirements. This leads them to a sense of responsibility and ultimately should lead to success in a real working environment.' Although preparing users to be a worker was the most common identity, very occasionally there was a hint about the need to prepare users for the identity of emergency homemaker: 'I try to make them self-sufficient in basic emergency cookery – being able to prepare for themselves if their parents can't do it for them. It depends on their abilities – some can't open tins and some can. I take them shopping for them to have confidence to go into a supermarket and recognise the foods they want.' But the homemaker identity was more complicated than the worker, and other potential identities within marriage or parenthood were ignored.

The possession of formal qualifications made little difference to the actual view of the staff task, but had implications for the strategies or means. Three distinctive strategies in working with the mentally handicapped were identified. The first might be called the 'counsellor' strategy and applied to those who said that they went about their work in order to form relationships with users. The second approach, the 'instructor' strategy, allowed instructors to set to their task by employing comparatively didactic methods: by imparting information to users. The third approach combined the first and second strategies: this amounted to varying degrees of joint counsellor-instructor strategies.

Unqualified instructors were more likely than the qualified to *talk* about counselling approaches as their main method of operating. They stressed the need to relate to the users – although in practice they said they spent no more actual time talking to the users individually than the qualified instructors. Qualified instructors either opted for the instructor approach or they combined both strategies together.[17]

Despite a verbal commitment to developing relationships with users, instructors organised their work in such a way that only half were responsible for the care of any special group of users. Very, very few – only 2 per cent – considered that the purpose of this grouping was to enable instructors to develop relationships with users. Most seemed to think that the purpose of such groupings was to allow them to execute a particular job skill, for example, 'to allow me to teach my skills in carpentry'.

Qualified or unqualified, the personal care of users had a low priority, judging from how little time instructors said they gave to it. Managers said they gave a higher priority to talking individually to users and their personal care. Although the managers estimated that they spent on average 60 per cent of their time each week on administrative duties, they calculated that next most time was spent either in talking to users or their families, or in the group or social care of users, for example, showing users how to do things. On the other hand qualified and unqualified instructors calculated that they spent most time in the week on 'general supervision' (defined as supervising users at work, leisure or meal times, or by controlling and reprimanding their behaviour). Next most time was getting on with the group or social care of users, perhaps by doing educational and leisure acitivities with them.

For instructors, issues of supervision and keeping order occupy considerable working time each week. How is keeping order in the training centre achieved? The views of managers and instructors about the rules were solicited. Although the actual restrictions and rules of the training centres are similar to those of other user groups, the penalties prescribed by staff for rule-breaking are uncharacteristic of the views of staff in other day services. The three most common sets of rules mentioned related to restrictions on behaviour, restrictions on movements in the centre and regulations on time-keeping. First, certain kinds of *behaviour* were outlawed (for example, 'no stealing' – 'no smoking' – 'no swearing'). Second, nearly as many rules restricted *movements* in the centre so that users, for example, were required to ask for permission to go out at lunchtime, or to leave the work section, or to go to the lavatory, and so on. A third kind of rule related to the *time-keeping* of users and included things like being in the unit at a set time in the morning, starting or finishing work at a set time or leaving the unit to go home at a set time.

The most common penalty in the adult training centres (quoted by over a third of staff) was reducing the 'pay' the user got for contract work. Mentioned more by those working with the mentally handicapped than by staff working with other users, in essence it meant reducing the 'pay' paid to the mentally handicapped person by the centre (an average amount of £1.00 per week).[18] The second most common penalty mentioned by staff was verbal criticism or reprimands of the user. 'Telling him off', 'putting her in her place', 'cautioning' or 'threatening' were examples. Verbal reprimands were more commonly mentioned by those in centres for the mentally handicapped than by those working with all other user groups except offenders. The third most common sanction invoked when rules were broken – a discussion between instructor or manager and the offending user – lagged well behind the amount it was said to be used by staff in other groups. It meant a two-way conversation and was described as 'having a chat about it', 'asking for an explanation to understand it' or 'giving a quiet reminder of the reason for the rule'.[19]

In summary, although more unqualified as opposed to qualified instructors talk about 'relating' to users, they appear to spend no more time at it than their qualified colleagues. In fact talking individually to users takes up less of the staff week than the time reported in supervising them. Other differences between qualified and unqualified staff were not significant except that qualified staff had rather different views as to the aims of their centres (but not the aims of their own jobs) and rather different strategies in the way they approached their job. The implications of this will be discussed later in this chapter.

REVIEW

If it is accepted that the community has delegated to those working in adult training centres the *community care* of the mentally handicapped, it is less commonly recognised that the community has delegated the *community control* of the mentally handicapped to the adult training centre as well. At earlier times in the present century, the mentally handicapped have been regarded as a significant affront to the social order, to the point where policies were designed for their social segregation and control in institutions. That time is over: the pendulum has swung to community care. But have policies of segregation and control been obliterated? In practice, although not intention, are mentally handicapped persons still 'segregated and controlled' away from the community? Do centres separate their users from the wider community unintentionally, creating a separation between community and centre?

All users in most centres are likely to stay there for the rest of their lives. The most common reason for leaving a centre is to go to another one.[20] As many users are admitted into hospital or long-term care as go to work in the open employment market. Yet we have seen that there are users in centres who want to leave. We need to ask again, what is training for?

Managers and instructors in training centres are in a difficult position because centres veer between the Scylla of improvement and the Charybdis of control. Historically, social interventions for the mentally handicapped have veered between these two extremes; on the one hand attempting to 'free' the mentally handicapped (by education), and on the other hand then trying to control their movements (by segregation). If this argument is acceptable, it follows that training centres are in a double bind. Put boldly, setting up adult training centres may actually *prevent* the integration of some mentally handicapped people into 'ordinary' society.

If part of the unspoken burden placed on training centres is the policy which implies that segregation of the mentally handicapped is the 'best thing' for the rest of us, the first question is whether there is much point in directing education at mentally handicapped users alone. Or whether there is a case for more vigorous education about the mentally handicapped outside the centre.

> The service has not been thought out! [said one manager] For the service to be meaningful it should have aims, total and individual. We have no place for the users who have acquired most of the skills necessary to progress to sheltered work, then hopefully to open employment. It must be decided rationally what training centres are trying to achieve and for whom? Employment or lack of it is one of the major drawbacks, both in open and sheltered environments.

It is also important to recognise that there is nothing particularly innovative in the current notion that education will improve the lot of the mentally handicapped. The first recorded social interventions into what was then called 'idiocy' were primarily educational but 'probably no field of education ignored its past as cavalierly as have educators of the mentally retarded' (Doll, 1967, p. 181).

First, take the famous Itard who nearly 200 years ago committed himself to a teaching programme for the young savage, Victor. This abandoned and apparently mentally handicapped adolescent was found living 'wild' in a French forest.

> He was a disgustingly dirty child, affected with spasmodic movements and often convulsions who swayed back and forth ceaselessly like certain animals in the menagerie, who bit and scratched those who opposed him, who showed no sort of affection for those who attended him, and who was, in short, indifferent to everything and attentive to nothing. (Itard, 1932, p. 4)

Itard opposed the prevailing pessimism which regarded 'idiocy' as 'a malady hitherto regarded as incurable ... not capable of any kind of sociability or instruction' (Itard, 1932, p. 6). His programme for teaching Victor (outlined in 1801 to the Academy of Sciences in Paris) was a series of reinforcements and rewards based on the principle of learning by social imitation. He promoted contact between Victor and others to increase Victor's social experiences and tried to arouse his awareness by intense stimulation. Although Victor learned to speak and spell only a few words, his social skills developed: he could eat a meal in a restaurant, dress himself and bath himself, and lay the table for a meal. 'He became sensible of the care taken of him, susceptible to fondling and affection, alive to the pleasure of well doing, ashamed of his mistakes and repentant of his outbursts' (Itard, 1932, p. 101).

After five years of working with Victor, Itard was disillusioned that the young man's later progress was not as dramatic as his initial gains, so it was left to Itard's student, Séguin, to refine Itard's learning methods. Séguin migrated to the United States and later adaptations of his work were made for classroom teaching. Some see him as the father of procedures now described as 'behaviour modification' (Baumeister, 1969). He aimed at the 'comprehensive harmonious development of the child, physically, intellectually and morally, based on individual observation' (Doll, 1967, p. 176).

In England the first services for the mentally handicapped appear to have sprung from an educational base. The Misses White started a school in Bath for four 'idiot' cases in 1846; and a small asylum at Highgate opened in 1848, a precursor to the large asylum Earlswood, at Redhill in Surrey (Jones, 1972). These developments interested Dr Tyerman, the mid nineteenth-century alienist at Friern Asylum in north London, a man much taken with the therapeutic properties of cricket for his suicidal patients. He became concerned with the need for proper training facilities for the mentally handicapped and dreamed of providing at Friern 'for the class of Idiot Patients with the requisite Tutors. [It] would be a delightful and interesting adjunct to this institution' (Hunter and McAlpine, 1974).

There is no available evidence indicating that educationally inspired programmes for the mentally handicapped became as widespread in the nineteenth century as 'moral treatment' for the 'insane'. Educational intervention for the mentally handicapped in the UK seems to have been idiosyncratic and fragmented. One wonders if it is coincidental that this early period of education for the mentally handicapped ended almost at the same time as the Education Act of 1870 conferred compulsory education on the populace at large. Did universal education imply a grading system which screened out and rejected more difficult educational propositions? For after 1860 there was a rapid growth in the development of large institutions, spurred on by the Idiots Act (1886) which empowered local authorities, if they wished, to build institutions for mental defectives. By 1881 there were 29,942 idiots in UK institutions, including asylums, prisons and workhouses. Only 3 per cent of these received training programmes (Jones, 1972).

In the early twentieth century came the 'eugenics' scare. A powerful social pessimism developed about the nature of mental handicap, and the belief that the subnormal were insusceptible to treatment and a danger to society became prevalent. Segregation within institutions and sterilisation of females were advocated as useful action. In England, Mary Dendy suggested establishing colonies for the mentally defective because 'only permanent care would be really efficacious in stemming the great evil of the feeble of the mind in our country' (Jones, 1972). In the United States, statements such as the following were common: 'The brighter class of the feebleminded with their weak and deficient will power are easily influenced for evil and are prone to become vagrants, drunkards and thieves' (Fernald, 1893).

These events mark a change. To return to the beginning of the chapter, the view of the mentally handicapped changed from viewing them as products of lack of socialisation to viewing them as products of bad, or faulty socialisation. Training and educational principles (or the development of 'full potential') gave way to the perspective which regarded mentally handicapped people as intrinsically 'bad', incurably and pathologically deviant, and a moral threat to national fibre. The Royal Commission of 1904–8 wanted to build more institutions (particularly for mentally handicapped women of child-bearing age) and a subsequent Act of Parliament in 1913 enshrined the duties of local authorities as those of 'supervision, protection and control'. But as it became obvious that institutions would never cater completely for all the feebleminded, it became possible in the 1920s to return mentally handicapped persons from institutions to the community under statutory guardianship. Thus the local authorities became responsible not only for 'supervision, protection and control', but also for 'training and occupation'.

Seeds of 'community care' came in the guise of occupation centres, set up after the First World War by local authorities. By 1938 there were thought to be sixty local authority and ninety-five voluntary centres providing about 4,000 places (National Development Group, 1977). The Royal Commission of 1954–7 endorsed community care and breaking down segregation, and in the 1960s, when the body called the Training Council for Teachers of the Mentally Handicapped was set up, a new phase of development in educational intervention for the mentally handicapped was established. Interim targets for training centres of 1.5 places per 1,000 population were established by *Better Services for the Mentally Handicapped* (DHSS, 1971). And now in the mid 1970s we estimate that there are about 46,000 places for mentally handicapped people in adult training and other centres in England and Wales.

Unlike other day services, day services for the mentally handicapped have an implicit 'universal' rather than 'selective' attitude to provision. That is, there seems to be the view that a place needs to be available for every mentally handicapped person – a philosophy which does not exist for day care for other user groups such as the elderly. But if an area provides a place for every mentally handicapped person within the four walls of a training centre, does it encourage new forms of segregation? To return to the beginning of the discussion, does this policy help each mentally handicapped person, or does it protect the community?

This chapter raised issues about training staff to work with the mentally handicapped. The small differences between unqualified and qualified instructors are not surprising, for unqualified instructors are in close touch with the qualified which means that they are a 'contaminated' group. Further, a one-year course is, by the standards of other professional 'socialisations' (such as school teaching or nursing), a bare beginning. The literature on professional socialisation tends to indicate that the longer the training course, the more homogeneous the graduates and the more they differ from other occupational groups. Instructors of the mentally handicapped are, as Chapter 3.2 points out, amongst the first to recognise deficiencies in their training.

Nevertheless, one asset of developing a training course for those working with the mentally handicapped has been to construct for them an initial sense of occupational identity, which has reacted sharply to the threat of being dismantled. This is often interpreted as 'vested interest', but there is an argument in favour of 'professionalising' workers with the mentally handicapped, because it is a route to public acceptability and recognition. This often (although not always) improves morale for the workers, which, it might be argued in turn, provides an insurance policy against perpetuating physical and social abuses against the mentally handicapped which years of institutionalising of patients (and their staff) have sown and then reaped (Howe, 1969; Jones et al., 1975). Many decisions about reorganising professional groups fail to consider questions of staff morale,[21] but in so far as work with the mentally handicapped is considered 'dirty work', maintaining high staff morale appears to be vitally important. Complaints about changes which turn 'teachers' of the mentally handicapped into 'counsellors' for the mentally handicapped should be carefully considered. As Chapter 3.2 points out, instructors already consider their teaching training to be inadequate and as they see it, they are being asked to exchange the identity of 'less than adequate teacher' for that of 'less than adequate counsellor', since many see this new qualification as that of second-rate social worker.

The short period of training implies that it is easier to teach a mentally handicapped young adult than, say, to teach a 'normal' young adult at a college of further education. However, the pioneer teachers found work with the mentally handicapped rather more difficult than teaching the 'normal' and a review of the relevant behavioural literature indicates that it is probably at least equally difficult to teach the mentally handicapped as the 'normal' (Mittler, 1973). This is not reflected in present staff recruitment to training centres. More instructors are recruited mainly from women who are early school leavers than from the now considerable pool of unemployed schoolteachers. A more fundamental question is whether *any* one training course can be expected to supply staff with a sufficient range of skills to meet the developmental needs of the young adult mentally handicapped person. If the arguments of history and staff morale are accepted, it may be reasonable for the core worker to remain a teacher, but day services for mentally handicapped adults might move to a multi-discipline basis.[22]

Managers of day units recognise this need. Three-quarters want the services of a speech therapist. Four out of ten want a social worker to be attached to the unit: at present only one has access to the services of a social worker for group work and work with families. A third would appreciate a part-time physiotherapist: only one unit has any arrangement with a staff physiotherapist. A third would like to work with psychologists: only one unit has an educational or clinical psychologist on the staff. A fifth would like more help from art and music specialists although one in five now have a qualified art teacher.

At present, the lack of multi-disciplinary skills inhibits planning individual training programmes for users. Only four out of ten managers say their unit plans for individual users. Further, the shortages and scarcity of therapy staff and psychologists makes the question of achieving better ratios of staff to users in the centre doubtful. So several authorities have begun to plan new services using the building as a 'home' base. An experiment is outlined in Chapter 19: other facilities to be used include the local adult education college for education classes, the community arts centre for specialist arts activities, and so on. One area experimented successfully with employing unemployed young people via Job Creation Projects to work with mentally handicapped young people (Millham, 1977). This venture might be explored further – even on a volunteer basis – as a way of assisting mentally handicapped people in day services to visit the shop, the library and the swimming pool more often, whilst achieving a practical orientation to mental handicap for a group of 'normal' young people.

Unlike the staff of the old institutions, present-day staff have hopes for their users. The problem is that their plans for action do not implement their hopes. Put more technically, the problem is that their everyday methods, that is, their skills or technology, lag behind their beliefs. This is a challenge, for if the gulf between beliefs and actions grows wider, staff in day services may grow disillusioned. Ill-founded and exaggerated claims made by Séguin's followers led to nearly a century of crippling pessimism about progress for the mentally handicapped (Baumeister, 1969). What day services for mental handicap need is effective action in developing and achieving plans for each user, whether within the centre or within the community: prototypes for this kind of planning have been developed in residential settings (Kushlick, 1975) and involve setting concrete behavioural objectives for each user.

It would be a mistake to leave the reader with the impression that policies for the mentally handicapped start and finish within the day unit. Rather they relate to influences emanating in the organisations of which the centres are part which are now large, hierarchically organised local government departments. Chapter 17 outlines the changes in liaison with their central administration wanted by those in training centres: mainly more detailed understanding of mental handicap and more interest. Consider one manager who reported that his attempts to introduce changes in the centre were continually frustrated by headquarters. It was, for instance, 'against departmental policy' to allow community clubs or societies (such as the Women's Institute) to meet on the centre premises during the day, even though this new centre offered adequate facilities and room space for this. Thus users were deprived of one more opportunity of meeting the normal community. It was 'against departmental policy' to have a public telephone box installed on the premises. Thus users were prevented from learning to make telephone calls themselves. It was 'against departmental policy' to encourage trainees to use public transport to get to the centre each day, even for trainees who were physically and socially capable of this. (The council paid a lump sum for the hire of special coaches and the numbers of users using transport had to be kept constant to justify costs.) Thus users were deprived of the social experience of catching public transport, timing the journey to the centre, paying for the fare and counting the change, ringing the bell to get off. The manager resigned. In this centre, the fact that bureaucratic procedures were more important than individual user training is a reminder that in the end, the question of including mentally handicapped people as part of 'our' community is as much a matter of commitment as educational method.

NOTES

1 Three-quarters of the managers of training centres estimated that no users at all were likely to leave their centres within six months of entry.

2 The information provided by staff in this chapter comes from 105 managers and staff working in the twenty-seven centres for the mentally handicapped in the interview sample.

3 Heads are usually called managers and staff are instructors in adult training centres. This is the terminology used in this chapter.

4 Two heads of units for the mentally handicapped who did not aim to train users were running voluntary units and the third was a 'special care unit' for multiple mentally and physically handicapped young adults.

5 Other images reported less often were about the way users 'adjusted' to the centre, ways of 'normalising' users, or questions of achieving 'stimulating environments' to enrich their lives.

6 As each of these images was endorsed by between ten and twenty-five people, one can see the variations in opinion amongst managers and instructors.

7 Further exploration of this might be fruitful. A number of managers mentioned the difficulties in working with families: one said 'there appears to be a gulf between the centres and the families even though they are given every opportunity to participate in the centres' activities'. If in the parents' view, by going to the centre their son or daughter has 'made it' into the 'outside world', this represents a considerable clash in perspective with those staff who see the centre as the 'inside' world and the broader world beyond as 'outside'. See Chapter 17.

8 The question 'What has coming to this centre done for you?' was answered by 100 users, but the examples discussed here over-represent users able to conduct a conversation (see Chapter 3.2). More information is given on the way this question was rated in Chapter 16.

9 In fact units with 'improved' users offered literacy classes to significantly more users on average than those with 'no improved' users.

10 There was some consistency in the way users assessed their units which implies that some units may be more conducive than others to user improvements. Users who improved were clumped together in the same units and came from different units to those who had deteriorated.

11 Users rated as 'improved' talked about the benefits of friendship significantly more than users who were 'maintained' or those who were disgruntled and had not changed.

12 The one dissenter felt there was not enough money in it to recommend the centre to others (he made £1.00 per week).

13 It is not clear whether improving educational skills of users leads to better relations with staff, or whether users with good relations with staff are more able to benefit from educational classes.

14 Interviewing users in the centre rather than at home may have affected this, but fewer of the mentally handicapped mentioned the effects of the centre on their outside life than either the physically handicapped or mentally ill.

15 An average centre contained ninety-six users and ten staff. If, for example, five users were taken to the library each trip, an individual's turn might only come up every three months.

16 At the time of writing the government plans to phase out the diploma in favour of a new course, the Certificate in Social Service.

17 Nevertheless, two-thirds of the people who stressed the joint counsellor-instructional strategies were managers – and here the 'counsellor' aspect of the strategy was directed towards the staff rather than the users, by an emphasis on the need for 'good communication' in the centre.

18 The other group where substantial numbers of users were paid for work in the centre – the physically handicapped – were only half as likely as the mentally handicapped to have their pay 'docked' for misbehaviour in the view of heads and staff.

19 Although the discussion here abstracts the punishment from the misdemeanour, it raises the question of whether misdemeanours in training centres are 'different' to those committed by other users. Because the study relies on interviews and not observations, the degree to which reported punishments represent linguistic differences between staff of different social classes working in day care rather than differences in their actual behaviour, needs to be explored.

20 Only 9 per cent of the 490 mentally handicapped persons who left training centres in the sample in the twelve months before the survey were placed in open employment. Four per cent went to sheltered employment, 9 per cent were admitted to hospitals or other forms of residential care, 5 per cent left to stay at home. Ten per cent moved to other areas, 5 per cent died, and the health of 3 per cent deteriorated. Forty-seven per cent were transferred to other ATCs.

21 The obvious arguments in favour of further government intervention to professionalise workers with the mentally handicapped thus, at present, rests fundamentally on issues of morale and social acceptability. However, this does not absolve the newly emerging profession from improving its technology and skills, which as this chapter indicates are at present difficult to define. The conventional view is that professionalism is granted as a result of an occupational group fulfilling certain 'traits' or 'attributes': knowledge, training, competence and ethics. But instead, 'professionalism arises where the tensions inherent in the producer–consumer relationship are controlled by means of an institutional framework based on occupational authority' (Johnson, 1972, p. 51). In other words, state mediation in the control of the occupation of teachers for the mentally handicapped is the critical variable in professionalising the occupation.

22 Kathleen Jones (1975) makes a similar point about those working with the mentally handicapped in hospital. Further work needs to be done on the contribution of staff with other training (19 per cent) in the centres.

REFERENCES

Baumeister, A. (1969) 'Much ado about operant conditioning – or nothing?', *Mental Retardation*, 7, 5, pp. 49–51.

Clausen, J. A. (1968) *Socialisation and Society* (Little, Brown).

Department of Health and Social Security (1971) *Better Services for the Mentally Handicapped*, Cmnd 4683 (HMSO).

Doll, E.A. (1967) 'Trends and problems in the education of the mentally handicapped 1900–1940', *American Journal of Mental Deficiency*, 72, pp. 175–83.

Fernald, W. E. (1893) 'The history of the treatment of the feebleminded', quoted in E. Balthazar and H. Stevens (1975), *The Emotionally Disturbed: Mentally Retarded* (Prentice Hall).

Howe, G. (1969) *Report of the Committee of Inquiry into Allegations of Ill Treatment of Patients at Ely Hospital, Cardiff*, Cmnd 3795 (HMSO).

Hunter, R. and McAlpine, I. (1974) *Psychiatry for the Poor* (Dawsons of Pall Mall).

Itard, J. M. G. (1932) *The Wild Boy of Aveyron* (Rapports et mémoires sur le sauvage de l'Aveyron), translated by G. and M. Humphrey (Century, New York).

Johnson, T. J. (1972) *Professions and Power* (Macmillan).

Jones, K. (1972) *A History of the Mental Health Services* (Routledge & Kegan Paul).

Jones, K., Brown, J., Cunningham, W. J., Roberts, J. and Williams, P. (1975) *Opening the Door* (Routledge & Kegan Paul).

Kushlick, A. (1975) *Some Ways of Setting, Monitoring and Attaining Objectives for Disabled People*, Research Report No. 116, Paper presented to a Conference on the Handicapped – Towards Independent Living, National Committee on Residential Care, Brisbane, Australia, 19–21 June.

Millham, S. (1977) *Springboard Sunderland*: an interim report on Community Service Volunteers (Dartington Research Unit).

Ministry of Health (1968) *Local Authority Training Centres for Mentally Handicapped Adults: Model of Good Practice* (HMSO).

Mittler, P. (ed.) (1973) *Assessment for Learning in the Mentally Handicapped*, Study Group No. 5 (Churchill Livingstone).

National Development Group for the Mentally Handicapped (1977) *Day Services for Mentally Handicapped Adults*, Pamphlet No. 5 (HMSO).

Chapter 7

'PREVENTING INSTITUTIONALISM': KEEPING USERS OUT OF HOSPITAL

> Personally, I have broken away from old-established ward practices with patients doing nothing. Here in the day hospital, we activate and stimulate people. Its satisfying to see the patients going to their homes each night and not regressing into vegetables. (Nursing officer, day hospital for the mentally ill)

INTRODUCTION

Day units, as Chapter 1 indicated, seem to be a specific twentieth-century development. The first recorded day hospital was the 'day statsionars', a dispensary developed in the Soviet Union in the 1930s which treated people outside hospitals and stressed their return to work. By 1941, there were thought to be 719 'day statsionars' treating psychiatric patients (Wortis, 1950). In the West, the first psychiatric day hospital was thought to be started in Montreal (Cameron, 1947) and in London, Joshua Bierer, a social psychiatrist, considered that day treatment avoided the trauma and the stigma of inpatient treatment, while keeping the patient with his family. His innovation, the Marlborough Day Hospital, started in 1946, still stands (Bierer, 1951).

Many day hospitals have developed since then, although, unlike the Marlborough Day Hospital, many are part of an institution. In the area health authorities nearly four out of five day hospitals are in the grounds of a hospital. Not only is their site most often in the shadow of the institution, but the largest group of staff in day hospitals have spent the longest period of their working life within the four walls of the hospital itself. Practically none of the workers in day hospitals at present have been given any intervening training before transferring from the institution to work in the day hospital.

Although the disadvantages of institutions were well known in the nineteenth century, these criticisms have, of course, been given considerable force by the recent work of social scientists. A new beginning of scrutiny of institutions began with Goffman (1961). Self-contained institutions, such as mental hospitals, prisons, concentration camps and monasteries, had many features in common. Fundamentally, these 'total' institutions were split in two, with a wide gulf between the largest group, the inmates, and the smaller group, the staff. There was relatively little contact between these groups, and what contact did occur was often hostile. Further, the organisation of such institutions was authoritarian, because the programme was imposed centrally by officials who belonged to a strict hierarchy. The inmates who spent twenty-four hours in each other's company were given very little choice in their activities: they proceeded to meals, toilets and baths in batches, and under strict routines. The implicit purpose of these procedures was to induce the inmate to lose his personal identity and to accept the institution's definition of reality.

After Goffman, many research workers detailed the negative effects of the institution, drawing attention to the excessive power and authority of officials, the relative impotence of the inmates, the heavy dependence on rituals and routines.[1] It may be useful to illustrate this kind of research. Wing and Brown (1970) looked at the management of schizophrenics in the mental hospital. They were interested to know how far the social environment actually affected patients' symptoms – whether it actually caused improvements or deterioration. They showed that there was an important connection between an impoverished social environment in the ward and what they called 'negative symptoms', that is, withdrawal and regression in the patient. The most important factor in 'improving' patients was to reduce the amount of time the patients spent doing nothing. Also, if the ward had a routine which restricted the freedom of patients, this seemed to play a part in the continuance of 'negative symptoms'. In other words, the more patients were free to choose their daily living practices, such as when they went to the shop or left the hospital grounds, the less likely they were to be withdrawn or regressed. The point of this work is to show that the social environment of an institution can exert a powerful influence on the progress or the deterioration of its patients.

While social scientists outlined the way that deficient social environments could handicap patients (and implicitly the staff), politicians became restive about the institution. The high cost of refurbishing the mental hospitals, which included some of the oldest and most obsolete buildings in the National Health Service, was noted (Ministry of Health, 1962). A decline in the number of hospital beds required for mental illness was announced in a plan to run down the mental hospitals. 'Because of the success of new methods of treatment combined with changed social attitudes . . .' 'there will be no place for many of the existing mental hospitals. Some can probably continue, if reduced in size and improved, but a large number will in course of time be abandoned' (Ministry of Health, 1962).

More recently, Sir Keith Joseph, then Secretary of State for Social Services, could say in support of his plans to phase out the mental hospitals:

The treatment of psychosis, neurosis and schizophrenia have been entirely changed by the drug revolution. People go into hospitals with mental disorders and they are cured, and that is why we want to bring this branch of medicine into the scope of the 230 district general hospitals that are planned for England and Wales.[2] (Joseph, n.d.)

The coincidence of political will, the findings of social science research and technological developments in drugs is often taken as an illustration of social progress in the development of community as opposed to institutional care. But is social progress the *only* reason for closing down mental hospitals?

It is one of the more interesting characteristics of the English in recent years to employ idealistic terms to describe certain branches of public policy . . . what some hope will one day exist is suddenly thought to exist already . . . all kinds of wild and unlovely weeds are changed by statutory magic and comforting appellation into the most attractive flowers. (Titmuss, 1961).

Some consider in retrospect that 'community care' is the state's attempt to achieve control of the escalating costs of health and welfare budgets. Economy, not beneficence is the guiding star (Scull, 1977). An anti-hero in Bernard Kops's novel *On Margate Sands* agrees. Discharged after twenty-six years from a mental hospital in Essex to a second-rate seaside boarding house in Margate, he said of his new lodgings to a fellow patient:

It's nice of them to send us to the seaside.
Nice of them be buggered. It's sheer economics, my old son. It's statistics. It boils down to this; it costs the National Health eighty-six quid a week to keep us in the looney bins; it costs them twenty-six quid a week to keep us here in Margate. (Kops, 1978)

Margate is one of a number of towns with an influx of discharged patients from mental hospitals in the mid 1970s.[3] Former long-stay hospital patients were taken in by landladies anxious for year-round custom to replace their former holidaymakers, who now fly to the Costa Brava. Put out of their boarding houses during the day, some wandered about the town aimlessly, sat on the steps of the Post Office, urinated on the railway station. Unwelcome at the nearby day hospital for the mentally ill, reserved for 'rehabilitation' cases, and excluded from the voluntary day centre for the town's retired elderly because of 'unsocial' behaviour (one ex-patient aged 68 insisted on burying her lunch leftovers in strategic places around the centre), these former long-stay mental hospital patients were pitiable; more so than when cloistered within their institution. Although a fictional day centre for the mentally ill was invented for the ex-patients of the novel – 'the place to pass the time. The place to pick up skills and companionships . . . his half-way house, his springboard', in real life the day wanderers of Margate had no such halfway house at that time.

AIM: TO KEEP PEOPLE OUT OF INSTITUTIONS

Chapter 1 made clear that services are neither entirely 'community' nor wholly 'institutional'. Day services are an untidy set of services, ignored, perhaps for this reason, by most contemporary writers on institutions and community care. Yet many day units themselves have very strong links with institutions. This chapter will explore a group of those working in day hospitals for the mentally ill, which are associated with institutions, since four of every five are in the grounds of a hospital. There is a group of heads and staff in day services – 15 per cent in fact – who say that one aim of their unit is to keep the users out of one type of institution or another, whether hospital, prison or residential home. Stating that the aim of the unit was to keep users out of institutions transected user groups, unlike some other aims, such as offering services which were practical (described in Chapter 5), or training users (described in Chapter 6).

Some heads and staff in nearly all user groups said that the unit aimed to keep users out of institutions. The largest groups were those working with the mentally ill, the elderly and the elderly confused. The proportions were similar for all three user groups: 26 per cent for the elderly confused, 32 per cent for the elderly and 34 per cent for the mentally ill.

'Keeping users out of hospital' was expressed more commonly as an aim by workers in area health authorities. The social services department exceptions were found in day units for the mentally ill.[4] But it appeared that the kind of professional training of a head or staff member related to whether or not a head or staff member propagated this view as an aim of the unit. For example, few untrained workers mentioned 'keeping users out of hospital' as an aim of the unit. Proportionately fewer doctors mentioned the matter than occupational therapists and nurses.

Why did heads and staff consider that users should be kept out of institutions? Some thought it had something to do with the public purse and practising economies, such as reducing the cost of keeping patients in hospital beds. The charge nurse of a psychiatric day hospital explained: 'The aims are to reduce the number of patients admitted to permanent hospital care and treat them here without admitting them: it saves beds. We can also reduce the length of stay.'

On the other hand, others wanted to save patients from the evils of institutionalism: 'The aims here are to prevent admission into psychiatric hospital and so to prevent institutional neurosis', said a 62-year-old nursing officer. 'We don't give the patient the impression he is sick. As you can see [this unit is in a mental hospital, but] I'm in mufti and it does not give the impression of being in hospital.'

'Basically', said a 56-year-old nursing officer, 'it's to delay hospitalisation and to keep people going in the community. It stops people becoming inpatients and thus too sheltered.'

This chapter could discuss any number of groups who saw the aim of the unit as keeping the user out of hospital. But for whatever reason, keeping patients out of institutions was seen as the aim by half the nursing officers in charge of day hospitals for the mentally ill, so the rest of the chapter will discuss the implications of their beliefs. Twelve out of twenty-one nursing officers in psychiatric day hospitals expressed the view that the day hospital aimed to keep people out of institutions and the twelve had a number of things in common. First, nine of the twelve worked in day hospitals located either in the grounds of mental hospitals, or else associated with a mental hospital which acted as a 'parent' hospital. Second, those nursing officers concerned that the unit aimed to keep their patients out of hospital worked in the 'older' day hospitals – those open for the longest time. (Nine of the twelve worked in day hospitals opened before 1970.) Third, those leaders were a little older than the rest (on average, 53 years old); and they had been at their jobs longer too: both on the wards and in the day hospital. They had worked for seven years, on average, in charge of the day unit, and before that they had spent an average of ten years on the wards of a mental hospital. (Four had spent twelve years or more on the wards.)

By comparison, the heads who did not discuss the aim of keeping people out of hospital could be considered junior in experience to those who did, because they had only spent two years, on average, at their job in the day unit, and five years, on average, on the wards. Most of them worked in day units in the newer district general hospitals, and they were, on average, eight years younger than the nursing officers aiming to keep users out of hospital. Table 7.1 makes this clear. From now on, the group of twelve nursing officers who aimed to keep patients out of hospital (the first group) will be compared with the other nine, who did not see this as an issue (the second group).

It must be said to begin with that the views of the heads were not shared by their staff. Heads who saw the unit as aiming to keep people out of hospital, the first group, had only two out of every ten staff who expressed the same view. The other heads, those who did not mention keeping the users out of hospital, worked with staff who more often mentioned this aim: four out of every ten staff mentioned that an aim of the unit was to try to keep users out of hospital. So the assumption made in discussing the views of the heads about the aims, that there is a relationship between the nursing leadership of the day unit and what happens within the day hospital, will be qualified later.

First, the heads in the first group, those who said the unit aimed to keep users out of hospital, offered more experiences to their users *outside* the boundary of the day hospital. They sponsored more visits by users to local facilities, such as the swimming pool, the library, local shops and local exhibitions. Twenty-one such visits in the previous month, on average,

Table 7.1 *Characteristics of twenty-one Nursing Officers in Day Hospitals for the Mentally Ill*

Characteristics	First Group Nursing officers who said the unit aimed to keep users out of institutions	Second Group Nursing officers who did not say the aim was to keep users out of institutions
	N = 12	N = 9
Day hospital situated in the grounds of a mental hospital, or associated with a mental hospital	9	4
Day hospital attached to a district general hospital	3	5
Working in a day hospital opened prior to 1970	9	2
Working in a day hospital opened after 1970	3	7
Average age of nursing officers	53 years	45 years
Average length of time at this job in day hospital	7 years	2 years
Average time spent on a ward of a mental hospital before this job	10 years	5 years

were arranged by the heads in the first group compared to those in the second who arranged an average of nine visits.[5] Further, more of the heads in the first group had contact with the world outside the day unit in another way. They made more systematic efforts to see families of more users on at least a quarterly basis. This may not be very much by some standards, but as most of the heads in the second group reported no systematic contacts with families and they saw them on only an *ad hoc* basis, 'as the need arose', the first group of heads had more contact.

When it came to who visited the day unit, however, there was very little difference. Both groups of heads reported that, on average, seven categories of professional people had visited the unit more than seven to twelve times in the past twelve months. It might be expected that the heads of the second group would report more visitors to the unit because more had access to the multi-disciplinary staff of the district general hospital, but this was not the case.

So much for the degree of contact between users in the day hospital and the outside world. What of the position of the users in units? What chances, if any, were users offered in running the unit? First, take the preparation and serving of food in the unit and the extent to which the user took part in this. Users in day hospitals where the head viewed the unit as keeping them out of hospital, were given more opportunity to help to serve food at either lunch or tea than those in the units led by the second group of heads.[6] Second, twice as many of the units where heads aimed to keep users out of hospital had a users' committee as the other group. It would be misleading to say that opinion about user involvement in the units where heads aimed to help users out of hospital was unanimous: some heads were firmly resolved against user participation. ('Well, its a medical decision for them not to, and this benefits the patient', said one head. 'No', asserted another, 'they don't come here to run the place, they come for a rest. We give a service here, and we don't expect the patients to help in any way.')

Third, there were some comparisons to be made in the extent to which each head of unit offered individual programme choices, 'tailor made' to each user. More heads who said the unit aimed to keep users out of hospital claimed that they made individual plans for their patients by arranging a special programme for each user's week, rather than expecting their users to fit into the preordained activities. They offered the users some choice of the activities available, but very few of the second group offered a choice. Then more heads of the day hospitals where heads said the aim was to keep users out of hospital offered their users freedom to leave the day unit at lunchtime without asking permission from the staff. But in the units run by the second group of heads, this permission was hedged around with restrictions. For example, 'we like to know where they're going first'.

TREATMENTS AND USERS

There are small differences in the 'treatments' offered by units where heads aim to keep users out of hospital. When the 'treatments' of both kinds of units were laid out side by side and inspected, they were similar, apart from the fact that those heads who said the unit tried to keep users out of hospitals used less of a medical component in 'treatment'. Perhaps this was underwritten by the fact that such units were not in 'proper' hospitals, the district general hospitals. Both groups of heads shared an 'eclectic' orientation and treatments in their units range from medical treatments, through occupational, individual and group therapies to social and community work. But there was a trend towards more of a medical component in the treatments listed by the heads in the units who did not mention that they tried to keep users out of hospitals (44 : 27 per cent). Perhaps a more 'medical' orientation in the second group of heads is expressed by the fact that although nursing care is offered by all heads in both groups, the units where heads see the unit aiming to keep users out of hospital offer it to fewer users.

Do intrinsic differences between the users more readily explain the different practices, than the attitudes of the heads? It appears that in units run by both kinds of heads, users had attended the day unit for comparable lengths of time, and few users in either group had attended other day hospitals before. But more users in the units run by heads aiming to keep users out of hospital said that they had *never* been an inpatient, and those who had, had generally spent less time in hospital than the users in the units run by the second type of head. Further, more users in this second group labelled themselves with a psychiatric diagnosis of mental illness than the users in the units run by the first kind of heads. Does this mean that these users see themselves as less mentally ill and are treated as such by the staff?

There were sixty-seven users in units where heads aimed to keep users out of hospital and fifty-five users in the second group. Both groups were comparable in the length of time their users had been attending their units; about a third had been there less than three months, and about another quarter had been there between five months and a year. And a third of the users in the group where heads aimed to keep them out of hospital and a quarter in the second group of users had been there for a year or more. Few users had attended other day hospitals before (about four-fifths of users in both groups were in a day hospital for the first time).

When it comes to their experience of psychiatric hospitals, half the users in the first group say they have never been an inpatient, compared with a quarter of those in the second group. Also, those users in the first group, where heads say the unit aims to keep them out of hospital, have spent shorter terms 'inside' than the second group. The users in the first group have also spent less time in any kind of institution in their adult life than the second group. Taken together – time in psychiatric institutions and time in *any* institutions – the findings suggest more chronic mental illness in the group of day hospitals for the mentally ill where their heads do *not* express the aim of trying to keep the users out of hospitals.

The users' view of themselves differ, too. Four out of ten users cared for by heads who consider the unit aims to help users keep out of institutions, report themselves to be free of complaints or disability. But one out of ten users in the second group reports complaints and disabilities and a higher incidence of self-reported schizophrenia, depression and non-specific mental and emotional disorders. It cannot be that they are in a more acute phase of their disorder, for as we have already seen, they have been in the day hospital for an equivalent period of time as the first group of users.

Are users more severely disordered in the second group, or do the first group see themselves as less mentally ill as a consequence of the different practices to which they are subjected?

Looking at self-reported depression alone, the differences are not great. Slightly more of the second group of users are more severely depressed. There seems to be more hopelessness amongst the second group of users, as over half say they have had thoughts of doing away with themselves the previous month, whereas only a third of the users in the first group say they have had such thoughts.[7]

COMMENTS

These comparisons are presented because of the potential interest in examining the differences, if any, between day hospitals run by heads who consider that an aim of the unit is to keep users out of institutions and those who do not express such a view. One potential interest of this is that more heads of the first group are in day hospitals associated with the 'old' mental hospitals and their work backgrounds demonstrate longer experience inside institutions. Yet they appear to be less institutionally minded and more aware of the dangers of 'institutionalism'[8] than the second group of heads who are less of a 'pure' group, although more are in day hospitals in the district general hospitals.

Nothing conclusive can be said on the basis of this chapter, other than the implication that this is an interesting issue in day services which deserves further exploration. Too many factors are left unexplored for one to be entirely certain that the differences shown relate only to different regimes sponsored by leaders who express different aims for their unit. For example, the orientation of the consultant psychiatrist is one unexplored issue. This is an unknown quantity since fewer consultants were interviewed than heads and this may have led to placing an undue weight on the views of the head as the leader. But we do know that one-third of the heads in both groups considered that they lacked support from their medical colleagues. Deficient medical involvement was interpreted as a result of being 'too busy' or as 'lack of interest'. Several put it this way:

> More participation by medical staff would be a great help. If only we had more support from our consultant.

> There is no real policy laid down for the day hospital, nor much involvement with medical staff, the consultants rarely come to see us. We have three, but only two come, and irregularly. I suppose they haven't the time, and the Registrars are always busy, they haven't the time either.

(Incidentally, the two psychiatric day hospitals in which it was most difficult to get permission from consultants to interview the patients were those day hospitals where nursing staff complained the most about lack of support from their consultant.) The influence of the consultant may be less than commonly supposed: further comments on this are made in Chapter 17.

Another omission is that we do not know the degree to which the views of the head are imposed on the unit with or without the co-operation of the staff. We do know that the heads who expressed the view that the unit should keep users out of hospital had fewer non-nursing and non-medical staff attached to the unit. The more multi-disciplinary staff in the second group is a factor which in itself might restrict the influence of the nursing leader. For example, we noted that more of the *staff* (as opposed to the *head*) in the second group than the first mentioned that an aim of the unit was to keep users out of hospital.

That fewer users in the first group had been in hospital and that fewer labelled themselves as mentally ill might be explained by a possibility that fewer users in the units run by the first group of heads were intrinsically disturbed than those in the second. There is no way of checking this. It is also possible that the differences in the type of patient referred led to the heads refining their view of the aims of the day hospital rather than the other way round: it may be easier to *aim* to keep patients out of hospital if the patients are intrinsically less disturbed. Although this needs further exploration, it does not sound convincing unless it can be demonstrated that day hospitals attached to the old mental hospitals attract more referrals of neurotic disorders and fewer referrals of psychotic disturbance than the rest.

However, if this chapter raises the issue of attempting to locate which day hospitals are more institutional and less community minded than others, it will be sufficient. It needs to be asked whether returning the day hospital to the more medicalised model in the district general hospital runs the risk of forgetting the expensive human lessons learned in the institutions of the past. Of course there may be no grounds for assuming that the district general hospitals of the present or future will be similar to the institutions of the past, apart from the uncanny way that historical patterns in the care of the mentally ill tend to repeat themselves. For example, in the mid nineteenth century there were moves in the care of the mentally ill which might be interpreted *post hoc* as 'keeping patients out of hospital'. A wide range of reforms were introduced to overcome 'institutionalism' in the asylum and it was well recognised that asylums could, by their practices, damage their inmates (Conolly, 1856). Reforms included early discharge, work and occupational therapy programmes, the exclusion of force by attendants and close attention to staff attitudes and involvement on the job. To take a specific 'community care' example, it was decided in 1856 to establish at Friern Hospital in north London a boarding out scheme for patients about to leave the hospital so they could stay with local families at weekends. In addition, a special rehabilitation villa was planned at Friern as it was considered that some patients needed the experience of living independently before their final discharge from hospital. Actually, this scheme never materialised. To introduce a current note, it was axed due to spending cuts, and the potential rehabilitation villa was turned into a nurses' home instead (Hunter and McAlpine, 1974).

That the lessons accumulated in the first half of the nineteenth century were then forgotten and buried for a century is now well known. If this chapter raises the possible danger of forgetting the experiences of those who have been through the institutional mill and their potential applications to the regimes of day units, it will have been useful.

NOTES

1 In Britain, the deficiencies of the institution have been detailed in studies about the elderly (Townsend, 1962), the mentally handicapped (Morris, 1969), mentally ill (Wing and Brown, 1970) and the physically disabled (Miller and Gwynne, 1972).
2 The exact role of psychoactive drugs in the de-institutionalisation of the mentally ill is controversial. Earlier discharge of patients and less restrictive regimes were already under way by the time that the psychoactive drugs arrived in the 1950s (Scull, 1977). Drugs may have reduced the incidence of florid symptoms amongst some patients, thus allowing for earlier management outside hospitals, but they reinforced a social movement of reform which had already started (see, for instance, Wing and Brown, 1970).
3 The evidence for this paragraph came from observations conducted by the researcher on the pilot phase of this project.
4 Other similarities between these units are discussed in Edwards and Carter, 1979.
5 The heads who said that the unit tried to keep users out of hospital had on average forty day places in their units as did the heads who did not mention this aim. The range of places was also similar.
6 The information about lunch and teas is based on observations in three-quarters of the units. In about half the units, where heads aimed to keep users out of hospital, patients were involved in serving lunch. But in only one of the units in the second group did patients help with preparing food. Staff and users ate together in both types of units. If staff mixed with users at lunch they often defined this activity as 'supervision' rather than interaction. However, the two units where staff and users *did* eat together were both units where the heads expressed the aim of keeping users out of hospital.
7 When it came to the point there were small differences between the two groups in the numbers of patients discharged from the unit in the previous twelve months. The day hospitals with heads who viewed the unit as aiming to keep users out of hospital discharged 876 patients (eighty each on average for eleven units) in the previous twelve months. Of these, fifty-five were admitted to hospital, an average of five patients per unit. In the second group, the units discharged 591 patients (seventy-four on average for eight units) in the previous twelve months. Of these, fifty-five were admitted to hospital, an average of nine per unit.
8 By institutionalism is meant the 'disease characterised by apathy, lack of initiative, loss of interest, submissiveness and resigned acceptance' (Barton, 1976).

REFERENCES

Barton, R. (1976) *Institutional Neurosis*, 3rd edn (Wright).
Bierer, J. (1951) *The Day Hospital* (Lewis).
Cameron, D. E. (1947) 'The modern hospital: an experimental form of hospital-

isation for psychiatric patients', *The Modern Hospital*, 69 (3) (September), pp. 60–2.

Conolly, J. (1856) *Treatment of the Insane without Mechanical Restraints*, edited by R. Hunter and I. McAlpine (1973) (Dawsons of Pall Mall).

Edwards, C. and Carter, J. (1979) 'Day services and the mentally disabled', in J. Wing and R. Olsen (eds), *Community Care for the Mentally Disabled* (Oxford University Press).

Goffman, E. (1961) *Asylums: Essays on the Social Situation of Mental Patients and Other Inmates* (Doubleday).

Hunter, R. and McAlpine, I. (1974) *Psychiatry for the Poor* (Dawsons of Pall Mall).

Joseph, Keith (n.d.) quoted in Scull, op. cit.

Kops, B. (1978) *On Margate Sands* (Secker & Warburg.)

Ministry of Health (1962) *A Hospital Plan for England and Wales*, Cmnd 1604 (HMSO).

Miller, E. and Gwynne, G. (1972) *A Life Apart* (Tavistock).

Morris, P. (1969) *Put Away* (Routledge & Kegan Paul).

Scull, A. (1977) *Decarceration* (Prentice Hall).

Titmuss, R. (1961) *Commitment to Welfare* (Allen & Unwin).

Townsend, P. (1962) *The Last Refuge* (Routledge & Kegan Paul).

Wing, J. and Brown, G. W. (1970) *Institutionalism and Schizophrenia* (Oxford University Press).

Wortis, J. (1950) *Soviet Psychiatry* (Williams & Wilkins).

Chapter 8

'BACK TO LIFE': AIMING AT CLINICAL ASSESSMENT AND TREATMENT

> They are trying to bring people back to life again, which they have done for me, because I was as good as dead after my stroke. Well, they seem to do things to stimulate your interest and abilities, and they are so kind, please put that down. Medically they seem very clever here.

INTRODUCTION

Many old people worry about the threat of ill health,[1] and for the old people discussed in this chapter the threat is now reality: half the patients in geriatric day hospitals are aged 75 or more, half suffer from strokes and half are depressed. An 85-year-old man who had a stroke two months previously made the comments above about the geriatric day hospital he attended, and also indicated that it was not so much death that was intolerable, but the interregnum dominated by physical incapacity and age. 'It is not death that is so grieving', wrote Ballanche, 'but decay.' Similarly the elderly man in T. S. Eliot's play was faced after a stroke with the prospect of a convalescent home ('with everything about it to suggest recovery'). Perhaps he spoke for many represented by this chapter when he said:

> I've not the slightest longing for the life I've left –
> Only fear of the emptiness before me.
> If I had the energy to work myself to death
> How gladly would I face death! But waiting, simply waiting
> With no desire to act, yet a loathing of inaction.
> A fear of the vacuum and no desire to fill it.
> It's just like sitting in an empty waiting room.
> In a railway station on a branch line.
> After the last train, after all the other passengers
> Have left, and the booking office is closed.
> And the porters have gone. What am I waiting for?
> In a cold and empty room before an empty grate.
> For no-one. For nothing.

(Eliot, 1969)

Imagine for a moment that elderly, ill people might be seen to share the waiting room at the railway station. Of two possible exit doors, one leads to the deserted station platform but the other door opens on to a corridor leading to the geriatric day hospital. This chapter will explore the route into the geriatric day hospital, but the exit to the equivalent of the deserted station platform remains open too and constitutes a fear for the users and a dilemma for the staff. For one reality of geriatric day hospitals – as arranged at present – is that they offer only a temporary stay to most users before they return them to where they came from – usually their homes. Three-quarters of the heads of geriatric day hospitals reported that, in the main, their patients would leave within six months of their arrival: [2] whether or not this departure symbolises a bleak return for patients through the waiting room to the melancholy of the deserted railway platform is a question asked by this chapter.

Although patients have visited inpatient wards by the day for many years, the idea of the geriatric day hospital is relatively new. A survey in 1961 found ten geriatric day hospitals in England, Wales and Scotland (Farndale, 1961), although not all of these would be classified as day hospitals today. It was estimated by another study in 1970 that 119 day hospitals for the elderly existed in England, Wales and Northern Ireland (Brocklehurst, 1970) and our estimates of England and Wales indicate that 246 day hospitals were operating in 1976.[3] What seems to have been the first official pronouncement, a Ministry of Health circular in 1957 (Ministry of Health, 1957), drew attention to the need to develop services for old people and mentioned the need for developing day hospitals to provide remedial therapy as a way of doing this. This chapter will examine the success or failure of this brief and, as very few accounts of geriatric day hospitals have looked at the service from the patients' point of view, this chapter will also attempt to correct this imbalance.

AIMS IN GERIATRIC DAY HOSPITALS

Eighty-one per cent of heads and staff in geriatric day hospitals suggested that one aim of the day hospital was 'clinical'.[4] Clinical aims appear to be based on the medical model. Oriented towards assessing and treating physical pathology, the 'experts' apply their diagnostic classifications in order to determine the appropriate treatment procedures and the prognosis. One sister-in-charge of a day hospital explained the unit's clinical perspectives in this way: 'It's rehabilitation of elderly people. The day hospital aims to mobilise them. We continue their medical care, their occupational therapy and physiotherapy, and do maintenance and supportive therapy.'

None of the heads and staff of the geriatric day hospitals suggested that the day hospitals aimed to incorporate a coherent view of the significance of life experiences, the past and present relationships of the elderly person, or the social consequences of his illness. Yet it is also clear that some found the clinical mode in itself alone to be inadequate; for over a third of the heads and staff proposed further aims. These have already been discussed in the two previous chapters in relation to other groups of heads and staff. For example, the aim of keeping the users out of hospital, 'not blocking beds', was mentioned by a third of those in geriatric day hospitals too. A woman clinical assistant explained: 'We keep elderly patients in their own home and investigate and rehabilitate them from there, as it prevents admitting them to hospitals where they become dependent and their home care arrangements often break down.'

A third of the heads and staff stated that the clinical mode was supplemented by issuing practical services to patients. This was not, however, the same thing as understanding patients' psychosocial circumstances, but it did imply dispensing food and company. Often heads and staff implied that this task was not really their job because these social matters were considered to be outside the day hospitals' terms of reference. Heads and staff accommodated social issues for pragmatic reasons and as a response to pressure from their patients. One nursing officer added a verbal footnote to her view of the clinical aims of the day hospital: 'Very occasionally we aim to relieve social pressure. Not more than three of our present patients are social cases though. For instance, there's one old lady diabetic who's a little slow and her old sister can't cope seven days per week, and also we check her urine here, so it's partly medical and partly social.'

How do clinical aims compare with other aims of other heads and staff looking after elderly people? Those in voluntary day centres for the elderly we have already discussed and they never mentioned clinical aims; instead, they singlemindedly offer services which are practical. Social services department staff speak of offering practical services to users to improve their psychological status. But three times as many heads and staff working in geriatric day hospitals talked 'clinically' as staff in day hospitals for the mentally ill or elderly confused (where there was significantly more competition about which aim predominated).

Although four out of five heads and staff of the geriatric day hospital attributed the aims of the day unit to the clinical frame of reference, the patients viewed the aims differently. First, only about a quarter saw the aim as purely clinical. 'I imagine it's to get you walking. We have treatments and exercise, and walk round with aids', declared one stroke patient. A second group viewed the clinical framework from almost an 'existential' perspective: while the heads and staff may not have seen the patients' life experiences and social relationships as crucial, a group of patients, comprising about a quarter, did, and they started from a feeling of a rather precarious hold on existence. Some patients felt doubtful about their present and future, and vulnerable about their worth. 'They help you to walk again, and that's everything. Being in a wheelchair makes you feel so old and unwanted', commented one 70-year-old woman. Further, patients were less able than the heads or staff to accept their own physical pathologies 'objectively': thus the physical conditions accepted without comment by the staff were viewed as quite abnormal burdens by the patients. In fact, patients often described a close link between the personal and the physical, and described this dramatically. 'Keeping people out of the grave' or 'bringing people back to life' or 'giving a brighter future' were some declarations of this.

A third group, about a fifth of patients, ignored the clinical frame of reference altogether. They considered simply that the purpose of the day hospital was to provide for their personal needs. Their comments indicated that attendance at the day hospital redressed the balance of adverse conditions at home. These adverse conditions were not so much material as personal. One woman who had come two days a week to the day hospital since her stroke three years ago said: 'It's given me something to live for. Sitting in four walls you soon get depressed. Well I mean for anyone who can't get out it's wonderful here.'

The aim of the day hospital for this group was 'trying to get happiness into the lives of elderly people', or 'making the old people happy', or even 'providing company'.

A final group, also about a fifth of patients, ascribed vague notions of helping to the day hospital, for instance: 'It's to do good to old people.' Few staff, with their emphasis on clinical precision, would recognise 'doing good' as a central aim in clinical assessment and treatment.

In summary, then, patients often saw the day hospital as an integral part of their personal existence and therefore appeared to be asking rather more of the day hospital than the staff. While many heads and staff indicated that they were well aware of the patients' extant non-clinical problems, their interpretation of the aims of the day hospital was such that these difficulties were considered secondary to their central task of treatment of, say, restoring physical functioning in an arm or a leg. No head or staff defined the unit's aim as dealing directly with any emotional challenges or changes which the impact of the patients' illness might represent, yet the patients saw their personal perceptions and emotional reactions to be of great importance. The exceptions were the few heads and staff who said they tried to prepare patients for a future of living inside an institution (Chapter 15).

USERS' PERCEPTIONS AND REACTIONS

By the criteria defined in Chapter 3, over half the patients in geriatric day hospitals considered themselves to be depressed. The immediate question is how day hospitals dealt with depression. We know that all day hospitals administered drugs to their users but if we assume that prescriptions of drugs are not an adequate way of treating those depressions which might relate, at least in part, to specific events in the patient's life, such as an unexpected overwhelming illness, or a long-term, limiting illness, it must be asked whether or not those in the day hospital avoid confronting the depression of their patients. Take the case of Mr F., who had a stroke at 73. He had been attending the day hospital for six months. A former agricultural labourer, he was now able to walk a little, but couldn't 'do' his garden: 'When I sit at home and see the wife out there working in the garden I sit and cry. I'm so depressed over this complaint because I've got the idea my wife has got fed up with me, and I sometimes wish the Lord had taken me off when I had this stroke and that would be the end of all my problems.'

Heads in two of the thirty-one day hospitals reported sponsoring meetings or discussion groups for users on any subject, so there were few opportunities for feelings of depression to be discussed legitimately in discussion groups, either of the 'stroke club' variety or therapeutic groups.[5] Apart from groups, the opportunities for patients to talk to staff about their depression seemed limited, since patients were assigned rarely to the particular 'pastoral' responsibility of one staff member in the day hospital itself. Perhaps the consultant geriatrician saw himself as undertaking this counselling role, but the impression is that few consultants talked to the patients in private. One sister-in-charge with apparently good communication with patients said, 'I'm in the middle, between the patient and the doctor. The patient will confide in me and I pass the messages to the doctor.' Two-thirds of users felt they could not approach staff to discuss really 'personal' problems, for a variety of reasons. 'Oh I'm too shy', or 'I keep myself to myself' were common comments. Yet most patients were full of praise for staff ability and kindness. Perhaps the apparent omnicompetence of the staff was a barrier when it came to users discussing their rather more intimate personal feelings, however.

Discussion of personal issues with patients and their families seemed to be given a relatively low priority by heads and staff in geriatric day hospitals. Over half the units did not have a social worker attached to the unit, and the time devoted to the actual personal care of users by staff – that is, the amount of time staff spent talking individually with users and their families – took up only a tenth of their week on average.[6] The physical, rather than personal, care of patients – activities like toileting, bathing and drying patients, serving lunches and feeding them – took up a quarter of the average week. Staff may, of course, talk to users while taking them to the lavatory or feeding them, but it seems that the users themselves do not always feel that these occasions allow for the expression of their personal feelings. The 70-year-old who mentioned that he had become so overwhelmed with gratitude and warmth that he kissed the nurse when he was in the bath was probably the exception to the rule.

Perhaps patients practised mutual aid and discussed their personal difficulties with each other? Certainly nine out of ten elderly patients said they had spent some time chatting to each other in the previous week: in fact one in five said they spent the main part of their time at the day hospital talking to each other.[7] However, three in every five users added that they could not discuss matters which they defined as 'personal' with their fellow patients. This did not seem to be in itself a consequence of being 'elderly', since twice as many users in voluntary centres and SSD day centres for the elderly said they discussed problems they defined as 'personal' with other users, compared to elderly in day hospitals. Nor can it be assumed that patients were able to deal with personal problems and depression outside the day hospital. Although significantly fewer of them lived alone than either the elderly members of voluntary or social services day centres, there was a tendency for fewer to feel that they could call in friends or neighbours to help out. For those who lived with relatives, as Chapter 10 discusses, the illness itself was likely to alter the relationship with relatives. For example, 'I get depressed because I can't do things for myself', said one stroke victim. 'My wife tries to do everything and I get angry with her.'

The most common way of spending time at home on those days when patients did not come to the day hospital was by 'doing nothing much, just sitting or sleeping', whereas the common way of attenders at voluntary and social services centres spending their time at home was in doing household jobs.

PATIENTS AND THEIR TREATMENT

How do patients react to the treatments they are offered? All geriatric day hospitals offer a physical treatment programme, based on medication, nursing care and sometimes occupational, speech and physiotherapy. Yet only two-thirds of patients considered that they had received such treatments from staff in the week before the survey. A partial explanation for this discrepancy can be found in the shortages of trained therapists in day hospitals in England and Wales; one out of every seven geriatric day hospitals surveyed – usually in the north of the country – had no trained occupational or physiotherapists at all.[8] And only about two in every five day hospitals (45 per cent) had what might be called 'adequate' numbers of trained physiotherapy and/or occupational therapy staff. In other words, on the basis of the presence or absence of trained therapists, there seemed to be three groups of geriatric day hospitals: first, those with 'adequate' numbers of therapy staff; second, those with 'inadequate' numbers of therapy staff; and third, those with no therapy staff at all. Further, whether or not a day hospital had an adequate number of therapists had a significant relationship to its size. In other words, those day hospitals with 'adequate' numbers of therapy staff were smaller on average than either the day hospitals with 'inadequate' numbers of therapists or those without therapists. The small day hospitals with 'adequate' numbers of therapists had on average twenty-four places, the medium-sized day hospitals with 'inadequate' numbers of therapists had on average thirty-four places, while the large day hospitals with no therapists had an average of forty-two places. Why smaller geriatric day hospitals have more trained therapists relative to larger ones is not clear.

Martin and Millard (1976) suggest that size is the important determinant for outcome in the geriatric day hospital; however, this chapter suggests that numbers of therapists is related to size as well as outcome, although the nature of this relationship in causal terms is not clear.

Whether or not a day unit had 'adequate' numbers of therapists, and its related size, had some impact on the way that patients viewed the geriatric day hospital. First, in the day hospitals with an 'adequate' number of therapy staff, which were smaller in size, patients had attended for a shorter time on average and there was a tendency for more patients to spend time at the day hospital on activities they defined as 'physical treatment'. Moreover, more of them tended to see themselves as having made progress at the day hospital.

Second, the larger 'no therapists' day hospitals had fewer patients who had come to the day hospital recently (in the last six months) and there was a tendency for fewer to consider that they spent the bulk of their time at the day hospital on treatment. Further, fewer patients in day hospitals without therapists tended to think that they had made progress since coming to the day hospital than in either the day hospitals with 'adequate' numbers of therapists or even those with 'inadequate' numbers of therapists: they were twice as likely as patients in day hospitals with 'inadequate' numbers of therapists, and three times as likely as patients in places with 'adequate' numbers of therapists to consider that their condition had not changed – or even that it had deteriorated – since coming to the day hospital. These issues will now be discussed in more detail, but a summary of these issues is provided in Table 8.1.

First, patients in day hospitals with an 'adequate' number of therapists (the smaller day hospitals) seemed to attend for shorter periods. For example, two-thirds of the patients interviewed in these day hospitals had been in the unit for less than six months. Only one-third of patients in units with 'inadequate' numbers of therapists (the medium-sized day hospitals) had attended for such a short term. But in the units with no therapists (the larger units), the number of patients with short attendance periods dropped to one in five. These differences were found to be significant.

Second, more patients in units with 'adequate' numbers of therapists seemed to define the time they spent at the day hospital as 'treatment'. In essence, half the patients in small units with 'adequate' numbers of therapists spent most (or second-most) time in the day hospital at treatment, but less than a third of the patients in medium-sized units with 'inadequate' numbers of therapists spent the bulk of their time on treatment. For patients in the day hospitals with no therapists, the number who spent most or second-most time on treatment dropped to just over a fifth.

Third, a few more patients (38 per cent) in hospitals with 'adequate' numbers of therapists tended to feel that they had made progress since starting at the day hospital.[9] Fewer (30 per cent) of the patients in units

Table 8.1   *Characteristics of Geriatric Day Hospitals and their Users[a]*

	'Adequate numbers of therapists' (N = 13 units) (N = 24 users)	'Inadequate numbers of therapists' (N = 12 units) (N = 30 users)	'No therapists' (N = 4 units) (N = 19 users)
Ratio of trained occupational and/or physiotherapists to number of day places	1 : 20 or more	less than 1 : 20	No trained occupational or physiotherapists employed
Average number of established day places	24 places	34 places	42 places
Average number of months users interviewed had attended day hospital	8 months	16 months	15 months
Proportion of users interviewed who spent most/second most time in the unit in 'treatment'	50%	30%	21%
Proportion of users interviewed who said they suffered from strokes	33%	60%	32%
Proportion of users interviewed who said they had not changed or deteriorated	8%	13%	26%
Proportion of users interviewed who were rated as depressed	58%	57%	37%

[a] One day hospital did not submit a return and another listed as a day hospital was excluded from the sample since it was purely a social day facility run by volunteers within the hospital.

with 'inadequate' numbers of therapists felt they had made progress (although about the same number in each group (47 per cent) felt they had been maintained or kept going). In day hospitals with no therapists, however, the proportion of patients who felt they had made progress was lower (26 per cent) and those kept going (42 per cent) was somewhat smaller than in the day hospitals with 'adequate' or 'inadequate' numbers of therapists, although these differences are not very striking. But one in four of the patients in units with no therapists at all thought they had not changed at all, or had even deteriorated at the day hospital, although the differences are not actually significant.

Patients in geriatric day hospitals suffering from the most common complaint, the stroke,[10] also reacted to their experience of the day hospital according to the distinctions of its size and the number of trained therapists. (Whether or not this relates to the tendency for more stroke patients to be short-stay and show immediate but not necessarily sustained improvement is unknown.) But whereas two-fifths of stroke patients in the small day hospitals with 'adequate' numbers of therapists and a third of the stroke patients in the medium-sized day hospitals with 'inadequate' numbers of therapists saw themselves as having made progress, in the larger units without therapists only a sixth of the patients described progress. Moreover, about three times as many patients said they had deteriorated.

Mrs S. And Mr B. attend two of the small day hospitals with 'adequate' numbers of therapy staff. Mrs S., aged 77, had a stroke in 1975, when she attended the day hospital first, and now she was back again with blurred vision. Three months ago she was unable to walk, but now she said: 'It's helped me to walk again. It's looked after me and helped me a lot. I've had stockings given me – white, probably elastic – and I've had new boots from the hospital. I didn't expect it to be so nice. I didn't expect to have had the help I do. They're all so kind to me.'

Mr B., a retired warrant officer in the RAF, was now 85. His wife, a trained nurse, had been looking after him since he had a stroke eight weeks before. He could still feed and dress himself, but needed help with bathing and walking. He said he had been rather muddled since his stroke, but said he was 'more than satisfied' with the day hospital: 'I came here for treatment and progress and I got it. It's improved me a lot, in my legs, my mind and my general health altogether.'

In units without therapists, the patients felt there was less feeling of progress, although they made it clear that the staff had 'tried hard' or 'done their best'. For example, Mr G., aged 67, was a master baker before his stroke three years ago and he had recently had a leg amputated after gangrene. Confined to a wheelchair, he appreciated the 'good dinner' at the day hospital, the fact that a doctor could come immediately should he 'take bad', and his jokes with ambulance men. But he said:

They can do nothing for me here. I suppose it hasn't done any harm coming either, put it that way. You mix with different people and the staff are all good. But I wish I could have physiotherapy: I used to have it [in hospital] but I suppose it was too much trouble for them here.

They had to hold me up and it took two people's time up, so they stopped it because it was too much trouble.

ASSESSMENT OF DAY HOSPITAL SERVICE

So far this chapter has established that elderly day hospital patients expect rather more of the day hospital in personal terms than the staff are prepared to acknowledge. The staff view the aims as more restricted to the clinical sphere, whilst allowing that the day hospital dispenses practical services, just as a pragmatic adjunct. In view of this philosophy, the depression of elderly patients was discussed in the light of the day hospital's current lack of capability for dealing with depression. Leaving the subject of patient depression aside, however, let us recapitulate on what the day hospital offered its patients. Day hospitals with 'adequate' numbers of therapy staff were significantly smaller than the ones with 'inadequate' numbers and those with no therapy staff at all, and also differed from them in that their patients stayed for shorter periods and there was a tendency for more patients to say they spent the majority of their week receiving treatment, and for them to feel they had made progress since coming to the day hospital.

However, in terms of influencing the self-perceived depression of its patients, there was not much difference between the different types of day hospitals. We have already noted that not much time was spent talking to patients: about the same amount of the week was spent by staff in talking to the patients in all three types of day units. However, in units with 'adequate' numbers of therapists, the emphasis of the way staff spent their time was clearly on physical care. The average time staff spent on the actual physical care of patients, such as toileting, feeding, washing and bathing, was the highest in those units with 'adequate' numbers of therapists.

All this evidence is highly tentative as the patients' views could not be corroborated by independent accounts. It does relate to other work, however, which suggests that the size of the day hospital relates to the length of time the patient spends there (Martin and Millar, 1976). But it suggests too that day hospitals, staffed by 'adequate' numbers of therapists and of small size, can discharge patients faster, offer them more treatment and make more feel that they are achieving progress. On the other hand, day hospitals without therapists seem to offer patients a longer stay, more non-treatment activities, give fewer a personal feeling of achievement from day unit attendance. But patients are slightly less likely to be depressed. Perhaps this is because day hospitals without therapists recruit less severe cases, although there is no necessary association between the severity of a stroke and the severity of depression. Or perhaps the nurses in day hospitals without therapists adopt a different role to compensate for the lack of visible therapy, or whether it is more that over longer periods of attendance patients become less depressed and more adjusted to their condition, is unknown. Or perhaps it is because the elderly patients in hospitals without therapists can feel more secure in the knowledge that they will not be summarily discharged? Whatever the reason, this appears to be a complex issue: another study found a positive relationship between depression and receiving treatment by a therapist (Brocklehurst *et al.*, 1978).

How effective the remedial therapies are in treatment of strokes is a debated question. But any inquiry into the effectiveness of a physical, psychological or social therapy which fails to measure progress subjectively and which ignores the potential impact of treatments on the morale of the patient and the family is ignoring important dimensions. This evidence implies that subjective evaluation of progress is separate from subjective feelings of depression and this is surprising since depression and low morale are usually considered to be associated. More attention needs to be paid to this area.

DISCHARGE

The co-ordinator of the day hospital, usually the sister-in-charge, found persuading old people that it was in their interest to leave the geriatric day hospital a continuing problem. Five out of every ten day hospitals faced this problem regularly, because they planned to discharge each patient within six months of their admission, and only an eighth of day hospitals catered for long-term patients to any substantial degree. So it was not surprising that three-quarters of the heads of day hospitals found that they had trouble persuading users to leave, most often because of the fears of the old person:

> Some patients become very attached to the unit and are therefore very upset about discharge. Some have been known to, for instance, aggravate ulcers so that treatment can continue.

> Patients are very upset when they complete their term of treatment. They have to be told they will return for a further course of treatment if necessary.

Heads of day hospitals would like to be able to refer patients on to a day centre, to reduce the distress and anxiety over discharge. But on average only one in twenty of the patients discharged in the previous year from geriatric day hospitals were transferred to a day centre. More day centres were wanted. Only one health authority in the north-east had day hospital heads who said there was no extra need for day centre places in their area. Even with the close liaison existing between day hospitals and day centres on the area, it was not always easy to persuade patients to go. The sister-in-charge of one day hospital in the area commented:

When patients have attended for a number of months, there is a tendency for them to become dependent on the day hospital. Presenting them with the idea of attending a day club after, often meets with disapproval. However, it is frequently overcome by commencing at a local day club while attending day hospital. After a period of two to three weeks attending both, discharge takes place.

In this particular day hospital, one in every four of the patients discharged in the previous twelve months had been discharged to voluntary day centres – a greater number than the national average of one in every twenty patients. Three times as many patients were discharged from this day hospital into either residential or hospital care as into day centres, but the largest group, over a third, was discharged without apparent further follow up other than outpatient attendance. Mr F., 84, a former trade union official, now blind and with Parkinson's Disease, who lives alone in a 'very isolated cottage', spoke up against his possible discharge, and appraised his need of the continuing help of the day hospital like this: 'I don't know what I should do without this place, it takes people out of themselves, they're not buttoned up. I should become a hermit on my own, do you know what I mean?'

The head occupational therapist at Mr F.'s day hospital, commenting on discharging patients, said this: 'It is so difficult to give an old person a physical, psychological and social crutch and then take it away.'

COMMENT

Metaphorically, then, for many old people the exit from the geriatric day hospital leads to the empty station platform and the recognition that the last train has gone. Nevertheless, geriatric day hospitals offer some old people a temporary route out of the waiting room: after all, until about thirty years ago there was sparse medical interest in the acute medical care of the elderly. The elderly ill, designated the 'chronic sick', were consigned to the long-stay ward of the poor law hospital, where the image was 'drab conditions, decaying surroundings, and inadequate staffing' (Felstein, 1969). The advent of geriatric medicine and the rehabilitation therapies has meant 'destruction of the static and hopeless attitude that tender loving care was the only therapy for a sick old person' (Felstein, 1969, p. 15). Countering the pessimism and disinterest of medical colleagues, the 'new' geriatricians have tried to demonstrate that clinical therapies and outcomes can take their place under the aegis of acute medicine.

Day hospitals may have contributed to raising the status of geriatric medicine (Brocklehurst, 1970). Most written accounts of geriatric day hospitals make a careful distinction between a day hospital and a day centre. 'In a nutshell, the aim [of the day hospital] is to dissociate the "hotel" element of hospital care from the therapeutic content, leaving only the latter . . . It is important to distinguish between day centres and day hospitals. Day centres provide social facilities, company, a cooked meal, possibly a bath and chiropody, but none of the remedial services found in the day hospital' (Brocklehurst, 1970, p. 11).

But some day hospitals do not provide remedial services; why do some geriatric day hospitals wish to dissociate themselves from the day centre 'image'? Within the context of clinical medicine in which geriatric medicine has struggled to gain recognition, the non-scientific accoutrements of the day centre, that is, the company and food, are considered a potential handicap to achieving status. Further, for geriatricians and 'scarce' therapists to dispense 'company and food' is also, if not a waste of expensive resources, at least a reduction of their potential clinical effectiveness. It would be a harsh critic who denied that achieving parity with clinical medicine was not of some importance: given our present structure of services and rewards, barefoot geriatricians are unlikely to catch on in the UK. But, on the other hand, as we have seen, many of the problems of the elderly are not medical, they are social and psychological. And of those that are medical problems, many are non-acute. So, although many geriatricians have been enthusiastic about day hospitals (enthusiasm being an attitude which follows many innovations in social and health services), questions need to be asked about the ability of day hospitals geared primarily towards delivering the benefits of acute medicine to deal with patients with long-term disabilities and social needs as well. One geriatrician comments:

> Saving [inpatients' beds] requires a high turnover and a short stay. This, however, is incompatible with relieving stress on relatives and physical maintenance treatment . . . increasingly I tend to send patients who I consider have a good chance of rehabilitation to the physiotherapy or other treatment clinics, while patients who need on-going care for social reasons go to day hospitals. (Millard, 1978, p. 13)

Area health authorities do not have explicit policies about the development or the operation of day hospitals, as Chapter 2 makes clear.[11] Before the reorganisation of the health service in 1974, geriatric day hospitals were started as a result of intiatives from individual consultant geriatricians. Little information is available on more recent planning mechanisms in health authorities, but initiatives stemming from consultant geriatricians will probably continue to be a primary factor in developing new geriatric day hospitals in the near future at least. While geriatricians appear to play a relatively small part in the organisation of what happens day by day itself, they emerge as major decision-makers about critical matters concerning patient admission.[12]

If the health problems of the elderly are accepted as long term and indivisible from the patients' subjective social reality, one question geriatricians will need to face is where the boundary should be placed between the knowledge and skills of the 'domain' of geriatric medicine and the 'domains' of the statutory social services and voluntary agencies. If it is accepted that separatism between medical and the social sides must be overcome, the following strategies could be considered as alternatives.

First, it is commonly argued that doctors should have more training in social and behavioural sciences and at an undergraduate level. But this is less rarely said of consultant training and at present consultant training in geriatric medicine, in its formal requirement at least, is extremely 'medical'. Whatever training a specialist in geriatric medicine picks up in social and behavioural science is *ad hoc* and unsystematic. The development of the speciality of geriatrics is sometimes compared with that of paediatrics, which in its early years was dominated also by the acute medical model. Training for paediatricians now acknowledges the sub-speciality of community paediatrics, the irreducible chronic problems of handicap and the socially induced disorders of childhood (compare Court, 1976). These are examples of a shift in the focus of interest of paediatricians towards the social 'domain' in recent years. But paediatricians have been forced to 'branch out' by contracting workloads due to the control of the childhood infectious diseases, the longevity of children with congenital disorders and the fall in the birth-rate. By contrast, geriatricians are faced with an expanding clinical workload, due to the increasing numbers of elderly people in the population. So, if the approach to training geriatricians improves medical recognition and intervention concerning the social and psychological problems of the elderly, the 'silting up' of expensive technical facilities would be increased rather than reduced.

A different approach for the geriatrician is to view himself less as a specialist in social and psychological issues than as an entrepreneur. He establishes other day facilities to act as outlets to the geriatric day hospital and he continues to control their policies and referrals. One example is a small day centre which opened on the same site as a day hospital, staffed by volunteers. This allows patients to be transferred from the day hospital to the day centre after their period of treatment ends, and successfully offers company and a good lunch to patients, but it does not overcome the expensive difficulty of transporting relatively frail old people from long distances. In an urban district in a different part of the country, geriatricians have fostered over years the growth of a comprehensive 'chain' of local day clubs in the area via the local old people's welfare association. Discharged patients are referred to volunteer-run clubs in church halls and community centres, and an example was given earlier in the chapter. Although our information on this is patchy, the impression is that patients transferred to voluntary day centres after periods of treatment in day hospitals find them unstimulating and dull; also there is the problem of transporting disabled elderly people to voluntary centres, which can often be done only once a week, on the 'housebound' day. Chapter 3.1 asked what this can be expected to achieve: to visit a day centre once a week is not much use to an 'at risk' old person who needs surveillance or whose relatives need relief or who needs any form of nursing or nutritional supervision. 'Once a week day care' can do little more than offer an interesting, stimulating day out but it cannot provide a lifeline in the same way that five days a week at the adult training centre might do for the family of a mentally handicapped person.

The strategies mentioned to date are intiatives made by consultant geriatricians. What of the role of primary health care? One development in a small town in a rural area is a two-day-a-week day centre in a cottage hospital. There is a local management committee and the scheme is backed in part by the local authority. Patients are referred via the group practice general practitioners and part-time social worker, transport and staffing are provided by volunteers and physiotherapy is available at the hospital 'outpatients'. The nearest 'proper' geriatric day hospital is 30 miles away, but the idea is for a consortium of local interests to provide a prevention, care and maintenance service locally. Difficulties have been found in the extent to which volunteer drivers will travel to collect patients and, of course, on the restrictions that volunteer transport places on the disabilities which can be collected. The most severely disabled cannot usually fit into a sedan car.

One other approach would be for geriatricians to act less as specialists in social issues, or as entrepreneurs or as co-opters of social services to the medical 'sphere', than as partners in joint efforts. This approach, which acknowledges the plurality of the services required by elderly and the need to harness relatively autonomous services together, relies on negotiation between representatives of health, social services and housing agencies to bring together a mosaic of services for a particular referral. At present, this method is used to assess intending applicants for residential accommodation in one area, but such a method might be extended to admission to day services, as long as a 'next friend' or 'named person' were available to help the old person use the mosaic of services (Chapter 3.3 provides a parallel suggestion).

On the other hand, it might be more sensible when setting up new day services for the elderly for a social services day centre to be the focal service. Such centres might serve old people who are at risk physically and socially or those with a high proportion of social needs. Regular health surveillance under the supervision of new 'community geriatricians' [13] who visit the social service centre could institute appropriate specialist medical and therapy referrals, often to the outpatient departments of hospitals, or to small day hospitals (staffed, of course, by adequate numbers of therapists!). Patients plus those who enter the day hospital after a medical emergency can be followed up at a less intensive medical and therapeutic level on the day centre site after their acute episode diminishes. Similar approaches in children's day services where social services have co-opted relevant health services are a model. A hard look at the functioning of some present day hospitals may lead to the acknowledgement that those day hospitals with inadequate numbers of therapists or no therapists at all might be more appropriately sponsored by social services.

Centring day services for the elderly around a social service base whilst calling in health services for special purposes would leave voluntary agencies or consortiums of voluntary and statutory services free to develop informal schemes which are neighbourhood based. These should stimulate the interests of those in a local elderly population who can get themselves to day centres and go as often as they wish.

Each of these schemes has merits and demerits and all could be tried and compared on an experimental basis. One main consequence of this chapter is to confirm the view that day hospitals for the elderly should not be planned *in vacuo*. Treatment and care for elderly ill people needs to be based on the assumption that the definition of problems needs to be inclusive and remedies specific.

NOTES

1 See for instance Hunt (1978). However, ill health 'is much more a source of complaint in the lowest income group' (p. 141).

2 Of the thirty-one geriatric day hospitals in the national sample, the heads of twenty-two units said that 70 per cent or more of users would leave within six months of admission, five heads said that 60 per cent or more of their users would never leave, and the rest catered in the main for patients who would stay an intermediate term of between six months and two years.

3 Thirty-one day hospitals were found in thirteen areas of England and Wales in 1976. A thirty-second was found to have been omitted from the sample after fieldwork terminated.

4 This chapter is based on postal information from the heads of thirty-one geriatric day hospitals and interviews collected in twelve day hospitals. Strictly speaking, two of these twelve units were additional to the stratified interview sample, but were included as 'extras' since they were said to demonstrate new developments in day hospital practice. Thus the interview sample of heads, staff and users of ten units plus two extras consists of twelve interviews with heads, thirty-six interviews with staff, and seventy-three interviews with users. Heads, unless otherwise stated, were sisters-in-charge. A pilot survey found that consultants spent relatively little time in the day hospital and the person nominated as head was the member of staff responsible for the co-ordination of the activities of the day and was usually the nursing officer or sister-in-charge.

5 Stroke clubs as self-help groups have recently been started for patients and their relatives (under the auspices of the Chest, Heart & Stroke Association). A stroke club met on the premises of one of the day hospitals in the evening, but day patients were not specifically involved.

6 This figure represents the mean number of hours that the random sample of forty-three heads and staff who had been in the day hospital in the week previous to the survey had spent on personal care activities.

7 The largest group of patients said they spent most time on arts and crafts (27 per cent). The next largest group spent most time chatting (21 per cent), and they were followed by those who spent most time receiving treatment (19 per cent).

8 Guidelines outlining 'appropriate' ratios of staff were issued by the British Geriatric Society (1977). Geriatric day hospitals with 'adequate' numbers of trained therapists were defined as those day hospitals with a ratio of at least one trained physiotherapist or

one trained occupational therapist to every twenty day places. Day hospitals with 'inadequate' numbers of trained therapists fell below this guideline. The presence or absence of speech therapists or chiropodists was not built into these criteria. Five out of ten of the day hospitals had the services of a speech therapist (nearly always part-time), and four out of ten had the services of a chiropodist, also on a part-time basis. As the information discussed in this section is derived from the 'census' rather than the 'interview' sample, it is legitimate to discuss 'day units' as well as the aggregate of 'heads and staff'.

9 Patients were asked, 'What has coming to this place done for you?' Their answers were rated on a three-point scale: 1 – *Progress*, statements which provided evidence of clear improvement since coming to the day hospital in physical and/or personal terms; 2 – *Maintenance*, statements which indicated that the day hospital had kept the user going personally and/or physically; 3 – *Deterioration*, where the user said the day hospital had done nothing at all, or that he had slipped back either personally or physically. Patients who had made progress in all three types of units were clear about the area of progress. In units with 'adequate' numbers of therapists personal and physical progress went together. This was also true in units with no therapists. In units with 'inadequate' numbers of therapists, physical progress was noted more often than personal or interpersonal progress.

10 Technically, 'stroke' is known as a 'cerebrovascular accident'.

11 This information was obtained in interviews with specialists in community medicine (social services) in twelve of the thirteen area health authorities.

12 Informal discussion took place with consultant geriatricians in four of the twelve hospitals. Formal interviews took place with five doctors who worked in geriatric day hospitals and who were selected in a random draw for interview. These were usually below the rank of consultant, that is, senior registrars and clinical assistants. In the thirty-one day hospitals in the census sample, consultant geriatricians were reported by heads as having the critical influence on admission. In three-quarters of units, the admission decision was made by consultant geriatricians alone. In the other quarter of units, admission decisions are made by consultant geriatricians with the involvement of staff in the day unit.

13 Considerable thought would need to be given to a potential role for a community geriatrician. The hospital geriatrician is a scarce resource anyway, and is better equipped for medicine practised within a hospital rather than a community setting.

REFERENCES

British Geriatric Society (1977) *Memorandum on Provision of Geriatric Services*, Report of a British Geriatric Society Working Party (unpublished).

Brocklehurst, J. (1970) *The Geriatric Day Hospital* (King Edward's Hospital Fund).

Brocklehurst, J., Andrews, K., Richards, B. and Laycock, P. J. (1978) 'How much physical therapy for patients with stroke?', *British Medical Journal*, 6123, 1, pp. 1307–1310.

Court, D. (1976) *Fit for the Future. Report of the Committee on Child Health Services*, Vol. 1, Cmnd 6684 (HMSO).

Eliot, T. S. (1969) *The Complete Poems and Plays of T. S. Eliot* (Faber).

Farndale, J. (1961) *The Day Hospital Movement in Great Britain* (Pergamon).

Felstein, I. (1969) *Later Life: Geriatrics Today and Tomorrow* (Routledge & Kegan Paul).

Hunt, A. (1978) *The Elderly at Home* (Department of Health and Social Security).

Martin, A. and Millard, P. H. (1976) 'Effect of size on the function of three day hospitals: the case for the small unit', *Journal of the American Geriatric Society*, XXIV, 11, pp. 506–10.

Millard, P. (1978) *Transport Problems of Day Hospitals* (National Corporation for the Care of Old People).

Ministry of Health (1957) *Geriatric Services and the Care of the Chronic Sick*, HM (57) 86.

Chapter 9

'A NORMAL LIFE': AIMING AT REHABILITATION

The aims are to get people's confidence back so that they can go back to work. They have no confidence in being able to work. It's to show them that life outside can be all right. It's to give them the confidence to sew and to get them back to being not afraid of the outside world. Like getting on a bus. (51-year-old domestic, day hospital for the mentally ill)

INTRODUCTION

Antonia White's autobiographical novel *Beyond the Glass* tells of the descent into madness of Clara, a gentle 22-year-old girl from a cloistered background, admitted to 'Nazareth Royal Hospital' in 1921. When she awoke, she was in a small, bare, white-washed cell with a heavy door without a handle. She lay on a mattress on the floor without sheets and, occasionally, nurses took her from the cell, dipped her into a hot bath, then ducked her in an ice-cold one before throwing her back on to the mattress in the cell. Later, she moved to a small, six-sided room where the walls and door were padded with rubber and then on to another cell where she lay on a mattress inside what looked like a great wooden manger. Over the manger was a stiff, canvas apron, fastened to the manger with studs. Clara wore a stiff, rough garment encasing her legs and feet and her hands.

One day she found that the sailcloth and straitjacket had gone. She had a rough nightdress on instead and she could stand up. She could even leap from the manger to the high windowsill and look out the barred window onto the garden. She was now allowed to visit a long, tiled washroom with a row of lavatories without doors and brass rods instead of chains. On other days, she was allowed to walk in an asphalt yard surrounded by high, brick walls. She learned what she must do to please the staff and how to avoid being punished.

Then, one day she found herself in a real bed in a small room with blue walls. There was a mirror and a strip of carpet and, best of all, a handle on the door. The room brought changes. 'We have good fun sometimes. Concerts you know. And twice a year we have a dance', a doctor said. Clara was allowed to have one book to read each week, to eat with the other women in a bare dining room and to visit the summer garden.

Some time later, the doctors decided that since she was much improved, her rehabilitation could continue if she were to go to a place in the country, with more freedom. She could have her own books and things. A nurse could take her to a cinema. There was tennis, good bridge and a thoroughly cheerful atmosphere.

Although it is not always easy to distinguish Clara's bad dreams from the reality, one implicit point is that Clara was treated in the hospital as if she were progressing along a snakes and ladders board. Progress up the ladder was rewarded by a more liberal regime but Clara slid back to where she began if she had an outburst of madness. So when she convinced the doctor that she could try life outside the hospital, she had mastered a sequence of rungs up the ladder. Nowadays, mental illness is treated differently. The unpleasant early steps that Clara underwent have been removed. Those who undergo treatment do not start off in the cold, comfortless cell, but in the equivalent of the blue room or even at the country house stage of tennis, bridge and chat. One question this chapter will address itself to is this: where does the day unit user move on to *after* the blue room or the country house? What are next rungs up the rehabilitation ladder?

REHABILITATION: THE AIM

This chapter will consider the place of the aim of rehabilitation in day services and our starting-point, as usual, will be the head and staff's view of the aims. Some synonyms for rehabilitation will be considered before discussing the way that people in day services view the *outcome* of rehabilitation, and similarities and differences on the subject between the staff and users will be outlined.

As an aim of the unit, rehabilitation was mentioned less frequently than other aims, such as keeping people out of hospital, or achieving clinical ends. Usually, staff who asserted that rehabilitation was an aim of their particular day unit were lone voices, unsupported in their contention by their colleagues within the same day unit. For instance, out of those interviewed in thirty units, only one staff member in each mentioned that the unit aimed at rehabilitation. In only fifteen units did two or more staff agree on this, and there were only four units where every staff member declared that the aim of the unit, as they saw it, was rehabilitative. These units were one family day centre, one unit for offenders, a day training centre and two employment rehabilitation centres. Unfortunately, the Employment Services Agency has refused to sanction the analysis and use of interviews collected in these units. This is a pity, as these centres provided valuable material against which to view the aims of other projects.

Overall, in all day units, one in seven of heads and staff thought rehabilitation to be an aim of the unit, as Chapter 4 points out. Many of this 14 per cent were found in day units for the mentally ill where over a quarter of the staff considered that one purpose of their unit was rehabilitative. Of these, a third were in day hospitals and two-thirds in social services day centres.

Rehabilitative *intentions* are hard to find in day services and, although it is not beyond the bounds of possibility that rehabilitation is practised where it is not preached, it is also apparent that even when the intention is there, the word 'rehabilitation' itself means different things to different people. Three examples from day hospitals for the mentally ill compare variations in the meaning of the word. Staff in one unit used the word 'rehabilitation' as a synonym for 'chronic'. Their day hospital was housed in one building, but split into two sections. The 'acute' unit looked after short-stay patients while the 'rehabilitation' unit handled the 'chronic' patients, many from the back wards of the mental hospital next door. Most of their 'chronics' had spent long years in hospital, and now, discharged to boarding houses and group homes outside the hospital, they came each day to the 'rehabilitation' unit to fill in their time by doing 'industrial work therapy' and having a 'good, hot lunch'. But this unit provided no individual programmes for its patients and there was little systematic individual contact between the day unit staff and patients. Nearly all patients were defined as long-stay, so the daily routines contrasted with the aim expressed by the head of the 'rehabilitation' section 'to rehabilitate patients: to socialise them to live in the community'.

So if rehabilitation was thought of as synonymous with 'chronic', it was also seen as coextensive with 'treatment'. The head and staff of a second day hospital offered a flat rate of six weeks in a day hospital to each patient, so that (in the words of the nursing officer in charge) 'patients could be made fit to go back into society as soon as possible. People from all strata of society have a breaking point, and many reach that breaking point, so we aim to give them six weeks' intensive treatment and hope they are cured for them to go back to their work and cope.' In between joining in with arts and crafts, patients were medicated, given electric shock treatment and attended relaxation classes. Although there were groups and meetings for patients to attend, there were no specially devised programmes for each user and each had to adapt to the standardised programme.

In a third unit, the word 'rehabilitation' was a metaphor for the word 'discharge', a process equivalent to the process of arranging a patient's exit from the unit. 'We rehabilitate patients for discharge from the day hospital', said the acting nursing officer. 'It's rewarding to see patients come for a short time, then get discharged into the community.' Few patients in this unit were short term (that is, likely to leave within six months of admission): rather, nearly all were likely to be in the unit for between six and twelve months. The programme offered was very similar to the second day hospital where rehabilitation was seen to be allied with treatment. Social and sporting activities took up the most time and 'classes' were held for patients, the most prominent being a current affairs class and a nature study group. Again, there were no individual programmes for users to follow, although a written programme outlining activities from week to week was pinned to the noticeboard.

OUTCOME OF REHABILITATION

If the semantics of rehabilitation vary, so do the outcomes attached to 'rehabilitation'. Although outcomes were referred to infrequently by staff, three need special mention. First, for some, the outcome of rehabilitation is concerned with returning people to work. One occupational therapist in a day hospital for the mentally ill summed this up. She started, 'Well, the aims in this unit are not set out' (a common comment) and then continued: 'But I *think* it's to care for patients living in the community, not needing hospital admission. The aim is rehabilitation, really, to retrain them for work. They need sheltered workshops as the next stage.'

One group who seemed united about the link between rehabilitation and work were those working in the employment rehabilitation centres. As one manager said: 'We try to get people back to work, but to the right job. We have a dual purpose, rehabilitative and assessment. We look at their abilities after disablement and assess them to find out what they can do. If they need retraining we send them off on a course.'

Aside from those who saw rehabilitation tied to future jobs for users, a second group saw the outcome of rehabilitation as that of getting people into the 'outside world'. This idea was the most common concept of rehabilitation amongst staff in the day hospitals for the mentally ill. A return to 'normality' and a 'normal' way of life was critical to this way of thinking, although normality as such was never defined, nor was it refined by class, sub-cultural or regional differences. 'This unit is to rehabilitate a person so that they can go out into the community to lead a normal life', explained a staff nurse. Another staff member, a state enrolled nurse in a day centre for the mentally ill, said: 'It's really to return people to a normal way of life, what they would have outside if they weren't ill.'

A few other staff hinged their view of the outcome of rehabilitation not so much as a return to work or as social normality, but as regeneration. For this group, rehabilitation was about a change or a new beginning. Particularly in the units for offenders (which are, of course, themselves relatively new), 'aiming for a new start' or 'setting the users on a new pathway' were ways in which this was expressed. For example, 'I think the main aim is to help the boys to learn to live a good life', said a cleaner who was very much a member of the staff in a day training centre for offenders: 'To give them a feeling of capability so that they can go out from here to do something they've never done before: painting, pottery, or woodwork. When they leave here, it's giving them an interest. When they come, they're only interested in gambling and crime.'

However, heads and staff did not commonly define outcomes to the aim of rehabilitation. The users had a more pronounced emphasis on outcomes, such as getting users back to work. The following examples suggest this: 'This place has the sole purpose of getting us back to a normal job', declared a 36-year-old former surveyor. 'Well, I think it's to get us fit again and going back to work', said a 59-year-old boot and shoe factory operative suffering from agoraphobia. 'It's to build you up to a normal way of living, to get you back to normal living again', said a depressed 39-year-old former postman. 'It's to get you back to living normal life in the community again', said a 49-year-old housewife.

Overall, however, not many more users than heads and staff in day units for the mentally ill (33 : 28 per cent) thought that one purpose of the unit was to rehabilitate the users.

REHABILITATION AND NEGOTIATION

How do day unit staff put across rehabilitation to their users? Taking the heads and staff in units for the mentally ill as an example, from what they said there was little emphasis on explaining the meaning of rehabilitation to users, prospective and present. Four out of ten heads asked the users to visit the unit for discussion before their time of attendance started and a third of the heads of units for the mentally ill said that the unit ran a 'general orientation programme' after the user had started coming to the unit. But none visited users at home before they started a period of attendance at the unit and only a couple were able to involve either relatives or friends before the user's commencement at the unit. Very few units assigned new users to particular staff members on the first day. In fact, only a third of the staff interviewed in units for the mentally ill considered that they were responsible for particular users for most of the day. The major reason they gave for undertaking this responsibility when it did happen was to give the staff member practice at exercising his or her job skills, for example, casework, nursing or art therapy. Does 'discharging one's professional skills' necessarily coincide with helping to rehabilitate the users?

There were some divergences between the views of the staff and users in the day units for the mentally ill. On the subject of the amount of talk about rehabilitation which took place in the units, about twice as many heads and staff as the users in the mental illness units considered that specific discussions took place about rehabilitation and training. Does this mean that the staff overestimated the amount of time they talked about rehabilitation or that their talk was not getting through to users?

For example, in the twenty-one day hospitals for the mentally ill, two-thirds of the heads and staff thought that there were regular discussions about rehabilitation and training, but only one out of five users claimed any knowledge of these. In the eight social services units, just under half the heads and staff claimed that regular discussions about rehabilitation and training took place, and a third of the users knew of these. However, we cannot be sure that staff and users' views corresponded unit by unit. Some support is given to the proposition that heads and staff, particularly in the day hospitals, do not discuss rehabilitation with their users, as only a third of the users in mental illness units considered that anyone on the staff had talked to them at any time at all about their future plans. On the other hand, it is just possible that heads and staff left having such talks until just before users were discharged, which would account for the low proportion of users indicating that heads and staff took an interest in their future. But the views of heads and staff in units for offenders coincided; half in each group indicated that rehabilitation had been discussed. This implies that heads and staff in day hospitals for the mentally ill are not getting through to many users on this subject.

However, some users hoped to leave the day unit at some stage. Five out of ten users in social services units for the mentally ill, and seven out of ten interviewed at the day hospitals for the mentally ill, anticipated leaving the unit, most to go to work. But, in practical terms, almost none of the users in the mental illness units (or in any type of unit) had made any concrete plans for this, and only about one-third had any plan, however vague, to occupy themselves after leaving. A lack of concrete plans to leave the unit has been interpreted as a measure of the institutionalising of the user (Wing et al., 1964). In this respect, it is important to note the tenuous connection between heads of most day units for the mentally ill and the employment services. Only one day hospital in the sample had its own disablement resettlement officer: but he was a rare visitor at most day units for mentally ill users: in only three out of ten units did he visit at least once a month.

THEORY OR PRACTICE OF REHABILITATION

It might be argued, then, that those working in day units are not geared closely to rehabilitation. If the charter of the day unit is rehabilitative, few recognise this as part of the aim. There is very little open discussion about rehabilitation and training. Do the characteristics of users militate against rehabilitation? We asked the heads and staff what made an ideal user. The ideal user for the largest group in day hospitals was dependent: one who accepted the views and succourance of staff. 'The ideal patient is someone willing to try to get better with our help. They have to be willing to accept our methods', said a charge nurse. But a second group of staff considered that the ideal user was motivated: 'It has to be someone prepared to look at their own behaviour and prepared to do something about it', said a young nursing officer. And a small, third group thought the defining feature of the ideal patient was that he was co-operative.

'The ideal user is one who is punctual and takes his medicine. He does what he is told to do in his interests', said a 35-year-old doctor, a clinical assistant. Similarly, a 37-year-old state enrolled nurse said: 'An ideal user is someone who comes here and gets straight on with what he is told to do.' So some see the ideal user as dependent, some as motivated to help himself and others as co-operative. Which images fit a user about to climb a rehabilitation ladder?

Rehabilitation involves a transaction between a staff member and a potential rehabilitee's personal, internal reality. Sometimes the untrained domestic staff expressed more understanding of the handicaps of the user facing rehabilitation. 'Really, until I came here I didn't realise that young people could be so lonely', said the cleaner in a day training centre for offenders where every staff member ascribed to and was formally involved in the rehabilitation process. 'I like to see the difference in the boys when they go compared to when they come. Malcolm was a real brute when he came, and when he went he was really kind.'

Many users are said to be in two minds about leaving the psychiatric day units. Two-thirds of the heads (more than in any other user groups except offenders) reported trouble in persuading the users to leave the unit. The biggest problem was said to reside in the users themselves: according to one nursing officer, 'Ninety per cent of them become attached and dependent, and some feign prolonged symptoms to try to manipulate the staff in regard to discharge.' For the rest, the problems were seen to reside not so much within the user as within the community. There was thought to be a lack of adequate support services after discharge, like evening clubs, and gaps in their social environment, such as lack of local employment. In the previous twelve months, about a third of the users from day hospitals and day centres eventually got back to open employment, although we do not know how many of these stayed. Another third of those in the day hospitals left the unit to stay at home and one of every seven discharges were admitted to hospital. On the other hand, almost the same number left the social services centres because they didn't like it. On this basis it is possible to be certain only that the users who return to work were, at least in part, rehabilitated, although some of the users who stayed at home may have been as likely to have taken up roles in the household, as sitting 'doing nothing'.

DISCUSSION

Over recent years, a tested wisdom about the process of rehabilitating psychiatric patients has developed: if by rehabilitation one means the ability to do a job and live outside a hospital with a greater or lesser amount of support from an outpatient department, or a social services department. For example, forty-five schizophrenic men patients with an average stay in two different hospitals of eight-and-a-half years attended a course the equivalent of an employment rehabilitation centre while they lived in the two hospitals. In one hospital, the men were extensively and systematically prepared for going to the centre beforehand, but at the other hospital preparation was hit and miss and rather haphazard. About half went on eventually to industrial employment, but the preparation and practice for work which took place before the patients went to the employment rehabilitation centres appeared to improve their attitudes to work and decreased the 'adverse reactions' common when a schizophrenic patient has a sudden change of scene and location (Wing *et al.*, 1964). 'The moral was drawn . . . that the skills and experience of rehabilitation which have been built up in mental hospitals might be just as relevant . . . in the community' (Wing *et al.*, 1972).

How many users in day care could benefit from a rehabilitation programme? In considering the users in day services for the mentally ill, there would appear to be very few whom one would want to exclude for rehabilitation on the grounds of the severity of their illness alone. For example, as almost all the mentally ill users were able to complete the interview and carry on detailed conversation about their everyday life and their views of the day units, there are few users who could be classified as 'severely' handicapped on the criteria of Wing *et al.* (1964).

As an example, consider those fourteen users who labelled themselves as 'schizophrenic'.[1] Thirteen of the fourteen completed the interview. Are these users who might be considered ready for a rehabilitative 'push'? Nine were men and five were women: all except the youngest (aged 25) had worked at jobs in the past. Ten of the fourteen came to the day unit on five or more days per week and, on average, each had spent three years in their respective day units. All these users had spent periods in psychiatric hospitals in the past, the largest group between two and five years.

Five of the fourteen lived with their parents and four in hostels: only one lived alone. As a group, they seemed to have considerable difficulty with practical everyday living activities. When compared with the parents who attended family day units, who were similar in age, only eight of the fourteen self-labelled schizophrenics said they could prepare and cook a hot meal without difficulty, but twenty-eight of the twenty-nine parents in family day care felt they could do this without difficulty. Schizophrenic users said they had difficulty with the daily routine of cleaning out their own room or living space, and also with doing their own laundry.

What essential conditions might be suggested to achieving rehabilitation in day services? First, concerted intention on the part of the staff. Some users may, of course, become rehabilitated, either by their own native efforts or by the fragmented work of the staff, but at a minimum there needs to be a shared view amongst the staff that rehabilitation must be a priority. Second, rehabilitation, whether conceived as returning people to work or normality, is not the same thing as keeping users out of hospital, or aiming at production, or restoring the failing function of an arm or a leg. Rehabilitation needs to be personalised to each user, so it constitutes a formidable intellectual and practical task. It means, first of all, being able to appraise a user's personal history, particularly his past roles, and statuses at crucial points of his life and the way she or he dealt with being say, a father, a worker or a friend. Also, it means being able to evaluate the irreducible minimum of primary impairment from which the user suffers: whether psychological, physical or social.[2] Gauging which of a user's handicap must be accepted rather than changed involves separating what has been called 'secondary handicap' from the irreducible impairment. Secondary handicaps might, for example, include the habits learned during a time in a day unit, for example, comfortable dependency or involvement, irresponsibility towards the programme or in running the unit. Another secondary handicap might be a reinforced lack of self-esteem as the user observes that the staff, for instance, appear to do things much better than he.

Next, rehabilitation will need detailed knowledge of the other 136 hours a week: the time when a user is *not* at the day unit. How does he use his leisure and conduct his relationships? It probably also involves a hope shared by staff and user that things could alter, and that eventually the user might aspire to, say, driving a bus again or starting an Open University course. Whatever the nature of this joint hope, it must have its roots in concrete reality for a specific user. Thus, it is not the same as a vague idea of returning a mass of users to 'normality', or to a mythical world where 'work' will be available. (At present, some of these who want their day units to rehabilitate their users view the outside world with millennial hope, similar to the Victorian view of the hereafter.) And it would also be a mistake to assume that rehabilitation in day services is only about preparing chronic, elderly long-term hospital patients for industrial work in factories. Nearly a fifth of users in day services for the mentally ill are parents with young children to care for: to what extent do units rehabilitate the skills of parenting? And half the users are young men under 40: what employment prospects exist for the bulk who are unskilled? Translating the cliché of rehabilitation into individual prospects for different users is a formidable task.[3]

In short, rehabilitation implies that the day unit is geared to achieving concrete aspirations for each user. Since the shared understanding is that users will need to alter or to develop, there needs to be built into the structure of the day unit a series of developmental stages for users to surmount. Returning to Clara at the beginning of the chapter we find that this notion of stages has almost disappeared from the treatment of the mentally ill. Many of the old stages involved unpleasantness that needed reform, but do units now offer a structure which allows a user to be dependent on the staff at the beginning, but at the end allows independence enough to cope without? This implies that the structure of the day unit should neither be entirely open ended nor entirely rigid, and that surmounting the rehabilitation ladder involves developing a time scale appropriate to the personal reality of each user. It also implies that the day unit will devote considerable attention to the complexities of preparing an individual user to leave the unit. There may be a member of staff whose job it is to help users leave the unit. This person may not be the user's counsellor or therapist.[4]

The Maudsley Day Hospital provides one of the few examples of a developmental ladder of day unit rehabilitation. The day hospital is next door to an industrial and clerical work centre. Users progress from the day hospital to the work centre next door and then an active job placement programme may place users in outside work or in a sheltered workshop. But this emphasis on development stages in rehabilitation is not at the expense of considering the individual timing and pace of the user, and each user can stay at one stage or return to an earlier stage without feeling that he has failed (Bennett, 1972; Bennett et al., 1976). Work is seen to be the central end of rehabilitation and in practical terms, work is viewed more in terms of the production than the craft ethic. Tasks are unskilled or semi-skilled clerical or manual tasks and stress values of good work habits, discipline and punctuality.

On the other hand, other approaches to rehabilitation emphasise different aspects of normality and work. For instance, the Barbican Centre at Gloucester, which caters for offenders and mentally ill, deals with the users' time at the centre by means of drawing up a detailed contract between a member and the centre. Members set their own social and work objectives and plan detailed activities to accomplish these. They record their own progress in a record system used jointly with staff. Planning job interviews and potentially uncomfortable work situations are part of employment preparation (MIND, 1978). The content of the task is seen as important and critical to the development of self-esteem.

These two rehabilitative approaches sketch different approaches to work and normality, but their common thread is that general changes in a social environment are 'no substitute for specific social treatment aimed at the individual and based on a detailed knowledge of his handicaps' (Wing and Brown, 1970). A further principle very apparent at the Barbican Centre might be added: staff-imposed goals are no substitute for self-help: the user needs to develop his own goals and ambitions. A third element common to both schemes is a sequential time-ordered series of stages for the potential rehabilitee to mount and an understanding by the staff that each rehabilitee has a personal and idiosyncratic view of time. The time scale of rehabilitation and its relationship to the clock and calendar is usually ignored: mostly, people see rehabilitation as more dependent on building, equipment and people than time (MIND, 1977).

Time and its interpretation is important to understanding rehabilitation in day units. First, the user's subjective perception of time needs assessing. Second, that a rehabilitee's progress in time can be erratic needs to be recognised. Thus, a rehabilitee can make a small advance, he can mark time, he needs to consolidate before moving on, if at all (Morgan, 1976). In other words, the rehabilitee's movement forward in time is largely unpredictable and erratic. So, producing a successful rehabilitation outcome depends, in part, on an accurate reading and handling of the rehabilitee's subjective responses to time. But this creates a problem: can the idiosyncratic progress of the user be reconciled with time scales in his day unit, since these may be related to quite different sets of requirements? For example, planning out the time of the day unit may, from a staff view, come to revolve around things like the efficient use of the transport (thus shortening or lengthening the users' day), or the calendar rotation of junior medical or nursing staff (thus removing continuity of staff help from the user whose progress does not fit neatly into the priority of staff rotation cycles), or the need to maintain a certain quota of discharges within a defined time sequence. So one difficulty is reconciling a user's erratic, idiosyncratic rehabilitative progress with the quite different requirements of the day unit. To what extent should a user's idiosyncratic time scale be tolerated by the day unit? Further, how does the day unit convey it expectations about the use of time? For example, are there 'average' standards of progress which might be expected from users within a defined time scale?

At present, heads and staff in day units appear to make an effort to deal with time in two ways. What each have in common is that they ignore the users' definitions of time. On the one hand, some heads and staff offer a flat, standardised time of rehabilitation to each user: this is a strictly 'time-bound' view of rehabilitation. A user is offered a predetermined term of attendance at a unit.

This standardised time course is adhered to quite strictly and the user has to leave when his time is up. The rationale for this approach is usually justified by a strict rationing approach: offering less time to more people. For instance, day services offered by employment rehabilitation centres (ERCs) specify a maximum length of stay. After this period the user is discharged and said to have completed the rehabilitation course. 'Fixed time' periods of rehabilitation are also offered by the new day training units for offenders, where offenders are sentenced by courts to day units for a period of ninety days (see Chapter 3.7).

Four day hospitals for mentally ill people and seven for the elderly offered time-bound rehabilitation. Each nominated a set period as the length of stay allowed: after this time expired, the user was discharged and the desires of individual users about this were not usually taken into account. Sometimes users indicated that their impending discharge was arbitrary and premature. A 25-year-old woman attending a 'time-bound' psychiatric day hospital said: 'I've seen people discharged from here and they're not better. God knows how they're going to cope when they leave here. I don't know what people say to you, but the ones I've spoken to are frightened and worried about what they're going to do, but that's the doctor's decision.' Two middle-aged patients with multiple sclerosis in a 'time-bound' geriatric day hospital described their process of 'faking' symptoms and distress to prevent discharge on the day that the consultant made his rounds.

On the other hand, other day units consider that the time for rehabilitation is limitless and infinite. The rehabilitation practices ignore the calendar and disregard the clock. 'Timeless' units are those which never make individual plans for users to follow because timeless units do not fret about the length of time the users might stay in the unit.

Getting users to the centre and giving them something to do on a timeless basis was occasionally considered to be rehabilitative in itself. One head of a unit for the physically handicapped explained that the purpose of the unit was to 'socially rehabilitate people. It is to get people out from their own homes and give them something to do, and put them in as natural a setting as possible. By coming here, you socially rehabilitate people as much as possible – it's getting them back into society.'

In timeless units, the day unit defines a user's needs for him and provides for them. Food, treatment, rest, work and leisure activities are offered to the user who 'fits in' to the orderly routines of the unit. The impression is that the everyday life in the unit consists of a number of routines, which have now lost their original social purpose. Thus 'social rehabilitation', in effect keeping the user occupied, indicates that the process of rehabilitation is the same as taking the user from his home to fit into the activity of the unit.

Timeless day units have a lot in common with the images of twentieth-century bureaucracies. Inefficiency, lack of urgency and devotion to routines ensures the survival of the unit itself, not the users. Of course the resource of limitless time may offer some 'refuge' to some users, but it may be damaging for others who have the potential but not the skills or confidence to escape. On the other hand, time-bound day units mirror an attitude to time found in the market place. Time is inflexible, valuable and regulated entirely by the clock. But unlike the products of industry, users of day units are human beings, frequently social casualties with idiosyncrasies and handicaps. The time and motion process applicable to the factory floor or office become inflexible and intolerant of individuality when transferred to the day unit.

These analogies are less fanciful than they seem, because rehabilitation practices in day units may be influenced by broad economic and political policies. For example, it might be argued that vocational rehabilitation – getting people back to work after an illness – has been emphasised more in societies one might characterise as time-bound: those countries which have a more pronounced market economy and a more stigmatising attitude to the unemployed such as the United States and Australia. 'Rehabilitation services that provide the means of avoiding the stigma of welfare can be expected to receive higher value in countries which impose a means test before granting cash benefits than in those which adhere to the principle of social insurance' (Noble, 1978). Great Britain, at present, might be characterised as having a timeless attitude to rehabilitation, an attitude likely to be reinforced by increasing unemployment. Perhaps introducing 'universalist' health and welfare services has masked the need for the more 'particularist' provision of special rehabilitation services. The rehabilitation services advocated by both the Piercy Report (1956) and the Tunbridge Report (1972) have not been introduced.

In theory, rehabilitation means 'that continuous process beginning with the onset of sickness or injury and continuing throughout treatment until final resettlement in the most suitable work and living is achieved' (Piercy, 1956). But in practice there is little link between day hospitals and day centres and little contact either with the employment services, if the statements of heads and staff are to be believed. No conscious effort has yet been made to sew together different shaped pieces of a potential rehabilitation patchwork: at present the user is left to go it alone through a fragmented fabric, which when cobbled together might constitute an effective rehabilitation mosaic.

NOTES

1 This group represents 8 per cent of those in day units for the mentally ill, probably an underestimate of those who would be labelled schizophrenic by the heads and staff.
2 This chapter adopts the outline given by Wing and Hailey (1972). Symptoms, for example, slowness or early morning waking in depression, are *primary impairment*. Attitudinal or behavioural reactions accumulate as *secondary handicaps*: for instance, lack of confidence or low self-esteem. A third element, illness or handicap existing independently such as lack of occupational or social skills, must be considered as a *tertiary handicap*, intimately linked to the other two.
3 Chapter 3 sets out the limitations of some current heads and staff for this task. For instance, most staff members in social services units for the mentally ill have no qualifications at all. Although there are more trained staff in day hospitals (there is a core of trained mental nurses), practically none of these have had any specific rehabilitation training, with the exception of occupational therapists. The lack of interest of consultant psychiatrists in rehabilitation in general is bemoaned in the current psychiatric literature. The lack of training in and understanding of employment problems of users by any particular member of staff is also a restriction.
4 Sometimes counsellors or therapists unwittingly maintain a user's dependency longer than necessary.

REFERENCES

Bennett, D. H. (1972) 'Day hospitals, day centres and workshops: general principles', in J. K. Wing and A.M. Haley (eds), *Evaluating a Community Psychiatric Service* (Oxford University Press).
Bennett, D. H., Fox, C., Jowell, T. and Skynner, A. C. R. (1976) 'Towards a family approach in a psychiatric day hospital', *British Journal of Psychiatry*, 129, pp. 73–81.
MIND (1977) *Better Prospects: Rehabilitation in Mental Illness Hospitals* by Joanna Murray (MIND).
MIND (1978) See Stephens and Nattrass (1978).
Morgan, R. (1976) *Rehabilitation* (unpublished: available from National Schizophrenia Fellowship, 29 Victoria Road, Surbiton, Surrey).

Noble, J. H. (1978) *Rehabilitating the Severely Disabled: The Foreign Experience* (unpublished paper, Department of Health Education and Welfare, Office of Assistant Secretary for Planning and Evaluation, Washington, DC, USA).

Piercy Report (1956) *Report of the Committee of Enquiry on the Rehabilitation, Training and Resettlement of Disabled Persons* (HMSO).

Stephens, A. and Nattrass, P. (1978) *A Study of Day Centres* (MIND).

Tunbridge Report (1972) *Rehabilitation Report of a Sub-Committee of the Standing Medical Advisory Committee* (HMSO).

White, Antonia (1979) *Beyond the Glass* (Virago).

Wing, J. K., Bennett, D. H. and Denham, J. (1964) *The Industrial Rehabilitation of Long Stay Schizophrenic Patients*, Memorandum 42, Medical Reseach Council (HMSO).

Wing, J. K. and Brown, G. W. (1970) *Institutionalisation and Schizophrenia* (Oxford University Press).

Wing, L., Wing, J. K., Stevens, B. and Griffiths, D. (1972) 'An epidemiological and experimental evaluation of chronic psychotic patients in the community', in J. K. Wing and A. Hailey (eds), *Evaluating a Community Psychiatric Service* (Oxford University Press).

Wing, J. and Hailey, A. (eds) (1972) *Evaluating a Community Psychiatric Service* (Oxford University Press).

Chapter 10

'I'M JUST A NUISANCE': AIMING TO RELIEVE RELATIVES

> The aim, because they are dementia cases, is to relieve the relatives. It means the younger ones can hold down jobs. (Staff member of a day hospital for psychogeriatric patients)
>
> We relieve social pressure on families. There's a lady with a stroke whose daughter looks after her, who also has a mentally handicapped child. The daughter is relieved if we have her here: otherwise the old lady becomes an inpatient. (Sister-in-charge, geriatric day hospital)

When the over 75 age group reaches 3 million by the mid 1980s, how will the families of the 10 to 20 per cent who will suffer from the dementias of old age manage? At present, some day units appreciate the problems of families because some heads and staff identify an aim of the unit as that of offering 'relief to relatives', particularly in units for the confused elderly and also in geriatric day hospitals. Chapter 8 discussed the consequences of infirmity for elderly people in geriatric day hospitals and this chapter will explore a further dimension of deterioration. Unfortunately, we have no direct information from the families of users or from others who themselves may look after them at home. So the discussion of this chapter will represent a one-sided view, the opinions of heads, staff and users in geriatric day hospitals, and – more particularly – those in day units for the elderly confused.

USERS AND THEIR FAMILIES

Sometimes it is assumed that elderly confused persons do not 'suffer' from the distress of the mental problems of old age, but their relatives do (Dechampsneuf, 1978). Because 'psychogeriatrics' are 'dements', they lack sentience and insight completely. But degrees of mental confusion are spread along a long continuum and care givers of the patient may affect the degree of confusion. Extremely complex but quite logical strategies have been adopted by confused old people to either compensate for, or defend against, 'the painful experiences of isolation, impotence and hoplessness' (Meacher, 1972). Painful feelings were experienced by some of the confused elderly in day services: about half admitted to being depressed in the previous month and over two-fifths said that they wished that they might have died. Both Miss T. and Mrs F. expressed the same wish quite independently of each other: 'I wish I could go off in my sleep and not wake up.' Mr M. commented: 'I wish I were dead but I don't think I'd have the courage to do away with myself.' Mr P., aged 71, had made a recent attempt to end his life: 'I thought there might be someone here at the day centre who could lay me out. I was very depressed about my situation at the time.'

The despair of the users in psychogeriatric units appears more self-directed than aimed at relatives, but users understood very well that a disruption had taken place in the family. For example, Mrs L., aged 78, felt that her family tried to keep visitors away from her: 'I'm such a nuisance to them.' A rather bitter Mr B. felt that he was 'just a bloody nuisance to my wife'. Miss J. worried that her confused behaviour, which she knew was quite strange, might prevent her brother from liking her any more.

On the other hand, elderly patients in geriatric day hospitals were more prone to dwell on the vicissitudes created by their illness for the immediate family than the users of psychogeriatric units. In particular, they considered that their recently acquired physical deficiencies reduced their ability to manage a role in the family. This had repercussions for other family members, for being a deficient spouse, parent or grandparent drastically altered the response of the other partner, children or grandchildren. It was deflating for elderly people to have to face up to this deficiency and other researchers have pointed out the importance of family roles for old people (Townsend, 1957).

For example, Mr B., formerly a master baker, used to be able to take a 'fair share' of the care of his adult spastic son. But the recent amputation of his left leg from gangrene following a stroke meant he was unable to help his son and left him totally dependent on his wife. He confessed that he worried mostly about his wife and the stress he imagined he put on her by requiring her to look after them both.

Mrs B., aged 83, a former midwife, was blind and also suffered from Parkinson's Disease. Unable to look after herself, she had moved in with her daughter. But she was grateful for the day hospital: 'If I had to be with my daughter all day, we should fall out.'

Sometimes users reached towards an uneasy accommodation with their family after illness dislocated 'normal' roles. Miss B., aged 79, a spinster formerly in service, lived with her elderly brother in a very old cottage without a bath. She could not prepare herself emotionally for the probability that 'he' would have to help her bath after she left the day hospital.

One actual *satisfaction* mentioned by staff working with the elderly confused was achieving the aim of giving relief to relatives. A middle-aged occupational therapist working with the elderly confused commented: 'Success is when you see somebody helped to live at home and coping with their problems. Success is in helping their relatives.'

Colleagues working in geriatric day hospitals mentioned relieving families rarely as an intrinsic satisfaction of the job.

AIMING AT RELIEVING RELATIVES

Overall, about one in seven heads and staff considered that relieving relatives was an aim of the unit. About a quarter of those working with the elderly confused and a quarter in geriatric day hospitals considered that one aim of the unit was to give relief to families.[1] For most, this emphasis tied together with the aims of keeping old people at home and in the community and out of institutions. The staff who mentioned these two things (relief of families and the need to keep users out of hospital) had spent the longest period of their working lives within hospitals and institutions. Transferring from work on the ward to the day hospital was seen to be progressive because the day unit represented interstices between the institution and community. Thus a nurse formerly employed in a long-stay hospital for the elderly who now worked in a day hospital with the elderly confused stated:

> This work is more progressive than long-stay geriatrics in hospital. There's only one result there – out in a box. Patients in a long-stay ward are like cabbages. Here you see them go home every night. You get a patient in like the one we had living at home for nine years with her son and never going out. Now you can see her laughing. She knows us now whereas before it was only her son she saw: here you see patients progressing.

Five out of ten of the 'elderly confused' came to the unit either for two or three days each week. Although three out of ten came for four or five days each week, these places tended to be as often taken by users who lived alone as users who lived with relatives. Thus, how much help is the day unit to the spouse or other relative who looks after the user? Chapter 3 suggests that, since most users are confined to two or three days' attendance, what the day unit provides for the relative is a break rather than the possibility of leading an individual life.

Of course, not all of the elderly in ill health who attend day units actually live with their relatives. About a third of the patients in the geriatric day hospitals and about half of the elderly confused live alone. However, in each group, nearly two-thirds had relatives or friends nearby, who were able to help them in an emergency with transport, shopping or when they were ill. But these old people were visited infrequently: the elderly in geriatric day hospitals only a couple of times a week and the elderly confused (on their own account) somewhat less.

Whether or not the user was immobile did not seem to relate to whether he or she lived alone: as many immobile old people lived alone as lived with their relatives. Although our measures of confusion, discussed in Chapter 3.5, could not be corroborated, there was no correlation between the degree of confusion evidenced on interview and whether or not the user lived alone.

Although offering day care to old people was seen by some heads and staff as a relief to relatives, this was not associated with actual contact between the unit staff and the relatives. In the main, such contact in geriatric and psychogeriatric day units was *ad hoc*, unplanned and infrequent. Nearly half the heads of the elderly confused units estimated that the unit 'saw' the families of users at least quarterly, but this applied to only a quarter of the heads of geriatric day hospitals. In the case of the elderly confused, the contact with relatives was sometimes attenuated. Several heads of units for the elderly confused explained: 'I try to involve the next of kin as much as possible but there is often little interest.'

'Relatives are encouraged to drop in whenever they wish', said another. 'Attempts to have regular family meetings either in the evenings or on weekends have failed.'

'Relatives' meetings were once a feature of this unit', said a charge nurse, who estimated that he saw only 10 per cent of the families of his patients. 'We intend to try a more informal approach in the future, giving tea, snacks and music.'

The gulf between some families and their elderly confused relatives was criticised by a few staff: 'Some families, frankly, do not want to know and do not welcome contact with the day unit', said the manager of a social services unit, while another was critical of the 'lack of insight' of relatives – 'they get angry about what they don't understand'.

Nevertheless, a reluctance by some families to get involved may be reinforced by the approach of day units themselves. When new users are introduced to units for the elderly confused and geriatric day hospitals, orientation procedures rarely include family members. One in twenty geriatric day hospitals made a home visit before admitting a patient and one in ten mentioned 'talking to relatives' as part of the orientation. In psychogeriatric day units, the home visit was also uncommon.

THE DAY UNIT AS A FAMILY

The day unit for the elderly confused affords opportunities for some users and staff (particularly nurses) to recreate family-like relationships. 'We're all a large happy family here', explained one nurse, and for another the most significant part of her job was contact between worker and patient and 'being father, mother and comforter' to an old person. Another 36-year-old pupil nurse declared that her job was similar to her previous experience as a mother of small children: 'You can either do it or you can't. Old people are very like children. If you bring children up all right you can cope with the old ones.'

Redefining the family group within the day unit seemed to make sense for some users who were often pleased that the day unit offered them a 'family'. Or, as one old lady explained, a 'home from home': 'Oh yes, it's a home from home here. Sister is so nice, just like a daughter. I've lost two daughters – the nurses are nice: even the cleaner is nice.' Mrs B. explained: 'I live alone and I do wish someone was with me. But here, we're just one happy family.'

The image of the family emerged more in the comments of staff in units for the elderly confused than in geriatric day hospitals. Perhaps this is because all heads of units for the elderly confused except two saw two-thirds or more of their users as long-stay, which was significantly more than the number of geriatric day hospitals with this view. As Chapter 8 discusses, there is a more vigorous investment in discharging patients home from geriatric day hospitals. Emotional attachments between staff and users hinder this, so in geriatric day hospitals similar emotional attachments between staff and users are reinterpreted and given a very different meaning. A statement from the nursing officer of a geriatric day hospital suggests this: 'Generally the busy atmosphere is enjoyed and social intercourse in the day hospital is stimulating for those who are housebound or live alone. Those who are psychologically immature have a tendency to become dependent if care is not exercised by senior staff.'

What happens to old people in day units: how long can the day unit sustain them? The most common route out of the day unit for the elderly confused led into hospital or residential care.[2] Twice as many were admitted to hospital or residential care as were discharged 'home' from the day unit. However, for the elderly in the geriatric day hospitals, the pattern was reversed, for twice as many were discharged to their homes as were admitted to hospital or residential care.

COMMENT

Some dilemmas arising between an old person who becomes mentally ill and his relatives can be illustrated by the case of the man who, as an octogenarian, decided to divide up his property between his two favourite daughters. After he had done this, both daughters rejected him. The old man interpreted his daughters' rejection and their refusal to make a home for him as thankless and opportunistic. Although his wits had begun to deteriorate before this particular family crisis, his mental decline accelerated when he was left to fend for himself. Once he was found naked, wandering around in the open air, muttering obscenities which included imprecations about his daughters. However, when the case was investigated from the daughters' point of view, they stated that they felt unable to cope with the unpleasant behaviour and habits of the old man, his 'laziness' and his poor judgement. One of them cited his unruliness, and noisy habits: the other, his descent into a second childhood. Both daughters wished to be free of the responsibility of his care so that they could lead their own lives.

This particular case became well known and public attention focused on the ingratitude of the daughters, sympathy being reserved for the plight of the mentally infirm and rejected father. The case belongs to an earlier period, certainly well before day care was available and a time when the obligations of children to their elderly parents were clearly delineated.

Social expectations of filial obligation to ageing parents have altered: 'Until the opening years of this century, provisions for old age was regarded as primarily a matter for the individual and his relatives' (Phillips, 1954, p. 3). But when the Phillips Committee reported in 1954 on the economic and financial problems of old age, far from assuming that children should sacrifice themselves to care for ageing relatives, the committee endorsed the notion that community services should help old people to stay in their own homes. Rehabilitative services for old age promised improvements 'in health and happiness and the relief to the heavy cost of looking after large numbers of the chronic sick. Moreover younger people now employed in looking after them can now be released for other work' (Phillips, 1954, p. 74). Thus, the 'right' of adult children to lead a social and economic life separate from their ageing parents was given public endorsement: a considerable social change. If Shakespeare had written about King Lear – the confused old man discussed above – in the mid twentieth century, there may have been greater public acceptance of the ungrateful Goneril and Regan. Even still, vestigial sentiment still rests with King Lear at the expense of his daughters (de Beauvoir, 1972), although many public services in theory recognise the position of children who do not want to take the responsibility of full-time care of ageing relatives.

Considerable changes in the size and, therefore, the function of the family over the past century have occurred. First, there has been a sharp rise in the number of women employed in the workforce, particularly married women. At the same time, the size of the average family has shrunk considerably. The average family in the middle of the nineteenth century had seven children: but in the mid twentieth century this number had shrunk to two, leaving fewer children to cope with ageing parents. At the same time, the number of parents actually reaching old age has increased considerably: in 1851, the elderly made up 14 per cent of the population, but in 1951 they constituted 41 per cent. The pool of potential caretakers has reduced while the number of ageing parents has increased (Moroney, 1976).

Creation of day units for old people in poor physical and mental health is, in theory, one social alternative for diminished family care for its ageing members. However, in practice, as this book has pointed out, day care does not appear to provide enough back up to families to allow relatives to pursue their own life in the same way that placement in residential care or hospital does. Thus there is little alternative for a relative who wants to continue to work and care for an elderly confused person: such a relative would need to seek a residential placement rather than help from day care.

This is of some importance because it raises the issue of the predicted increase in numbers of ill elderly people over the next decade and the problem of how day services will cope with this. Are day units to increase in number, so as to take on the role of providing substitute family care for the aged who cannot manage alone? This is at bedrock a political issue, but it needs to be examined now. Social research could refine alternative strategies. For example, we know that most of the elderly confused go from day units to long-term care: which are the group which do *not* get admitted to hospital? If they are the group who live with their children, perhaps these are the group which day units for the elderly confused in the future should aim to support? (Bergmann *et al.*, 1978)

If this is the case, a second question relates less to the extent of day care than to its quality. How can day units relieve families and shore up those gulfs which illness exacerbates between the elderly patient and the family, without 'taking over' the user and fracturing tenuous and fragile connections with the family on the one hand, or overloading the relatives on the other? If we assume that care of the elderly is neither a totally private nor a totally public responsibility, the lack of positive contact between heads and staff of day units and relatives both at admission and thereafter seems to reduce the possibility that the different sets of interests and expectations existing between day unit staff and families can be bridged.

Day units for the elderly confused need to develop more conscious partnerships with relatives. Special groups for relatives as a forum for discussion, negotiation and modification of discrepant expectations could, in the right hands, be helpful. Such groups have been used occasionally with relatives of stroke patients in the day hospital (Mykyta *et al.*, 1976) as well as for relatives of the elderly confused (Whitehead, 1970), with apparent satisfaction for both relatives and staff. Although groups for relatives are not the same thing as psychotherapy groups, the skill required to develop such groups has been underestimated in day units. Clinical experience indicates that friendly social contacts are extremely important but are not a substitute for discussing the social and emotional upheavals in the family of users with chronic physical and mental illness (Carter, 1976). These upheavals raise questions about personal philosophy and causation of illness – 'Why has it happened to him?'; alterations and adaptions of everyday roles within the family; special problems of communication with the patient resulting from the illness: these are some issues for discussion. At present, few day units have the internal expertise or staffing to offer this kind of service. But field social workers or even clinically experienced social workers, now administrators, could consider adopting a project in a day unit. Given the isolation of day units and the regret of many administrators that their practice days are past, groups for relatives are an ideal way to keep in touch because they offer a regular,.

time-limited practice commitment. There is also a potential role here for the clinical psychology services.

At present, the aim of supporting relatives with the care of their elderly confused person rests on the good will and perception of the heads and staff of day units rather than on a deliberate policy at an area or even national level. This implies that although the pendulum has swung towards the idea of allowing relatives to lead their own lives if they wish, in practice this is difficult if they also want to actively assist in the care of their elderly relative rather than place him or her in a residential institution. The statement of the staff member at the beginning of this chapter – 'The aim . . . is to relieve the relatives. It means the younger ones can hold down jobs' – is rarely fulfilled in the day units of the present.

NOTES

1 Additionally, about a quarter of the staff working in the day care part of residential homes for the elderly nominated giving relief to the relatives as an aim.
2 Forty-two per cent of those discharged from day units for the elderly confused in the previous twelve months had been admitted to hospital or residential care. Eleven per cent 'resumed activities at home' and 3 per cent were transferred to other units. Seventeen per cent died. (These figures exclude the one psychogeriatric assessment unit.)

   Thirty-six per cent of the elderly in geriatric day hospitals left to resume activities at home. Five per cent were transferred to other day centres and fifteen per cent admitted to residential or hospital care. Nine per cent died. (The most common prediction offered by patients about the way they might spend days at home when not at the day hospital was 'doing nothing much, just sleeping'.)

REFERENCES

Bergmann, K., Foster, E. M., Justice, A. E. and Matthews, V. (1978) 'Management of the demented elderly patient in the community', *British Journal of Psychiatry*, 132, pp. 441–9.
Carter, J. (1976) 'Parents' meetings in a hospital day centre', *Child: Care, Health and Development*, 2, pp. 203–12.
de Beauvoir, S. (1972) *Old Age* (Deutsch, Weidenfeld & Nicholson).
Deschampsneuf, P. (1978) 'Old, demented and rejected', *The Listener*, 26–7, 2 March.
Meacher, M. (1972) *Taken for a Ride* (Longman).
Moroney, R. M. (1976) *The Family and the State* (Longman).
Mykyta, L. J., Bowling, J. H., Nelson, D. A. and Lloyd, E. J. (1976) 'Caring for relatives of stroke patients', *Age and Ageing*, 5, pp. 87–90.
Phillips, T. (1954) *Report of the Committee on the Economic and Financial Problems of the Provision for Old Age*, Cmnd 9333 (HMSO).
Townsend, P. (1957) *The Family Life of Old People* (Routledge & Kegan Paul).
Whitehead, A. (1970) *In the Service of Old Age: The Welfare of Psychogeriatric Patients* (Penguin).

Chapter 11

'A USEFUL LIFE': OFFERING PRACTICAL SERVICES FOR THERAPEUTIC IMPROVEMENT

> This place exists to provide a place for the physically handicapped.
> They have available here various outlets to express themselves fully
> in craft situations they would never normally get a chance to do. It
> gives them a sense of well being, gives their lives a greater fulfilment.
> (Head, social services centre for the physically handicapped)

In Chapter 5 we introduced people working in day services for the elderly
who considered that an aim of the day centre was to offer the users
services of a practical nature – things like company and food. These
services were offered with no particular end in view, so that (in a manner
of speaking) staff cast their bread upon the waters as well as on the lunch
table. But Chapter 5 also referred briefly to a group of staff in social
services centres for the elderly who offered practical services to users, but
this time as a means to an end. That end was seen to be achieving a
therapeutic result – the well-being of the users. In all, sixty-three heads
and staff, about 12 per cent, thought this to be an aim of the unit.

As one example, the head of a social services centre for the physically
handicapped, said: 'The centre is to occupy people, really, to give them a
sense of belonging and to be useful.' A third of those who offered
practical services for therapeutic results worked with physically handicapped people and this group of twenty heads and staff will be the focus
of this chapter. Excluding two who worked in sheltered workshops, these
twenty are just under a quarter of those working with the physically
handicapped – not a very large group. Half of the group worked in units
where they alone expressed this view of the aims and they were spread
equally across social services and voluntary-sponsored units. Two of
every three were untrained.[1]

It will be recalled that those heads and staff who said that the units
aimed to dispense services which were practical, named company, food,
activities and information or advice as the main content of their offerings.
By contrast those staff who are the subject of this chapter did not
emphasise serving food or imparting information. Instead the central
services offered were the company of other users and activities to occupy
the users' time. This chapter will concentrate on the second of these
services and will examine the role of 'activities' in the thinking of heads
and staff.

As the heads and staff saw it, the main function of activities was to 'occupy' the users. Providing a stimulating interregnum to punctuate the users' life outside the centre was the main point. At home the handicapped users led a narrow, constricted, lonely existence. For example:

> We take them out of their four walls. You hear cases of people being alone and only having the district nurse to visit.

> We provide a service for handicapped people who would otherwise be forgotten. Some are prisoners in their own home, incarcerated.

> We motivate them away from being cabbages and thinking of suicide.

> They just sit at home on their own.

'Occupation' nearly always meant doing arts and crafts to these staff, but some added a modicum of industrial and contract work. Its purpose was to provide a means to an end. The end was bringing about therapeutic improvements in the well-being of the users, a contrast to the philosophy of Chapter 5 – where practical services were an end in themselves. In Chapter 12, the next chapter, another activity, work, was promoted as an end in itself. In contrast the approach of the staff discussed in this chapter is almost a 'human relations' approach. Activity is the means; the ends are making users feel useful, restoring human dignity and offering a chance to identify with a social group. A less prominent end was to help users adjust to their difficulties. These comments illustrate this:

Making Users Feel Useful
> We help spastic people to feel useful members of society. If we help adults start to lead a useful life again, they feel of use to themselves and the community.

Restoring Human Dignity
> It's to make people feel they are loved and cared for and never to patronise them. They all have a gift or talent and in discovering this, they regain their self-respect.

> We help them to realise the good things about themselves.

A Chance to Join A Group
> This is a community that people are very happy to come to. Socialising makes life more satisfying for the members.

> We consider the atmosphere here to be paramount: a cordial atmosphere is passed from above to the staff and from them to the clients.

Helping Users Adjust
We help them to come to terms with their difficulties.

We try to keep them comfortable and happy.

THE STAFF AND THE TASK

For heads and staff to achieve these ends occupation was devised. About half the group of twenty thought that this was a matter of helping a person to be creative and to develop new skills. The most forceful advocates of this outlook were these few with art or craft training. They made the extra point that ability to stimulate the user was related to a teacher or a staff member's ability to enjoy his or her own work. 'The more I'm with them myself the more they respond. Because I enjoy the work myself, they sense this', said one 27-year-old woman with an art diploma. 'I try to bring out the creative aspect of the person; pottery, copper and jewellery. I talk to them as I would to my friends.'

The other half saw occupation as more a matter of filling in time: for example, 'It gives them something to do with their hands: so they don't just sit.' In contrast to those who advocated developing the users' creativity, the staff who viewed occupation as a way of filling in time spoke of their concern about having the 'right' atmosphere. The right atmosphere was seen as something to be constructed socially:

The atmosphere has to be good. When you can walk around with a visitor and you sense the congenial atmosphere, that's success.

We consider atmosphere to be paramount: a cordial atmosphere is passed from above to the staff and thence to the clients.

On the other hand the trained art diplomates considered that 'a good atmosphere' was generated by creativity and that a harmonious social atmosphere inevitably followed creativity. Thus manufacturing a good atmosphere was not necessary.

FRUSTRATIONS FOR THE STAFF

What frustrations did heads and staff members speak of in trying to bring about therapeutic improvement? For a few, the community's lack of interest in the users was a source of disappointment. It is also worth noting that amongst all staff working with the physically handicapped, nearly eight in ten considered that users had special needs to which the community had failed to give attention. This was frustrating to the few heads and staff who were the subject of this chapter.

It's a *dream* factory here. We play at work, we set up a situation as much like work as possible but we know that the majority of people here will never return to work.

We don't aim to retrain them here as such, we do try to get some into open employment if this is indicated, but it doesn't happen very often.

Other staff felt uncertain about how to meet the gap they considered existed between the users' disability and the staff task.

Physically handicapped staff don't seem to have the courses to go on that are available to mentally handicapped staff [commented a former electrician, now head of a large centre]. I know how to design and make aids. But I would like to know more about the clients. There are some frustrating moments when you don't seem to be getting through. You tend to get exasperated when some clients take a lot of things for granted: some are quite lazy and they have a bad effect on others: they tend to wallow in their handicap. More in-service courses would be very useful. It keeps the staff interested and together: it makes them feel they are not forgotten. Staff often get the idea they are thought of as highly paid babysitters; courses help to dispel that idea. Even if the subjects discussed are not particularly relevant, it helps keep up staff morale.

This and other evidence implies that it may be the meaning attached to the task rather than the task itself which contributes to job satisfaction. In other words, the function of courses is not so much to change the task as to change the conception a staff member has of himself from a 'babysitter' to 'specialist worker with the physically handicapped'. By what might be a similar process, these twenty staff members had translated the aim of the unit, from 'giving practical services' to 'giving practical services for therapeutic improvement'.

All these heads and staff were either 'very' satisfied or 'fairly' satisfied with their work. One head of centre, a former tradesman, said: 'I'm in the lucky position of being able to help people all the time – and I'm being paid for it – this must be the ultimate! It's fantastic – the ultimate in job satisfaction.' Another staff member, 64-year-old former telephone operator, now widowed, said: 'It's my life, this work. I have nobody to worry about so I find every little thing satisfying about this job.' Half of this group of twenty staff considered that users helped to run their day unit. The most frequently mentioned avenue was a user's committee. 'They have a small committee of their own. If they don't like a thing they make it awkward and things have to be done to suit them', explained a former nurse. The other half were either equivocal about whether their users helped to run the unit or they thought that users did not contribute to this. 'Frankly, they aren't mentally capable of it', said a former dental nurse. 'Personally speaking, I think that none of them have the educational background to do so', commented a former greengrocer.

Turning now to the users of voluntary and social services centres, we find that half thought they were not given enough say in running the place. Enjoyment of being in a day unit was highest amongst those in the oldest age group. For example, almost every physically handicapped user over 60 would prefer to continue to come to the day centre ahead of doing anything else. It would be inaccurate to describe the younger age groups as dissatisfied, but one in every ten users would much prefer to be doing something else; usually a job away from the centre. More young and middle-aged users, that is, those aged 59 or less, than older ones stated that what the centre had done for them was to provide them with either work or occupation. This may imply that occupation is not only a matter of filling in time to users, but doing it in a way that can be viewed as socially legitimate is important too. (Of course, it needs to be remembered that these users were not necessarily confined to the unit where the staff under discussion in this chapter worked; it will be remembered that these staff were scattered across the units.)

DISCUSSION

One value of the day unit is to construct a timetable to interrupt a vacuum of uninterrupted time. It is not only physical limitations which imprison users, it is the mental consequences of the physical facts. For example, one aspect of this is enforced loneliness: away from the centre many physically handicapped users lack the mobility to seek out their own contacts. The reverse of this is that at the centre, users are forced to mix with people they cannot necessarily get away from. One middle-aged woman, who lived alone and who was unable to walk, did not mind mixing with other users who were physically handicapped: 'I think the centre has helped me most mentally, otherwise I would live on my own seven days a week. I don't think you can be on your own that long. It does people in my position good to get out of their homes and mix with people in a worse situation.'

The second mental consequence is that the day centre seems to provide a framework within which physically handicapped users can view their handicap. For instance, the day centre provided an object lesson for some users by displaying people worse off than themselves. 'It's given me a grateful heart', answered a 69-year-old grandmother, crippled with arthritis and unable to walk. 'I've got twenty-four grandchildren and nine great grandchildren and they're all normal. Some people who don't come here moan a lot and it would do them good to come here and see others that suffer worse.' Locating 'someone worse off than yourself' and being 'grateful for what you've got' were common comments. It was almost as if filling in time by moaning and feeling sorry for oneself away from the centre could then be transcended, by filling in time in the unit and noting that others were worse off.

However, dealing with one's own handicap by locating users who were worse off than oneself did not seem to apply to all users. Another framework for viewing personal handicap suggested a stronger identification with fellow users than the detachment of observation. 'I hoped coming here would help my depression and it did. I have a rapport with a young patient here who can't talk, I can understand and help her.'

This raises the matter of helping each other. One in ten users in centres for the physically handicapped said they helped other users and that this was one way they liked to feel they helped to run the centre. At the same time four out of ten staff in centres for the physically handicapped said that 'helping users' was one of the rewards of the job. The impression is that it is more often the staff than the users who are able to get satisfaction out of helping each other. Day units are geared more to allowing the staff to discharge their tasks than they are geared to encouraging users to help each other as a matter central to their occupation at the centre.

Could more users help each other? Do some feel inhibited either by the staff or the structure of the unit? This matter is discussed again in Chapter 18. When Tolstoy said that disease should not be a source of division amongst men but that, on the contrary, it should be a source of loving good fellowship, he might almost have been referring to centres for the physically handicapped.

NOTE

1 A second small group who offered practical services primarily for therapeutic results and to improve the well-being of users were heads and staff working in social services centres for the elderly. These were discussed in Chapter 5.

Chapter 12

———◆———

'PUSHING FOR PRODUCTION': AIMING AT INDUSTRIAL PRODUCTION

> We provide maximum employment for the Section 2 disabled at minimum cost to the ratepayer. A secondary endeavour is to provide a maximum job satisfaction but providing maximum employment can't always provide maximum job satisfaction which doesn't matter so much. You can employ any industrial objectives like any other business. (I personally believe we should train our people to progress to employment in open industry. But they are pretty low in IQ and don't wish to progress.)

INDUSTRIAL PRODUCTION

This view of the aims of his unit comes from a manager of a sheltered workshop for the physically handicapped, but actually nine out of every ten managers and staff in sheltered workshops identify the aim of the unit as achieving industrial production. This aim is an end in itself.

This chapter will explore this particular approach to work but it should be noted first that other units provide work for more pragmatic reasons: more as a means than an end. For instance, work may serve the purpose of attempting to rehabilitate (Chapter 9). If a head said a unit for the mentally ill offered work (and about half did), the heads saw the aim of the unit as rehabilitation of users. In these units which did *not* provide work, more heads and staff aimed to keep users out of hospital. Work was even offered to a few elderly people. In three work centres for old people users worked a half-day shift, perhaps three times a week, at packing, labelling and assembling work. In two day hospitals for the elderly, work was offered to a few patients in a centre away from the day hospital (this was thought to be 'therapeutically' helpful). Half the units for the confused elderly provided work for users: these units were staffed by a consultant psychiatrist, rather than a geriatrician, and shared premises – or staff – with a day hospital for the mentally ill which also offered work.

Two-thirds of the mentally handicapped in adult training centres say they spend most time at work, but very few staff in these centres consider that the purpose of work is to achieve industrial production. Most saw work as a method of training users.

Three-quarters of physically handicapped people spend most time at work. This chapter will discuss the group largely confined to the sheltered workshops,[1] where in the view of the heads and staff the rationale of work was production. However, outside the sheltered workshops, others offered work for its psychological benefits, or its occupational value. But achieving these latter aims did not hinge on offering work alone: since work was usually seen as one of a variety of activities.

SHELTERED WORKSHOPS

If work, and work alone is all that is offered in sheltered workshops, what do workers do?[2] Chapter 3 established that 'work' usually means factory work. This random selection of comments comes from sheltered workers about the previous week's work:

I solder and twist wires so they don't fray. Also I'm stripping wires on a machine.

I was supposed to be assembling hearing aids but I sat around waiting for work.

I was fitting [brush] bristles into stocks, then mitring, knot making and selecting.

I put spokes on to the hubs of wheels. It's done by hand for wheelchairs.

I was finishing off the mattresses [for divans] with a tape wedge.

I make 'staybars'. I cut, clean them, bend them, tie them and send them off. Then I clean up the whole workshop; I do that as well.

I took soap from the conveyor belt to boxes.

These comments and disclosures of managers indicate that work in sheltered workshops also includes unskilled factory work: assembling, sorting or packing; or perhaps working with simple handtools. There is some machine work: more sheltered workers work with machines than workers in other kinds of day units. Sheltered work is also service work such as sweeping up or brewing up tea, although managements never mentioned this. And 'waiting around' for work is also part of a working week as far as the workers are concerned.

Sheltered workshops are either self-contained, 'one off' operations, connected to a local authority social services department, or are part of a national quasi-statutory group. Sheltered workshops sit uneasily in day services because most are seen as 'commercial', not 'care' enterprises. There are no instructors or nurses; instead there are chargehands, foremen and possibly an accounting department, dispatch, stores and production divisions and, depending on the size of the operation, perhaps an advertising account. One workshop was departmentally structured, with sales and technical divisions. It made toiletry items and several workshops made their own 'branded' product: kitchen or bedroom furniture, or toys and toiletries formed part of the range of products.

Pay for sheltered workshops was quite variable: in one workshop, according to managers, workers were paid 97p per hour, but others paid a weekly wage ranging from £42 to £60. These wages are much higher than the amounts paid for 'work' in centres for the physically handicapped where two-thirds of users earned less than £2 per week. For the rest of this chapter, staff and users in nine sheltered work units will be compared with staff and users of twenty-one units for the physically handicapped. The amount it was possible to earn distinguished users of sheltered workshops (hereafter sheltered workers) from users in centres for the physically handicapped, who were paid for work within the limits of the statutory benefits disregard limit of £2 per week in 1976.[3]

Who used sheltered workshops? Eight out of ten sheltered workers were men, nearly half in their 50s and on average they had been at their work benches for over six years. By contrast, the users of the centres for the physically handicapped were mainly women, they were both younger and older than the sheltered workers and had attended on average for rather less time.

By their own descriptions, sheltered workers suffered most often from visual disabilities, including blindness; with neurologically based disorders ranging from migraine, epilepsy to cerebal palsy accounting for the second largest group. Mental and emotional complaints came third, along with diseases of bones and joints like arthritis. This implies that the disabilities of sheltered workers can be mental and emotional as well as physical, and that their handicaps leave them reasonably mobile. Certainly more sheltered workers say they can climb stairs or walk outside the house without help than the physically handicapped group. (They also relied much more on aids and appliances to achieve these activities.) But the most marked feature of the physical independence was their ability to travel alone: nearly nine out of ten of the sheltered workers could travel alone compared to only four out of ten of the physically handicapped.

Who staffed the sheltered workshop? All managers and three-quarters of the staff were men. As well, over half are aged over 50, they tended to be older than staff working in units with the physically handicapped or in any other type of unit. Twice as many staff in sheltered work (that is, half) came from a skilled manual background, as those working with the physically handicapped. Also there was a tendency to show less enthusiasm for training or obtaining qualifications by sheltered work staff than by those employed in any other user group.

Differences in motivation between staff in sheltered workshops and other day service staff for coming to work in the unit exist. More of those working with the physically handicapped were idealistic: five in every ten said their application for their current job was a general interest in either services or problems of handicapped people. But only one in ten managers and staff in sheltered workshops gave idealistic reasons: the most common reason was that they 'needed a job'. Many were out of work and unable to find a job in industry:

> Well, I had no choice really: the employment exchange sent me round here and that was it.

> I gave up my previous job because I wanted to change. I was on the dole: there were two jobs vacant and I had to take one, otherwise I would get my dole stopped. This was a foreman's job so the choice was more or less made for me.

Aside from expressed interest in handicapped people, there are marked differences in the style in which the two groups work. To start with, the average sheltered work staff member spends most of his time on duties that he defines as 'supervisory' activities (activities like watching workers and their movements, giving instructions, reprimanding workers, and so on). By contrast, the average staff member in physically handicapped units was much more concerned with 'social care activities' (things like playing games with users, showing them how to do something new, sitting at table, eating and talking to users in groups, and so on). Use of work time connects with what most of those in sheltered workshops see as the most important function of their job: providing quality control of their 'product'. As an illustration, a 45-year-old dispatch supervisor explained: 'The most important thing in my job is to ensure that the orders are put up properly and to watch the economy of the deliveries, by putting each lorry out to its full capacity. The most important thing really is inspection of the work: it's quality control, you can't pick out just one thing.'

More staff working with the physically handicapped nominated forming relationships and getting to know the users by talking to them as the most important use of time.

So fundamental differences exist in the focus of the task. In sheltered workshops most managers and staff view an 'ideal' user as the user who makes a good worker.

> Intelligence is ideal and so is conforming to discipline, their willingness to work wherever you put them.

> The will to work to the best of his ability for eight hours a day and someone amenable to reasonable discipline.

> A person who has worked in outside industry and has had a physical and mental breakdown, he will make the best worker.

One that works every day, comes on time and gets on with the work without any fuss or bother.

Heads and staff working with the physically handicapped concentrated less on the ideal of a good worker and more on an ideal personality: extroverted and happy, cheerful and companionable users are ideal. The next most common ideal preference was for a user to be dependent; that is, in need of help from the staff and appreciative, grateful or receptive of help.

WHAT ABOUT THE USER-WORKERS?

What do sheltered workers feel about their work? They have a greater opportunity of doing machine work and of making more money than users of physically handicapped units. Despite this, more sheltered workers express less enjoyment of the day-to-day task, and more want to leave the workshops. More make substantive complaints about the workshop and say they are not given enough voice in how the unit is run. In sum, there is considerably more dissatisfaction than was found in users in units for the physically handicapped. The latter express more enjoyment, more desire to stay in the unit and less in the way of complaints.

Despite work on machines and more pay, over a quarter of the sheltered workers would rather be doing something else: another job outside the workshop or a change of work inside the unit. This is twice the number of users in physically handicapped units who wanted to be doing something else. These comments come from workers who wanted a change.

'I'd like more productive work', said one worker in his mid-50s who had been inspecting wiring for six months. 'I don't make an end product here. I'm getting on a bit. I used to think I'd like to do office work but I've got used to this and it brings money in.'

'It's a necessity to work but I don't enjoy it', said another worker aged 60.

'They could have had more interesting work to start with', a man in his mid-30s commented (he spent most of his time assembling switches and sockets).

'They mean well and all that. But these places are dead end', said a man of 35.

Five in ten sheltered workers filed complaints about the workshop and the way it was run, compared with one in seven of the physically handicapped. The largest group of sheltered workers complained about the building the factory was housed in, and the facilities, matters discussed in Chapter 17.

Lack of liaison between the staff and the users was criticised and other complaints by users attacked the apparent insensitivity of staff to the feelings of handicapped workers. It was clear that although the strongest criticisms were confined to three particular workshops, sheltered workers in general were less inclined to talk to staff about their personal problems than users of physically handicapped units.

> The staff are not interested in people, just the output.

> The staff treat you as if you were mentally handicapped ... Occasionally they have visitors round here but first of all they take them aside and give them a lecture and say things like we're all mentally disabled, but we're not. There's the bloke ... from social services and he ought to know better, he stands behind our chairs talking as if we're mental or in a zoo – it makes me furious.

Workers in one unit defined the major problems as stemming from the attitude of the manager. His aims are described in the quotations at the beginning of the chapter and the following comments are randomly selected.

> The manager doesn't care about us and all he wants to do is to get us to the benches and sweat hell out of us. I think he is the wrong man in the wrong job.

> Get rid of the general manager, he doesn't seem to understand the needs of blind and disabled, he only recognises we come here to work.

> A bit more tolerance with workers and you'd get more out of them.

In a second workshop, the manager's 'distance' was mentioned again:

> The manager here is unfriendly. [He] could create a situation where people were more relaxed. The pace here is rather greater than in normal industry: they are always pushing for production here without the normal labour-saving devices and a cynical attitude creeps in.

> They need a welfare officer you can go to, like a padre. They should be more interested in disabled people.

Are management of sheltered workshops so anxious to establish their production credentials that they forget the legitimate personnel function and welfare amenities that industry regards as normal? Other complaints centred on the workers' influence and poor communication between staff and workers. For example, nearly twice as many sheltered workers wanted to be given more say in running the unit than users in units for the physically handicapped. One user put it this way: 'It would be nice to have a bigger say in things. One thing they could do is send out a questionnaire and find out what we could do to improve things for them. They could take a bit more interest. If we have any ideas of our own, they could benefit by listening.'

The paradox is that all but one of the sheltered workshops had (on paper) mechanisms to facilitate 'joint consultation' between management and staff, usually a shopstewards' committee: 'to maintain efficient industrial relations in the factory by exchange of information, ideas, grievances, etc.' In theory, then, user representation was more common in sheltered workshops than in units for the physically handicapped. But clearly these formal structures of consultation did not mean the same thing to managers as to workers, since two-thirds of the sheltered workers viewed their participation in the unit as inadequate.

Do more sheltered workers want control of their work activities because they have higher aspirations than users in physically handicapped units? Or do users in physically handicapped units have the compensation of informal rather than formal participation, which makes them feel rather less dissatisfied subjectively, even if in objective terms their actual participation is less? The first question cannot be answered, tentative evidence supports the second, since more physically handicapped users than sheltered workers considered they had 'choice' about their activities in the unit. Further, more implied that they had more positive informal relationships with the staff: more were able to talk to the staff about personal difficulties than the sheltered workers.

When it came to the point, though, four-fifths of sheltered workers were prepared to say that they were more satisfied than dissatisfied. Satisfaction was not a 'black and white' issue. Sometimes it seemed to be a highly qualified pragmatic judgement based on a prudent assessment of the available options. It ranged from patient resignation ('I'm not satisfied but I'm willing to accept the situation') to adjusted neutrality ('everyone can find complaints: it's just a day's work. I'm satisfied') and unqualified satisfaction ('I'm satisfied').

Nevertheless, unqualified and unequivocal satisfaction was rare among sheltered workers. Even the one in four who indicated they had 'improved' since coming to the unit had complaints or suggestions for improvements, although notably these were never complaints about the staff. 'Improvement' for these people was mostly about self-esteem, then about straightforward financial improvements before physical improvements: but sometimes these things all went together. A middle-aged man explained the interaction between money, health and self-esteem for him and his wife like this: 'It has relieved me of the problem of having to count my money continually. I no longer have to worry about whether I can afford to buy odd things. I can save money comfortably each week in the Post Office. It's given me a feeling of making a contribution in work. Physically the occupation with my hands helps me to forget the constant pain in my forehead.

A contradiction of the sheltered workshop is that more sheltered workers (23 per cent) felt they had improved since coming to the unit than users in centres for the physically handicapped (18 per cent). But, again, more sheltered workers said that coming to the unit had done nothing (17 per cent) while this applied to few users in units for the physically handicapped (4 per cent). Fewer sheltered workers (43 per cent) were inclined to say the centre had maintained them and kept them going than the physically handicapped (70 per cent). Does sheltered work hold within it the powerful potential for improvement or deterioration of users, while the provision of other day services for physically handicapped people offers more neutral and safer 'maintenance'?

COMMENT

The initial guess was that more users in sheltered workshops might be more satisfied than those in centres for the physically handicapped because they were paid more, they worked with complex machinery and they had more formal access to consultation with management. However, this was not the case.

Does dissatisfaction amongst sheltered workers relate to particular management policies about staff recruitment: for example, employing staff without particularly strong motivation to work with handicapped people? Or, does the more mechanised work in the sheltered workshop alter the aims of the unit and thus the atmosphere, independent of 'interest' of the staff in the workers? Although this research cannot answer these important questions, other evidence suggests that, once day units adopt production aims ahead of pragmatic aims for work, the significance of the users is bound to change. A sheltered worker becomes a means towards fulfilling the production quotas and making a profit for the unit. The 'distance' between the staff and the workers is increased, the staff define the contact with workers as primarily supervisory, because the staff's job is to control the quality of the product. The user's job is to deliver the work performance to fulfill this. And thus the sheltered worker sees little variety in work activities and little discretion or choice about what he does and when he does it. So it cannot be assumed (in terms of worker satisfaction) that 'promotion' of a user from a day centre or day hospital to a sheltered workshop is an unqualified good. There is no present way of judging whether the aspirations of users rise if they are transferred to the sheltered workshops from centres for the physically handicapped, or whether sheltered workers are just more ambitious.

Three further points need to be made about work in day services. First, it appears to be easy for the aims of work programmes to change over time. Some staff in adult training centres using work for training purposes found themselves more concerned with production targets: this is discussed in Chapter 6. Second, the practice of work in day services has a very narrow definition, when judged by the variety offered in other parts of the programmes of day units. What tasks are defined as 'work' are extremely limited conceptions of the possibilities. The *status quo* – 'work is unskilled manual work in a factory' – is rarely challenged. One of the few examples of non-manual work is Kelvedon Programmers, a small venture of the Spastic Society, which deals with sub-contract computer programming work. But clerical work is never used and while arts and crafts are offered widely in day units for the mentally and physically handicapped (although never in the sheltered workshops), such activities were rarely defined as 'work' (nor were users paid for it).

So a user who makes a pot or a macrame wall hanging is not 'at work' nor is he paid for his product. But a user who counts envelopes or packs sanitary towels is paid a small amount for the work he does.[4] Yet, the common assumption that users are to be prepared by factory work for jobs outside the unit in industry takes on less credibility year by year as the number of jobs in the production sector contracts.

Reactions of sheltered workers are akin to other studies of factory work which described it as boring, tedious and repetitive (Fraser, 1968; Terkel, 1975; Shaiken, 1977). The skilled factory worker has been described as a cog in the production process, a 'baby sitter' for a machine who feeds his subject, watches it and cleans up after it. Shaiken writes:

> We are left with an enormous contradiction between the unique and varied intelligence that constitutes a person and the 'hand' that industry wants to carry out its work. A machinist may require constant supervision by management to produce the bare minimum during his shift at work giving the impression that even stricter supervision would be necessary for more production. Yet the same worker goes home and works until two o'clock in the morning in the garage making parts for his motor cycle at a rate of speed that would displace half the machinists at work, (where it applied), and with a quality that would virtually eliminate the need for an inspection division. (Shaiken, 1977, p. 117)

It is not so much the *content* of the work as the relationship of the user or sheltered worker to his work and the degree of discretion he has over it which is at issue. At present, work in the sheltered workshops follows classic 'scientific management' theories, assuming that work is an end in itself, that the product is achieved aside from the feelings of the workers and that what is required from the worker is obedience. In comparison, more staff in units for the physically handicapped consider the finer feelings of workers, thus approximating 'human relations' management by emphasising group togetherness. Are low user aspirations the result of this approach?[5]

The sheltered workshop approach to work is close to the 'low discretion' view of work (Fox, 1976). Of several characteristics, the first is basic to explaining the rest: subordinates cannot be trusted of their own free will to 'produce' to management goals. So – the job needs tight definition, close supervision, rules and procedures to monitor the workers' performance. This leads to a declining trust between the supervisor and a worker because the supervisor sees the worker as essentially unmotivated and untrustworthy. Being watched and directed arouses the worker's ire, so the rules become stricter, bringing about 'low trust' relations. Informal contacts between workers is restricted and free-flowing suggestion and criticism is discouraged. Failures of performance are dealt with by enforcing sanctions rather than by encouraging either 'internalised' standards of quality performance or by promoting a more personal identification of the worker with that organisation's particular goals. Finally, conflicts between management and workers are handled through a system of bargaining and agreements are based on coercion rather than on a recognition that each side is mutually indispensable. So, Fox thinks, there is little incentive to the worker to offer much more than minimal terms.

If a 'low discretion' worker is also a worker in the sheltered workshops one might not expect a sheltered worker to be very identified with management goals. Yet, the officially presented view of the advantages of sheltered work for the disabled (*Guardian*, 1978; International Seminar on Sheltered Employment, 1975) indicates that sheltered workers' views have not yet been taken into account. The ensuing comments aim at widening work choices for disabled sheltered workers, although the assumptions underlying the suggestions are humanitarian rather than economic and about 'value for money' by subsidy rather than non-subsidy.[6] Work for disabled workers will continue to need subsidies and it would be dishonest to pretend that the savings suggested below would be economic rather than human.

First, can there be more variety in sheltered work? Why not specialist arts and crafts products? The most important reason for considering arts and crafts as potential 'product' is that it would change the relationship of the sheltered worker to his product. Craft workers have much greater control over the product, because they form and shape it, they also 'own' it psychologically. The 'high discretion' syndrome implies a higher worker commitment because of more discretion and choice in making decisions (Fox, 1976). Rather than eyeing each other with mistrust and bad will, management and staff in high discretion settings 'continue overtly to define each other as responsible agents doing their honest best in a difficult shared situation. Such mutual compliments are rarely exchanged between top management and low discretion employees' (Fox, 1976, p. 32).

The assumption in craft work is that the worker is motivated to achieving a quality product by self-discipline, rather than by rules and coercion. To get the work finished, he or she has to be able to make decisions which control his immediate work, decisions which could relate highly to potential worker satisfaction.

Second, who should manage sheltered workshops? Most sheltered workshops are managed by the 'able-bodied' for the 'handicapped'. Worker control or workers' co-operatives might be considered: 'control' perhaps by the government of a worker-elected management committee, of which the manager may or may not be a member. The labour force may choose to become shareholders and shareholding offers voting rights and differentials in the share out of profits. If the government is prepared to support sheltered work for disabled people (Remploy, and so on) as well as workers' co-operatives (as in the example of the Meriden Motor Cycle Company), two such schemes might be experimentally tried together. One example is Rowen (Onllwyn) Ltd, which started from a charitable base as a self-managed company employing disabled ex-miners (funded by public appeal and the National Union of Mineworkers), and became a commercially competitive common ownership company (Hadley, undated).

A final question needs to be asked: why sheltered workshops? If the disabilities of sheltered workers allow them to get to work independently, could more in sheltered workshops move on to jobs outside? Sixty-one per cent of employers (including many government and local authority departments and the nationalised industries) fail to fulfil the quota of the Disabled Persons (Employment) Act 1944 that all employers with twenty or more workers should employ 3 per cent of 'registered disabled' persons. Recent policies for the employment of disabled people in the workforce include urging employers to consider disabled people for all types of vacancies, use of special 'job introduction' allowances, employment trials to workers who are paid by special government subsidies and increasing help with fares to work. Also retention of newly disabled employees in general employment is urged by offering help with fares, adaption of premises and modifications to equipment under special grants or free equipment loans (Manpower Services Commission, 1977, 1978; Employment Services Agency, 1977).

'Integration' into normal employment is the approach in line with the aspirations of many disabled people and that of recent civil rights thinking.' The United Nations Declaration (1975) claims that disabled persons 'whatever the origin, nature and seriousness of their handicaps and disabilities, have the fundamental rights as their fellow citizens of the same age which implies first and foremost the right to enjoy a decent life, as normal and full as possible'. As William Morris said, happy people means people happy in work.

NOTES

1 Sheltered workshops are usually classified administratively as units for the physically handicapped – even though in practice other user groups such as the designated 'mentally ill' may use workshops.
2 Only one unit offered workers other activities: a social programme.

3 The disregard limit has now been raised to £4 per week.
4 (In fact in over half of the units for the mentally handicapped and physically handicapped, contract work and arts and crafts together were part of the programme: users were paid most often for doing 'simple' packing and sorting jobs but almost never for making crafts.) Arts and crafts are thought to be less marketable. But the assumption is that industrial or contract work is 'real' work and somehow intrinsically 'better' for users than making a product which is also an art or craft. This view remains unsubstantiated while the rewards of work and arts and crafts remain dissimilar.
5 The founding father of modern Scientific Management, Taylor (Taylor, 1947), saw the purpose of work as the maximising of productivity. His task was to adapt the rationality of the worker to the task defined by technology, that is, the machine. In the interests of efficiency, any discretion of a worker over his task should be eliminated. A fundamental common interest between management and worker should be rewarded by financial incentives.

On the other hand, the so-called 'human relations' school of management still persuades the worker to adopt values defined by management and considers that people are motivated by feelings which might be at odds with the management goals. Thus management should promote good communication and the participation of the workers to 'ensure the stable equilibrium of the workplace' (see Argyris, 1960). But both the 'scientific management' and 'human relations' schools define the interests of the workers in the light of the interests of the management.
6 It has been disputed that the 'economic savings' argument for reforming services is effective: see, for instance, Macintosh (1977) on policies for the elderly and the Office of Health Economics (1977) on policies for disabled people. The Remploy group of sheltered workshops was subsidised to the sum of £2,500 per annum for each of its disabled employers in 1976-7.
7 See for instance the film 'Like Other People' (Mental Health Film Council: Concord Films, Ipswich); the report of the Snowdon Committee (Snowdon, 1976); United Nations General Assembly Declaration (1975) on the rights of disabled persons.

REFERENCES

Argyris, C. (1960) *Understanding Organisational Behaviour* (Tavistock).
Employment Services Agency (1977) *Outlook – The Rehabilitation and Resettlement Services Magazine*, No. 3 (November).
Fox, A. (1976) *Beyond Contract: Work, Power and Trust Relations* (Faber).
Fraser, R. (1968) *Work: Twenty Personal Accounts* (Penguin).
Guardian (1978) *Special Report: Sheltered Employment*, 24 January.
Hadley, R. (undated) *Rowen: South Wales* (The Society for Democratic Integration in Industry).
International Seminar on Sheltered Employment (1975) *British Council for Rehabilitation and Remploy Ltd. in association with the Vocational Commission of Rehabilitation International*, Guildford, England, 8–15 September.
Macintosh, S. (1977) 'Old age as a social problem', in R. Dingwall, C. Heath, M. Reid and M. Stacey (eds), *Health Care and Health Knowledge* (Croom Helm).
Manpower Services Commission and Employment Services Agency (1977) *Positive Policies: A guide to employing disabled people* (HMSO).
Manpower Services Commission (1978) *Developing Employment and Training Services for Disabled People* (HMSO).
Office of Health Economics (1977) *Physical Impairment: Social Handicap* (Office of Health Economics).
Shaiken, H. (1977) 'Craftsman into baby sitter', in I. Illich (ed.), *Disabling Professions* (Boyars).

Snowdon, Report of the Working Party (1976) *Integrating the Disabled* (National Fund for Research into Crippling Diseases).

Taylor, F. (1947) *Scientific Management* (Harper & Row).

Terkel, S. (1975) *Working* (Wildwood House).

United Nations (1975) *Declaration of the Rights of Disabled Persons*, General Assembly, Thirtieth Session, 3447 (xxx), 2433rd plenary meeting, 9 December.

APPENDIX TO CHAPTER 12

The differences between the users of units for the physically handicapped and sheltered workers have been assessed as statistically significant by the chi-squared test throughout this chapter. Differences *not* significantly different are introduced by the phrase 'there was a tendency' or 'a trend'.

The comparison between physically handicapped and sheltered workers around the dimension of work implies that the physically handicapped spend most of their time in centres at a work programme. This is not, in fact, the case, as only 42 per cent of the physically handicapped not in sheltered work spend most time at contract work. However, the only significant difference between physically handicapped users who spend 'most time' at work and those who didn't was found to be in their perceptions of choice of activities. Physically handicapped users who did *not* spend most time on work considered they were more able to choose what they did in the unit. There were no significant differences between the number of complaints, the numbers of users who would prefer to be doing something else or the type of improvements they wanted for the centre.

Chapter 13

———◆———

'WE ALL HELP EACH OTHER': AIMING AT THERAPEUTIC SETTINGS

I'd recommend this place to others in the same situation as me because you're not treated as a patient here, we're all treated the same, even the staff. (44-year-old woman with four past admissions to mental hospital)

INTRODUCTION

What is the place of the therapeutic setting in day services? What *is* the therapeutic setting? It has been seen 'not as a place where patients are classified and stored, nor as a place where one group of individuals (the ... staff) gives treatment to another group of individuals (the ... patients) ... but as a place which is organised as a community in which everyone is expected to make some contribution to the shared goals of creating a social organisation that will have healing properties' (Rapoport, 1960, p. 10). In other words, the therapeutic setting 'is distinctive amongst other comparable treatment centres in the way the institution's total resources, both staff and patients, are self-consciously pooled in furthering treatment' (Jones, quoted by Clark, 1977, p. 559).

Those creating a therapeutic setting are less concerned about diagnosing, treating, teaching or in any way 'doing to' their users, than in communicating with them, by releasing their therapeutic potential and expanding the status of users from relatively passive recipients to that of active participants in their own and other users' therapy.

Twenty-four staff members considered that the aim of their unit was to create a therapeutic setting and most of these staff were bunched together in eight day units. These account for both 5 per cent of day units and 5 per cent of day service staff. Seven of the eight units classified as therapeutic settings opened after 1970. One of these units was found in the health service: the rest were spread between local authority social services departments, the probation service and voluntary agencies. Of three units for the mentally ill, one for the elderly confused, one for offenders and three for families, three-quarters were located in London with half within just one inner London borough. Details are provided by Table 13.1.

This chapter will look at the growth of the therapeutic setting in day services and examine the themes and values implict in their aims and the ways they clash with other aims. Much of the chapter will compare different kinds of therapeutic settings located in day units. When at least half the staff interviewed considered that the aim of their unit was to provide a therapeutic setting, we called that unit a therapeutic setting. In each of the eight units, we interviewed at least half the staff and usually half the users. This chapter discusses therapeutic settings in day units (an exception to the rule identified in Chapter 3).

While declining in the traditional mental hospital (Manning, 1976a, b and c), ideas similar to the therapeutic community have taken root in user groups other than the mentally ill; for example, in services for families and offenders. In day services, more therapeutic settings are sponsored by social services and voluntary agencies than the health authorities.

LOCATING THE THERAPEUTIC SETTING

A social survey is an unusual method by which to explore a therapeutic setting. Neither an intensive field study nor a clinical review, a survey has the disadvantage of collecting what people say rather than observing what they do. But it allows a basis for legitimate comparisons between different kinds of therapeutic settings. For example, there are 'therapeutic communities' and 'therapeutic milieux' (Clark, 1977). 'Therapeutic milieux' use some, but not all, of the ideas and activities of the 'therapeutic communities'. Only one of the eight therapeutic settings described in this chapter approximated to a therapeutic community and the other seven were similar to therapeutic milieux.

The unit approximating a therapeutic community was a social services department day centre for the mentally ill and we called this a 'complete' therapeutic setting. The seven other units used some – but not all – of the ideas and activities of the therapeutic community so they were called 'incomplete' therapeutic settings. Much of the rest of this chapter will compare the 'complete' and 'incomplete' therapeutic settings, using the therapeutic setting as a kind of reference point. The method by which the units were classified is described at the end of the chapter (Appendix A) and Table 13.1 identifies the eight therapeutic settings.

AIMS AND IDEAS

Certain ideas seemed integral to the aims of the therapeutic settings. Take the 'complete' therapeutic setting first, the day centre for the mentally ill. The heads and staff talked about three central ideas, each of which could only be achieved within the context of the 'group', that is, the staff and users within the unit. First, there was the need for users to take an active part in the government of the unit and its activities. Second, there was the need for the users to have considerable licence in exploring and exercising personal choice and autonomy. Third, there was the need for users to face up to problems within themselves, their relations with the staff and with other users.

To illustrate these themes in the words of the heads and staff, first,

Table 13.1 *The Eight Therapeutic Settings*[a]

'Complete' Therapeutic Setting

No. 1 A day centre for mentally ill users in Innerborough (London) sponsored by the local authority social services department.[b]

'Incomplete' Therapeutic Settings

No. 2 A day centre for elderly confused clients in Innerborough and again sponsored by the same social services department.[b]

No. 3 A community centre/day nursery for 16 under 5s and their parents funded partly by Innerborough social services department but sponsored by a voluntary neighbourhood group.

No. 4 A drop-in neighbourhood centre for 15 isolated parents with practical or child-care problems in Innerborough, sponsored by a family service unit and open three days per week.[c]

No. 5 A psychiatric day hospital for 24 patients in London's Northborough sponsored by the area health authority.

No. 6 A drop-in centre open seven day per week, catering for members in London's Outerborough, sponsored by the local association for mental health.

No. 7 A day training centre to which offenders are sentenced by the court for ninety days. The centre is situated in Steeltown and is the only unit in the survey at which attendance is legally compulsory.

No. 8 A day centre for 'multi-problem families' reckoned to accommodate 6 families and their children three days per week in a new town of Midshire and sponsored by the local authority social services department.

[a] The average ratio of 'direct service' staff to users was 1 : 4: average number of places was 16.
[b] Numbers are attendance on day of the survey 1976.
[c] Units are open five days per week unless otherwise specified. On average users come to the unit for four-fifths of the time it is open.
   Note: Two more units organised as therapeutic settings opened after the survey and could not be included. One was a unit for ex-offenders in Southshire and the other a day unit for battered children and their parents in Midshire.)

there is the question of users taking an active part in the government of
the unit and its activities. In practical terms, the staff insisted that they
operated as a collective without a head. One said:

> They [the users] help to run the place by planning our activities on a
> weekly basis: the programme is run by them and guided by us [the
> staff]. We all take turns in doing everything. All rules are negotiable,
> they are made by the members and for instance they decided that being
> here before ten o'clock entitles them to a free lunch. Also, no physical
> violence is allowed. If users break the rules, the group decide what to
> do: their free lunch might be docked or they are asked to modify their
> symptoms.

Second, there is the question of providing licence for users to explore
and exercise their personal choice and autonomy:

> The centre aims to give users back responsibility for themselves.

> It's to help people take back the autonomy that has been taken from
> them by becoming mental patients.

Third, there is the question of enabling the users to face up to difficulties and problems within themselves. The staff see a dialectical relation
between personal change in the user and his relations with other users and
the staff, since personal change was nearly always seen in relation to the
other people *in* the unit, rather than related to the wider context of family
or workmates.

> The centre aims to help them become more aware of themselves and
> what's gone wrong and why they can't cope [said one staff member].
> Through that it's to improve their relationships with other people in
> the centre.

> Hopefully, to improve their relationships with other people in the
> centre.

Yet facing up to one's own problems meant growth, rather than
exclusively exorcising or reducing personal psychopathology: 'It's to help
people use their own energy [in the group] and to stretch people's
experimental horizons.'
Within the 'incomplete' therapeutic settings, these ideas were mentioned by fewer staff, partly because staff were working with colleagues
who – consciously or unconsciously – disowned the intentions of the
therapeutic setting and also because some pursued aims in addition to
therapeutic ones. This multiplicity of aims might intentionally – or unintentionally – dilute the therapeutic setting ideals.

For example, a collision between the therapeutic settings aim and other aims can be illustrated by one 'incomplete' therapeutic setting, the day hospital for the mentally ill (No. 5). Here the themes of the therapeutic setting such as user and staff government and user autonomy and choice were constrained by another aim, that of clinical assessment and treatment, which requires users to co-operate with their treatment by clinical experts. The sister-in-charge explained this ambiguity: the purpose of group and community life was 'to help them explore some of their problems – bearing in mind, of course, that they must co-operate fully with the [drug] treatment'.

A nurse spoke of the decision-making of the unit as follows: 'Yes, the users help to run this place by their committee, they organise some of their activities and just by interacting with others in community life. They also make the rules here with the staff.'

But other statements implied that the authority of the unit was vested in the hands of the staff, rather than in the members of the unit as a whole: the doctors defined the rules and prescribed the punishments: 'Patients must attend when they are supposed to and not take medication unless prescribed by a doctor, they must not drink alcohol, and they are to try to behave in an acceptable manner. If they break the rules, they are given a counselling session by medical and nursing staff and reprimanded, whether in a group or as an individual.'

So the intention of the therapeutic setting can be diminished by other aims, in this case the clinical frame of reference. At other times, an aim appears to be less of a threat to the therapeutic setting than an expansion of it. For example, at the day training centre for offenders, the combined view of the staff about the aims of the unit was very complicated, for they included offering a therapeutic setting to a user, training a user by providing him with skills to get jobs, rehabilitating a user in the community by working on improving his behaviour before his 'sentence' was complete, and also providing him with relevant practical social services. Said one:

The centre aims to help users avoid further convictions, to work through [group] discussion towards insight into their problems by having a wide range of settings in which to examine their behaviour. For instance, we give clients the opportunity to find out things they don't know about: how to find a job, or how to use their leisure time. Really it's to make them aware of their own potential to provide a viable alternative to prison. It relates to peer group pressure, and the building up of group identity and feeling so that clients make decisions about a wide variety of things and carry them out and experience the results of things.

Here, the aim of offering a therapeutic setting to users within the unit is combined with the aim of rehabilitation. So the therapeutic setting becomes more of a means than an end: primarily intended to meet the end of rehabilitation of users in the community. This contrasts with the 'complete' therapeutic setting, where the emotional interactions which take place might be regarded as an end in themselves. For example, one of the workers in the complete therapeutic setting, described what he most enjoyed about his work: 'It [the unit] provides an environment where rare emotional interactions take place between me and other people.'

OF DEMOCRACY, PERMISSIVENESS AND REALITY

Three themes found in the views of the staff of the 'complete' therapeutic setting can be summarised: first, user involvement in the government of the unit, that is, democracy; second, user licence in expression of choice and autonomy, that is, permissiveness; third, user self-awareness of personal problems, that is, the degree of reality confrontation.[1]

Democracy was assessed by looking at two specific questions. Did the heads, staff and users make the rules of the unit together, and did users play a prominent part in helping to run the unit? Permissiveness was assessed by gauging whether users and staff considered users had choice over their activities in the unit, and whether users were free to leave the unit without permission – for example, at lunchtime. To assess reality confrontation we asked if users had discussed personal problems with staff in the past fortnight, and also whether staff had talked with users about their future in terms of rehabilitation and training.

Where did the heads, staff and users of therapeutic settings stand on each of these matters? Did they have substantially the same views or radically discrepant opinions? Also, where did the staff of therapeutic settings stand compared to the other staff in day units: were they noticeably more democratic or permissive than the rest? Third, did the users of the therapeutic settings have any distinctive opinions about these matters which might mark them off from attenders of other day units?

In summary, the heads and staff of therapeutic settings saw the practices of the day unit as significantly more democratic and confronting of personal reality than the users. Users, in turn, saw the day unit as significantly more permissive than the heads and staff. Differences between the heads and staff of therapeutic settings and those of other day units were not significantly different; but there was a tendency for those in therapeutic settings to be marginally more democratic, permissive and 'reality-confronting' in their views.

There was, however, no doubt at all that the users of therapeutic settings saw the practices of their day units differently to attenders of day units in general, as significantly more democratic, permissive and reality-confronting than the rest. A detailed outline of these findings is given in Appendix B at the end of this chapter.

THE USERS AND THEIR VIEWS

There were three women for every two men in the therapeutic settings and as most users were in their 20s, they were significantly younger than the average users of day units. Most users were married, although a minority lived alone. Although nearly all users lived conventionally in a house or flat, a few lived in 'alternatives' such as a squat or a commune. Three out of four were without formal educational or vocational qualifications (not significantly different to other users), but at the same time there were significantly more users with higher educational qualifications such as nursing or teaching qualifications.

This chapter has already established that more users of therapeutic settings saw their units as democratic, permissive and reality-orientated more frequently than other users in the survey. Additionally, more users of therapeutic settings said they were satisfied, making them (aside from the elderly) a most satisfied group attending day units. Ninety-four per cent were satisfied with their unit and there was franker enjoyment of the activities of the unit than was found by users in other individual groups, such as the sheltered workers of the previous chapter. However, satisfaction was not simply acquiescence: there was a careful appraisal of the unit in terms of possible future personal progress. This was different to the criticism or negative comments of the sheltered workers, or the more uncritical acceptance of, say, the elderly. The views of the users about the benefits of the centre imply that the idea of 'reality confrontation' – the view that users should face up to problems within themselves and with each other – is practised.

The largest number of users spoke first of the difference the unit had made to relationships with others in the unit and the second largest group detailed the difference the unit had made to the way they felt about themselves. For some users, of course, these two things went together. From the complete therapeutic setting, a 32-year-old man who lived in a London squat, whose exact disabilities were not known because he 'had taken a stand against categorisation', asserted: 'I didn't have any expectations, but coming here has meant activating, even resolving some problems together. It's good company and a free lunch.' Another user, a 36-year-old woman who had a nervous breakdown in 1960 and who had been at the 'complete' therapeutic setting for seven months, said: 'I didn't expect to be so happy here. I thought it would be more like a hospital. I've made many friends – it's smashing the way we all help each other by joining in things.'

At the day hospital for the mentally ill, some users implied that being labelled as 'mentally ill' had provided them with an opportunity for learning about communicating with others, an experience which their background had previously denied them. For example, a 27-year-old woman who said she suffered from depression and a 'confused state of mind' said:

It's helped me meeting people and sharing experiences they've had in life and seeing the other person's point of view. I thought I was going to be locked up. sort of strait-jacket and things. I was ignorant about these places. It's broadened my outlook about different people and what goes on. I've also found out quite a bit about myself I didn't know before. I also found a few things I could do which I didn't know about before I came here.

Even the elderly confused spoke about the benefits of relating to others. 'It's taken me out of myself', declared a 72-year-old woman who said she had suffered from a nervous debility since 1960 which made her muddled and unable to remember things. 'It's helped to cheer me up: talking to people and meeting them helps to pass the time away and I like [the staff] Anna and Harry.'

Five of the six offenders in the day training centre described 'improvements' since they came to the unit six weeks before. 'Talking easier' to people and feeling 'less shy' were important, in the context of having 'no one on your back all the time'. 'It's opened me up – I was very shy and it's helped me to be able to talk to people', said a 26-year-old who had spent fourteen months in prison. 'I've only been here three weeks. Imagine what I'll be like after a couple of months!' 'The court sent me here to try to keep me out of trouble. I can talk easier to people since I came here', commented a twenty-three-year-old youth with experience of two remand homes, borstal and four years of prison.

They saw getting on better with people as it related to 'keeping out of trouble'. 'It's made me discuss things with people', said a 31-year-old single man living with his mother. 'The problems you get into with the police: it's made me think about the future.'

In the three family centres, the parents (mostly mothers) echoed the need to relate to others and to explore themselves but also to improve their abilities in parenting their children. A 35-year-old graduate mother, who attended the community nursery, said this: 'I had certain ideals about the nursery I wanted for my daughter and I have been helping to bring the place about. It has provided a family atmosphere for my 4-year-old which has been a great benefit as I'm bringing her up on my own. It's provided a group of friends for me as a focus for my life working with other people in the group.'

On the other hand, a 25-year-old mother with two sons, separated from her husband and on social security, said of the drop-in neighbourhood centre: 'It's done a lot for me in seven months. I can make 'phone calls on my own which I couldn't do before. I can even help others which I couldn't do before. No one laughs when you can't spell to fill in forms. It's given me confidence because I can say more what I think now and tell people when I don't know what they're saying.'

A 21-year-old single mother with two children, who said she had been 'very depressed' before coming to the family centre, spoke along the same lines as all the other users when she commented:

When Michael [the head] came down for me first, I said I had a cold, I was too scared to come . . . But it's helped me cope with the children better. When I first came here I was very bad with nerves. But I don't need my nerve tablets any more, my nerves don't bother me. I've met some friends – before I came here I couldn't mix with people but since coming here I can speak to anybody. They [the staff] help you and there are other mothers and you have discussions, this helped me more than anything. For instance, if you have a problem, you come along and tell them. They are awfully good and listen and help you in any way they can . . . they do everything they can to help you, you only have to ask. You get a break from the children too because they take them over.

STAFF AND ACTIVITIES

Differences existed between those working in therapeutic settings and other heads and staff, regarding their perceptions of democracy, permissiveness and reality confrontation. Implementing these approaches are not, as other chapters indicate, everyone's chosen way of working. One obvious difference between the staff in therapeutic settings and those in other day units relates to their qualifications. There were significantly more qualified staff in the therapeutic settings: three out of every four of the heads and staff in the therapeutic settings had tertiary academic or vocational qualifications, compared to one out of two in other settings.

University degrees in social sciences or social work-related qualifications were more common than nursing qualifications, the latter being the most common qualification of heads and staff in day services as a whole. Five out of eight heads were university graduates, all but one in social sciences. Only ten heads in the sample were graduates so this means that the therapeutic settings – a mere one in every twenty day units – cream off half of the graduate heads.

Only one centre offered industrial or contract work: meetings and groups were the most frequently offered activities. The 'complete' therapeutic setting had the most comprehensive system of groups – community meetings, discussion and therapy groups, as well as the planning meeting and co-counselling groups. In some units, however, the overlap between discussion and therapy groups was close: 'Our groups with parents in a family day centre are seen as halfway in between [therapy and discussion groups]. Groups of two staff and six to eight parents are led by a social worker with the purpose of airing the problems of parenting.'

Apart from regular community meetings and therapy groups, there were other variations in groups. The 'complete' therapeutic setting held a planning meeting at the end of each week to enable staff and users to review the successes and failures and design a programme for the ensuing week. In other units, 'complaints' meetings were called when grievances or grumbles built up. A few units had 'user only' meetings, to discuss common issues, and the 'complete' therapeutic setting sponsored co-counselling groups which grouped users in twos and threes to counsel each other.

'Talking' groups are the core activity but group approaches are implicit in other activities too. For example, after meetings and groups the most common activities were painting (arts and crafts), group games like table tennis and cards (social/sporting programmes), 'survival' groups like shopping expeditions, domestic training, music classes (education) and relaxation groups and keep fit classes (treatments). Thus the activities in therapeutic settings seem often to demand a skill of the user and invite him to communicate with others at the same time.

Is there a contradiction between a unit seen by users to be relatively self-governing when most users are uneducated and the staff highly qualified? Users indicate that they see their staff as highly approachable. Day units provide a situation where the staff and the users are consistently and continually exposed to one another, but one user put it this way: 'Well, they treat us the same as them.'

DISCUSSION

Earlier research indicates that if staff and users are recruited from widely different class backgrounds this can lead to a clash of frames of reference between the two groups. Mutual bewilderment and misunderstanding results, and social and psychological 'distance' is reinforced (Mayer and Timms, 1969; Brill and Storrow, 1960). But social distance between staff and users does not *necessarily* increase in linear fashion in day care as the staff qualifications increase, for the most qualified heads 'lead' the most democratic day units, that is, the units where social distance is least. This implies that the beliefs of the heads and staff about democracy may be important and, of course, some education favours the inculcation of certain beliefs. This issue will be returned to again later in this chapter.

Therapeutic settings run counter to and challenge some of the hierarchical assumptions of other day units, but even their sternest opponents could hardly object to their present operation in day services. Considerable checks and balances operate on the freedom of therapeutic day settings: first, from the organisation of which the therapeutic day setting is a part, and second, from checks and balances in the unit itself.

First, there are the constraints on a therapeutic setting from the organisation in which it operates. None of the therapeutic settings were independent of sponsorship by 'head office' – even the voluntary family centre was funded by the local authority. In the carefully graded establishment, hierarchical accountability and scrutiny by local politicians are potential constraints on the therapeutic community. Other checks exist because the unit is a day service, rather than a twenty-four hour hospital or residential home. There have, of course, always been isolated, if well-known, examples of therapeutic communities in day settings, such as the Marlborough Day Hospital and Paddington Day Hospital. Despite this, many consequences of transferring therapeutic settings from a residential to a day setting are still unexplored. Users visit a day therapeutic setting only for a maximum of thirty-five hours weekly, compared to the 168 hours in a week of institutional life. What happens in the 113 hours per week that each user spends outside the therapeutic setting?

Other checks within the unit itself on the freedom of therapeutic setting have already been implied. First, some staff see other aims for the unit. Second, there is the more complicated issue of whether one staff member can pursue multiple goals. If the aim of the therapeutic setting is to explore the dimensions of personal contact and personal change between its members, other aims of whatever sort might impede this. On the other hand, if the balance is adjusted so that the aim of the therapeutic setting is to discharge its members to everyday life outside, the therapeutic setting becomes a means rather than an end, and the ultimate in the exploration of personal contact and personal change between its members may of necessity need to be curtailed.

When the therapeutic setting provides an alternative world for a group of users, it may not matter whether or not staff have multiple aims. But if the aim is to return users to everyday life, then 'complicated' rather than 'simple' sets of aims on the part of the staff may produce better rehabilitative results. This was found to be the case in hospital rehabilitation and long-stay wards (Coser, 1963). The conflict between the aims of various staff groups kept people on their toes.

The important study of the archetypal therapeutic setting at Belmont (now Henderson) Hospital, started by Maxwell Jones, indicated that the therapeutic community faltered when its members returned to the outside world (Rapoport, 1960). The assumption that 'everything is treatment, all treatment is rehabilitation' was pointed out to be insufficient and contradictory because the values of this therapeutic community were quite different to those of, say, the factory floor or the office:

> Such ideas and values may be therapeutic in the sense of bringing about better social relationships and better understanding of behaviour while in the hospital community . . . the same values and attitudes applied to the outside world may produce serious conflicts on return to the wider community . . . The follow-up data indicated that those patients who tended to change their values in the direction of the values of the unit community showed less satisfactory adjustment outside than those who did not. (Rapoport, 1960)

However, this criticism and others imply the value judgement that being in the outside world is 'better' than being in a therapeutic community. For some people this may be true, but not necessarily for all day unit users. Many users in day units will never leave the unit to enter the work world: for the elderly confused, for some of the middle-aged mentally handicapped, or for mothers of 'multi-problem' families and others, aspects of the therapeutic setting may provide an enriching satisfaction and investment for members which might need to be calculated as an end in itself.

How have the ideas of the therapeutic setting, born in the institution, got through to day units? Often it is assumed that therapeutic settings have come from social psychiatry and the mental hospital, particularly from Main and Jones, whose work with servicemen during the Second World War led to two distinct groups of therapeutic community practices in mental hospitals after the war. One theory is that the subsequent development of 'community care' emasculated the principle of inpatient treatment in a mental hospital and led to the closure of beds, so that the therapeutic community became an innovation which subsequently 'diffused' its beliefs to organisations other than mental hospitals and user groups other than the mentally ill (Manning, 1976c).

But at least half the therapeutic day settings contained workers without any past formal record of work in the field of social psychiatry, so it may well be that alternative sources of ideas have inspired therapeutic settings. First, there is education in the social sciences. Heads of therapeutic settings have had an above-average exposure to either social science concepts which analyse organisational issues or to social work theory, with its bias towards notions of democracy, permissiveness and confrontation of emotional issues. These approaches are still largely ignored in other forms of training represented in day services, such as nursing, medicine or teaching the mentally handicapped.

Second, there is also the relative youth of the users in therapeutic settings. This is important because of the revival of interest amongst younger people in the 1960s in promoting non-hierarchical social arrangements in the institutions with which they associated. One aspect of those was the growth of what might be called 'Utopian' movements. Many communes of the past and present have strong resemblances to therapeutic settings: in fact, some claim to be therapeutic settings. Synanon, which deals with drug addicts, provides its members with sets of alternative living arrangements and offers 'services with a mission' to addicts. A rapport between the 'counter-culture' and therapeutic communities has been noted (Clark, 1977) but there has been no systematic exploration of this interchange. (It is probably no coincidence that the few users who lived in squats and communes attended therapeutic day settings rather than sheltered workshops!)

One of the ideals of the commune which relates to the therapeutic settings is the idea of human perfectibility (Kanter, 1972). This can only be achieved in the 'perfect society', not in the chaotic disharmony of the outside world. 'Perfectibility' can only be achieved within an internalised small society like a commune – or a therapeutic community. This may explain why there is so much reluctance in therapeutic settings to get their members to accept the standards of the outside world and why therapeutic settings are poor at rehabilitation. If the standards of the outside world are second rate compared to those of the 'community', the reluctance to get members to re-enter is understandable. This suggests that unless therapeutic settings in day units are prepared to modify their aims to include other aims, the most obvious value of the therapeutic day setting lies in its ability to provide a protected, concerned setting for those who need the day unit on a long-term basis.

NOTE

1 These themes are very close to the 'ideology' of the therapeutic community described by Rapoport at the Belmont Hospital (Rapoport, 1960) with the exception that our data contained no mention of 'communalism'.

REFERENCES

Brill, N. Q. and Storrow, H. A. (1960) 'Social class and psychiatric treatment', *Archives Gen. Psychiatry*, 3, pp. 340–4.
Clark, D. H. (1977) 'The therapeutic community', *British Journal of Psychiatry*, 131, pp. 553–64.
Coser, R. (1963) 'Alienation and the social structure: case analyses of a hospital', in E. Freidson (ed.), *The Hospital in Modern Society* (Free Press).
Jones, M., quoted by Clark, op. cit.
Kanter, R. M. (1972) *Commitment and Community* (Harvard University Press).
Manning, N. (1976a) 'Values and practice in the therapeutic community', *Human Relations*, 29, 2, pp. 125–38.
Manning, N. (1976b) 'What happened to the therapeutic community?' in K. Jones (ed.), *Year Book of Social Policy 1975* (Routledge & Kegan Paul).
Manning, N. (1976c) 'Innovation in social policy – the case of the therapeutic community', *Journal of Social Policy*, 5, 3, pp. 265–79.
Mayer, J. E. and Timms, N. (1969) 'Clash in perspective between worker and client', *Social Casework*, January, pp. 32–40.
Rapoport, R. (1960) *Community as a Doctor* (Tavistock).

APPENDIX A TO CHAPTER 13

1. *Aims*

Chapter 4 describes how the statements made by staff about the aims of their unit were inspected for evidence that the unit was arranged as a therapeutic setting. Twenty-four staff members described the aims of their units in this way. If at least half or more of the staff interviewed in a unit considered that the aim of their unit was to provide a therapeutic setting, we called that unit a therapeutic setting. In this way, eight units were identified, accounting for nineteen of the twenty-four staff. All the staff of three units agreed that the unit aimed to provide a therapeutic setting.

2. *Groups*

Within these eight therapeutic settings, activities available to users represented the staff intention of running a therapeutic setting. Evidence of whether 'the community' – staff and users – met in 'community' groups for discussion and/or therapy groups and what proportion of users were eligible to attend these meetings was considered. All eight units had discussion groups. Nearly all had community meetings and just under half held therapy groups.

3. *Shared decision-making*

Even if half the staff aimed to offer a therapeutic setting and the unit offered all users meetings, or groups, how can one assess the communal status of the unit? One indicator was which individual or group gave permission for the researchers' visit to the unit. If this decision was made by the heads, or senior staff, this did not seem to demonstrate shared decision-making. But if permission was given by the staff and users, this seemed a reasonable test of the shared decision-making in the unit.

To summarise then: the intention expressed by staff that one of the aims of the unit was to offer a therapeutic setting was confirmed by determining whether communal meetings for all were part of the practices of the unit. Further, the communal nature of the unit could be assessed by observing whether or not the 'community' had decided to allow the researchers to visit the unit.

These three criteria discriminated between two different kinds of therapeutic settings, leaving a residual group of individual staff. The first kind was called the 'complete' therapeutic setting. Only one unit, the social services department day centre for clients who were labelled as mentally ill (No. 1):

(i)   scored 100% agreement between all the staff concerning the aims;
(ii)   had offered community/therapy/discussion groups in the previous week which all users were said to attend;
(iii) users and staff gave communal permission for the researchers' visit.

The second kind of therapeutic setting was called the 'incomplete' therapeutic setting. In these seven units, all three criteria were never met in one unit. If agreement about the aims was total, a full range of groups was not offered to users. Many staff in these units worked with colleagues who saw the unit pursuing different aims. In about half the 'incomplete' therapeutic settings, staff and users were not consulted about the decision to make the research visit.

There was a residual group of five isolated staff members who expressed their intention that the unit should aim at therapeutic setting ideas but each was unsupported by their colleagues in this. These staff were called 'sporadic social therapists'. None of them was head of a unit, and three of the five worked in area health authority day hospitals for the mentally ill.

In the therapeutic settings there were some agreements and some disagreements between the views of staff and users. Taking 'democracy' first, proportionately three times as many staff as users said that staff and users together made the rules of the unit (staff, 59 per cent; users, 19 per cent). Also, more staff (33 per cent) tended to consider that users played a prominent role in helping to run the unit than did the users themselves (19 per cent). Thus on the whole staff, more frequently than users, saw the unit as 'democratic'.

Turning to 'permissiveness' next, fewer staff than users were inclined to consider either that users were free to choose the activities they did in the unit (staff, 59 per cent; users, 82 per cent), or that users had freedom to come and go from the unit, for instance at lunchtime (staff, 55 per cent; users, 82 per cent). In other words, more users than staff thought the unit was 'permissive'.

Concerning 'reality confrontation', there was a reverse of opinion. Over half the staff (52 per cent) but only about a third (31 per cent) of users agreed that there was regular discussion in the unit about such issues as rehabilitation and training. And significantly more staff than users (staff, 78 per cent; users, 50 per cent) said that the users had discussed personal problems with them in the last fortnight. Thus in broad terms staff in therapeutic settings more frequently than users saw the unit as 'democratic' and 'confronting reality', while more users said the unit was 'permissive' using the indicators described.

It also seemed important to assess staff in therapeutic settings compared to staff in other settings. Taking first the indicators for 'democracy', staff in therapeutic settings were twelve times as likely to say staff and users jointly made the rules of the unit as their colleagues in other settings (59 : 5 per cent). There was also a strong tendency for more staff in therapeutic settings to agree that users played a prominent role in helping to run the unit (staff in therapeutic settings, 33 per cent; staff in other day units, 18 per cent).

In relation to 'permissiveness', while staff in the two kinds of settings did not significantly differ over whether users chose the things they did in the unit, they did differ in their opinions as to whether users were free to leave the unit. Over half the staff in therapeutic settings said users were free, while under a third of staff in other settings agreed (staff in therapeutic settings, 55 per cent; staff in other units, 32 per cent).

A similar split occurred in relation to the two indicators of 'reality confrontation'. The staff in the two kinds of settings did not significantly differ over whether users had discussed personal problems with them, but did differ over rehabilitation and training discussions. Again, over half

Table 13.2 *Users in therapeutic settings compared with other day units*

Proportion of: Users in Therapeutic Settings	Users in Non-therapeutic Settings	Who Said:
19%	2%	'Staff and users make the rules of the unit together.'
19%	5%	'We [the users] play a prominent role in the helping to run the unit.'
83%	59%	'We [the users] choose the things we'd like to do in the unit.'
82%	51%	'We [he users] feel free to leave the unit.'
31%	10%	'There is regular discussion in the unit about such things as rehabilitation and training.'
50%	24%	'We [the users] have discussed a personal problem with the staff in the last fortnight.'

the staff in therapeutic settings said there were regular discussions about rehabilitation and training compared to just under a third of staff in other settings (staff in therapeutic settings, 52 per cent; staff in other units, 32 per cent).

Thus the staff of therapeutic settings tended to view their units as more 'democratic', 'permissive' and 'reality-confronting' than their colleagues working in other day settings.

But the most consistent differences on these indicators came between the users of therapeutic settings and the users of other day units. In all cases, significantly more users of therapeutic settings saw their units as 'democractic', 'permissive' and 'reality-confronting' than their peers in other settings, as indicated above. These results are set out in Table 13.2.

Chapter 14

---◆---

'LISTENING TO USERS': AIMING AT RELATIONSHIPS

> We help them get a relationship with someone. This enables them to
> feel reassured, and makes them realise they're part of the community
> as well as us. (Staff member, adult training centre)

AIMING TO 'RELATE'

A small group of heads and staff considered that one aim of the unit was
forming personal relationships with individual users. Their views did not,
of course, entail academic dialogue about whether it was feasible for an
organisation like a day unit to 'relate' to individual people: perhaps they
understood a day unit to be the sum of its people, we do not know. But
these heads and staff considered it important enough to mention that an
aim of the unit was to relate to users; whether or not their words and their
behaviour synchronised is another question. However, those who considered that relating with users was an aim of the unit claimed that they
spent more actual time talking to users than in doing any other of the
things – professional, domestic or bureaucratic – that comprised the data
of a staff member's week.

As only twelve heads and staff members emphasised this personal
relationship between user and unit, they represent a minute fraction of
the staff. Like the biblical disciples the twelve represented specialist
backgrounds, although instead of being fishermen four of the twelve
represented offenders and six the mentally ill. In proportion, though, one
of every three of the staff working with offenders espoused the aim of
relationship between unit and user, whereas only one in twenty of those
working with the mentally ill did so. Amongst the twelve, professional
qualifications were, perhaps, over-represented, since three of every four
had been through a recognised course of training, as against only about
half of the staff at large.

ASPECTS OF RELATING WITH USERS

Although what distinguished this small group was their belief that
relating to users could be seen as an aim of the unit, this is not to say that
the rest of the staff (the other 96 per cent after all) did not consider that
communicating with users was an important part of the job. One out of

every three staff saw the most important thing they did personally on the job as talking with or relating to users.

What distinguished the twelve? First, some – although by no means all – rejected firmly groups and group techniques, which were seen to be almost humiliating in their emphasis on public confession. One psychiatric registrar who felt strongly about this said: 'This unit helps people who need help to cope with the strains and stresses of everyday life. Hours and hours of listening and individual conversation is involved, and I resist the pressure to conform to the group therapy vogue.' Second, relationships were seen to be based on certain humanistic values. A former lawyer, now working in a day centre for the mentally ill, said: 'We used to be industrial, but now it's more therapeutic. We're trying to give them more self-respect and dignity – to give them more choice and feeling for themselves.' Third, relationships were seen to be the product of applied skill: 'This unit provides therapeutic support to patients', said a social worker in a day hospital; 'that is, I help and develop casework relationships with patients.'

How did these heads and staff set about their jobs? Within this small group two particular approaches could be discerned: what might be termed the humanistic as against the technocratic approaches to relating. The humanistic approach implied that relating was fundamentally a matter of innate personality. One staff member said this: 'Be honest, be genuine, and keep the "self" under control. It relates to the interaction between people, and its achieved mostly through verbal communication.' Another worker put it rather more earthily: 'I'm very ready to listen to parents or children, being interested in their problems. I'm basically a shoulder to cry on, and a Mum to both parents and kids. I have to be able to take a lot without rejecting them.' On the other hand, the technocratic approach implied that relating to users was more a matter of applying an acquired skill. At one end of this scale, a staff nurse in a day hospital spoke as if applying counselling and bandaids had a lot in common: 'The most important thing that I do in my job is to do psychotherapy. I try to apply it daily even if it's only for five minutes.' A more moderate if traditional view which implied that 'relating' could be, at least, a learned skill: 'I used my skills as a social worker – skills in individual counselling. If I have a client with a particular problem I try to co-ordinate the people involved by forming a working relationship with them.'

RELATING WITH OFFENDERS

A quarter of those who talked about relationships between unit and user worked in centres for offenders. A third of the users in centres for offenders had approached a staff member in recent times to talk about a personal problem – rather more users proportionately than other groups apart from family day care. More offenders than other users said that they expected help with a personal problem when they started coming to the centre. This was a relatively unimportant expectation for members of other user groups, again aside from those in family day centres. Further, more users in centres for offenders had views on the qualities they felt desirable in staff members: more offenders considered an ability to communicate personally with users the most important attribute of a staff member in a day centre. At the same time, after the elderly, offenders were the group least likely to complain about their staff. Very few users overall complained about the staff who worked in their particular centre, but even fewer offenders were dissatisfied with their staff. It was not that offenders enjoyed day centres unequivocally, for half of them – more than most user groups – would have preferred to be doing something else than coming to the centre and more of them were dissatisfied than other user groups with the centre.

What aspects of the units for offenders went some way towards facilitating the development of relationships between staff and user? For a start, the ratio of staff to offenders was relatively favourable – on average one staff member to every five offenders, compared with, say, one staff member to every eleven physically handicapped users. Nevertheless, other sectors had ratios which were similar to the centres for offenders – for example, the day hospitals for the mentally ill and the day hospitals for the elderly.

In centres for offenders staff relied more on the humanistic strategies described earlier than technocratic approaches to relating with the users. By contrast, their peers in day hospitals for the mentally ill and elderly were much more geared to using technical approaches with their users than humanistic ones. Four out of ten staff for offenders described humanistic strategies and approaches to their job, compared to two out of ten of those working with the mentally ill.

DISCUSSION

Should you be in need of a relationship with a professional should you enrol at a day unit? If you do, you may not find that the focus of the day unit is towards helping you with your relationship problems. Very few day units allocate staff members to work with particular users, and when they do the reason is not one which facilitates relationships: the most common reason for allocation is to suit 'administrative convenience'. You will not either, by and large, find a great deal of expertise in day units in the practice of the various 'therapies'. There is one day unit which offers hypnotherapy here (in the north-west) and another which deals in behaviour therapy there (in the midlands), but by and large the spread of technical therapeutic skills in day services is parsimonious. No day unit employed a trained psychotherapist and only 7 per cent of day units which offered *therapy* groups to users had a mental health professional such as psychiatrist, psychologist or social worker with conventional mental health credentials on the staff. These traditional professional qualifications vary a great deal, of course, between and within disciplines in terms of the amount of actual 'relationship' work with people involved, and in the degree of therapeutic skill their graduates acquire. There is some limited evidence that people without psychotherapeutic training claimed to be doing 'psychotherapy', as the statement from the staff nurse earlier in the chapter indicated.

In sum, very few staff of day units see the question of the unit (whatever that may be) and its potential relationship to users as a fundamental issue of the aims of the unit. Nevertheless, there is a lot of *informal* emphasis by heads and staff on relations with users, as over a third from all user groups take relating to users seriously in their individual work: this one-third mentioned that relating with or talking to users was the most important part of the job. Should relationships between staff and users become then a part of the formal aims of the unit, rather than the idiosyncratic purview of individual job holders?

What models of approaches to relationships are current in day services? On the one hand, some blueprints for the day care of the future, for example, the Certificate in Social Service, imply that skills in interpersonal relationships can be acquired and that ability to relate to users is a fundamental requirement of all workers in day units. This, of course, contrasts with the old approach which employed a worker in a day unit because of his trade skill or his craft: this new approach implies that the technical man must be able to 'relate', because relationships are fundamental to other methods in day care – instruction, recreation, treatment and organisational skills (CCETSW, 1975).

Another model advocates a division of labour: some staff remain technicians, while others became specialist 'relaters'. For example, the employment rehabilitation centres employ tradesmen to teach or supervise work skills, while social workers are employed presumably, at least in part, to relate. We cannot comment on how this works out in the employment rehabilitation centres, but in general terms one danger of such a division of labour is often that relating becomes a secondary function, to serve the technical aim of the unit. This model has, of course, been highly criticised in hospitals for years – the 'human relations' staff, such as social workers and counsellors, usually lack prestige and influence, and decisions about patients remain primarily technocratic and relatively uninfluenced by human relations considerations.

A third strategy might be to turn the 'relaters' into technicians, in other words, to 'technicalise' the relationship between a staff member and user. This happened in a few mental illness units when relationships between staff and users are reinterpreted as treatment therapies.

A fourth approach is that used in those family day centres which were described in Chapter 3.6 as concentrating on mutual aid. In this view you do not need to be a specialist to relate to users; neither can the qualities fundamental to helping other people – warmth, genuineness and empathy – be inculcated by training. Thus all those in a day unit, whether staff or users, have something to offer from their own personal experience and what counts is the ability of a staff member or user to share with others.

Thus of the four models, the first and the last are two different 'generalist' approaches to relationships. The relationship is primary and other matters secondary. The second and third approaches assume that relationships are specialist matters, achieved by those who have been trained in these fields. Of course, in practice these models overlap and it is possible that several models may be found in any day unit at once.

But before any of these approaches can be advocated, an empirical question needs to be answered: what is the point of developing relationships between staff and users in day units? As a confirmation of the 'existential human condition' which would suggest that all adults, whether in day care or not, need to be 'in relationship' with those about them? Or should relationships between staff and user address the 'problem component' of those in day services? To argue that relationships alone can solve the problems of users in day units seems shortsighted; to see a spastic 25-year-old as only a target for a relationship ignores many social aspects of his life: a job and weekly wage may improve his self-esteem as well as a therapeutic relationship!

In day services at present, most relationships between staff and users are viewed as flowing in one direction: 'relating' flows from staff member to user. This attitude prevents users from helping each other and traps the staff into considering that their skills are superior ones. Even if they lack formal counselling expertise, the unit structure supports their assumptions of superiority. Might it be worth considering training users to be counsellors as well as staff? Accounts of people who are handicapped or 'deviant' stress over and over again that their appointed helpers find it difficult to empathise with their predicament and to understand their feelings of stigma. The idea of suggesting that helpers share the same predicament or label, tried as part of the New Careers movement (the attempt to provide users with a ladder to penetrate the professional career structure), has now been tested in several day centres (NACRO, 1978; Barbican, 1978). Whilst presenting some difficulties, particularly for younger people, the success of the *approach* justifies its extension to other groups.

REFERENCES

Barbican (1978) *The Barbican Centre Now* (Gloucestershire Probation and After-Care Services).
Central Council for Education and Training in Social Work (1975) *Day Services: An action plan for training*, CCETSW Paper No. 12 (CCETSW).
NACRO (1978) *The Hammersmith Teenage Project* (Rose).

Chapter 15

'LIFE IN A HOME': PREPARING USERS FOR INSTITUTIONS

> We give our day people a change from their own homes: get them out of their house. It's a sort of stepping stone before permanent residential care so we give them an insight into what life is like in a home.

Chapter 7 established that many heads and staff in day services aim to keep their users *out* of institutions. This chapter will discuss the aim of those few heads and staff – only 2 per cent – who, far from aiming to keep people *out* of institutions, actually see the day unit as a bridge *into* the institution. Thus attending a day unit is seen to offer the user a transition from living at home in the community, to life inside a hospital or a residential home.

Most of these staff worked in units whose chief job was to care for the elderly and all worked in day units attached to a residential institution. For example, five of the ten worked in two day care centres for the elderly and one mixed centre attached to local authority residential homes for the elderly. Three worked in day hospitals for the elderly which were in the grounds of long-stay hospitals for the aged. Another two worked in the day centre attached to a hospice, for dying patients.[1]

In preparing the user for living in an institution, the day unit provided a kind of orientation course, almost a training programme for old people, before their admission to home or hospital.

> It prepares people for when they have to come into residence. (Staff member, day care in social service residential home)

> We rehabilitate people to part three accommodation. (Sister, day hospital for the elderly)

> [This day centre] gives a more gradual introduction into what will ultimately become their permanent home. (Staff member, day care in residential home)

> Basically, it's to get patients to us early – to give them care before they come in as inpatients. They know us, we know them: there's some form of relationship. (Nurse, day centre attached to hospice for terminally ill patients)

The rest of this chapter will present two case studies of two day units where at least half the heads and staff thought the unit aimed to prepare the users for institutions.[2]

ST MARK'S

A voluntary organisation runs St Mark's, a hospice for the terminally ill. Built on heathland on the outskirts of a northern city, its day unit was established by default in 1975. Funds were not available to extend the fifty-bedded inpatient unit so it was decided to start a thirteen-place day centre instead. A separate day room, bath and toilet facilities were built at the other end of the attractive single-storey building which contains the hospice.

Attracting staff to St Mark's is no problem. Although the health service units in this area have inadequate numbers of remedial therapists and social workers, there are no shortages at St Mark's. Senior medical and nursing staff, including a community nursing sister, link the hospice and day unit with the community by caring for patients in their own homes. The community sister also teaches district nurses and general practitioners to care for terminal cancer patients at home. She says:

> We teach pain control plus keeping an eye on the fistula lesions. We offer patients a *choice* about where they die, here [in the hospice] or at home.
>
> We find that the day unit has proved that patients don't need to come into [the hospice] as inpatients as fast. They aren't coming in as inpatients through physical deterioration brought on by anxiety and fear. Many of our day patients don't need to come into the hospice at all. The day centre gives them great security and they can make a choice about coming into the hospice or dying at home. Dying at St Mark's is second best to dying at home . . . The day unit can provide a stepping stone to the inpatient unit . . . I get great job satisfaction from offering something good and knowing that people get quality and dignity at the ending of their life. Their [the patients'] fear is a stinking dying death with pain: out emphasis on quality and dignity is so positive.
>
> We offer patients a day place in a caring atmosphere where the kettle's always on and there's always time to talk and chat. Nothing must be rushed. The day unit must be flexible: its important that the patients have people to talk to. You have to be prepared to spend time to win people over. The day unit provides a break from patients with pre-terminal diseases. A break from home, their depression and boredom.

The users attending St Mark's day centre are described in Chapter 3.8. All places on three days each week are taken by those with terminal malignancies. On two days a week some people with long-term deteriorating conditions such as multiple sclerosis attend. Users are offered one or two days per week. The most common reason for discharge from the day centre is death: nearly two-thirds of the fifty-six users who left the day unit in the previous twelve months had died.

CIRCLE HOUSE

The other day unit, Circle House, is in a residential home for the elderly in an area of private housing. Built in 1970, it provides no special facilities or staff for its day attenders, who join in with the residents of the home, by sharing two day rooms, a dining room and toilet facilities. Circle House is described in Chapter 3.1. The head of unit, the warden, is married to the matron, and the deputy head and deputy matron are also a married couple. Ten care assistants work on a rota but they do not work particularly with either day or residential patients. As the deputy warden explained: 'We provide sustenance for people to live in their own community. It brings outside interests in for the residents. It prepares people for when they have to come in as residents.'

All the users at Circle House are able to feed themselves and get to the toilet alone and walk. Users come once a week; there is very little turnover: only two users had left in the previous year, because they did not like the unit.

STAFFING THE CENTRES

At St Mark's, nursing staff and volunteers are allocated by rota to work for six weeks at a time with the day attenders. Then they are transferred to care for the residents in the hospice. The rationale for this is that it allows staff to get to know the patients in the day unit and then follow them up when they are admitted to the hospice for terminal care. Arts and crafts programmes are provided and users each day choose from a range of about ten activities. There is a daily social programme of bingo and games and also a treatment programme: medication, physiotherapy, occupational therapy, general and special nursing care.

By contrast, at Circle House the staff work with both residents or day users and divide their time each day as best they can between them. Circle House places much less emphasis on the users doing things than at St Mark's. About two users each day bring knitting from home, there is a weekly bingo group and medication and nursing care is provided for one or two users. All users interviewed at Circle House had spent most of their time 'doing nothing at all' in the previous week, whereas most of the users at St Mark's spent most time doing arts and crafts.

TALKING TO USERS

The most striking difference in the approach of the staff in the two centres was the amount of time they spent each week talking to the users. At St Mark's an average of over a quarter of the working week was said to be spent by staff talking to users. At Circle House the average time in the working week spent in personal talks between the staff and the users was very slight (7 per cent). In fact, at St Mark's, talking to users was the activity at which staff spent the *most* time: this ranked ahead of injections and other treatments or administration. At Circle House, talking to users was the thing at which the staff spent *least* time. Administration, domestic and physical care activities, supervising the users, all came before spending time talking with them.

CONTACT WITH FAMILY AND COMMUNITY

The day centres at St Mark's and Circle House have heads with very different attitudes to the world outside the unit. For example, the head of St Mark's claims that the unit has contact with the family of each user at least monthly. Families are invited to visit the day unit (particularly when the user first comes to the day unit) and also to keep in touch with a member of staff specially designated for that purpose, the community liaison nursing sister. Once the day user is admitted to the hospice, the family can help care for him or her. But at Circle House, however, contact with the families of users is rare: for example, of the fifteen current users, the family of one is known to the unit and this contact takes place only intermittently. In fact the head of Circle House nominated 'relatives' as one of his chief frustrations and complained: 'Relatives can be a problem, usually they have a guilt complex.'

Apart from families, outside visitors are much more common at St Mark's than at Circle House. Visits from the area specialist in community medicine, district nurses, students, chaplains, visitors from other parts of the country or overseas and local volunteers are regular and at least monthly. At Circle House in the previous twelve months some schoolchildren and the district nurse paid regular visits. But aside from a visit from a student and a local councillor, no one else had visited Circle House from the outside world.

THE USERS AND THE CENTRES

One factor absent at St Mark's and present at Circle House was conflict between the day attenders and the residents. At St Mark's, where the day users had separate staff and facilities, no such conflict was mentioned. Day users were encouraged to visit the inpatients and talk to them and vice versa: but each group had its own defined 'territory'. At Circle House, however, there was a clash between users and residents, as the following comments from the head of Circle House indicated: 'Basically we are *residential* and the place is geared more to them. It is difficult when you are a combined centre [day and residential]. Residents tend to resent the day people . . . We discourage quarrelling . . . We haven't enough experience really of day care.'

At St Mark's, on the basis of comments made about what the centre had done for them, three of the five users interviewed were rated as 'improved' (that is, the attendance at the unit enabled the user to do some activity or meant he had progressed by attendance at the unit). By contrast none of the Circle House users were defined as having improved. Four of the six were 'maintained', that is, the unit had kept them going, and two had not progressed: in fact they had *deteriorated* since coming to the unit. The following comments compare a user rated as 'improved' at St Mark's with a user rated as 'maintained' at Circle House. A 63-year-old widow who lived alone (her only daughter was in the USA) suffered from cancer of the breast and the brain. She had been coming to St Mark's for twelve months and she said:

Before I came to the day centre I tried to commit suicide. I didn't know what to expect here, I thought I'd be out in a box, I said I don't want to be shut away, I thought it would be geriatrics. But it's given me a new lease of life, it's given me a life, I wait for my day here to come. On Tuesday we do modelling, it's given me something to live for and nothing is too much trouble for them. I was going to drown myself, that is all over now. Working for this place is the most important thing we can do. I'd do anything for this place. I made progress in my health, I've gone from wheelchair to calipers to a stick. The [church] services here are lovely, they encourage you and give you hope . . . I was telling a nurse I was frightened of dying and they were really reassuring. I've seen three people die here and its nothing, they just go to sleep: that was very comforting.

A 76-year-old woman who lived alone and described her problems as 'poor memory' could not remember how long ago she had come to Circle House. She said:

When I'm by myself I'm sort of confused, I go to the shops and forget my way home and have to ask somebody. I like coming here: I meet people and talk to them. It's helped me quite a lot, it's a change from sitting alone.

DISCUSSION

Day care which shares the site of an institution can offer a service which is either 'integrated' or 'segregated' (Edwards and Sinclair, 1980). An 'integrated' service is that where day attenders share services, especially space and staff, with the residents. In other words, if the day attenders share the lounge, the dining rooms, the toilets and staff with the residents, leaving only the bedrooms as the residents' private space, the service is 'integrated'.

By contrast, a 'segregated' service offers day attenders separate facilities from the residents. Where the day attenders had a separate sitting room and a separate place for the midday meal, where there were separate toilet facilities and separate staff allocated to the day attenders, the service was said to be 'segregated'.

This cleavage between segregated and integrated facilities developed from examining the patterns of care in residential homes in local authorities (Edwards and Sinclair, 1980). But it applies to other day facilities too. Thus Circle House, the day unit in the residential home, is 'integrated', whilst St Mark's, the day centre attached to the hospice, is 'segregated'. These case studies amplify the information discussed in Chapter 3.8 on mixed centres which indicate that when the facilities of two user groups are separate there are fewer difficulties between the user groups.

The aim of preparing people to live in an institution is a complex matter. No conclusions can be drawn from such abbreviated case studies, but one issue which distinguishes the two centres is the degree of choice that users have, first, about what they do in the day centre and second, about whether or not users are admitted to the institution. At St Mark's the user has an active choice about his activities in the centre and also about whether he would prefer to be nursed at hospital or at home. Equal effort is invested in supporting these choices by keeping a user at home (if he wants this) or in admitting him to the hospice (if he wants that). No such choices are available at Circle House. A further implication from the case of St Mark's is that preparing old people for entering institutions cannot be separated from the aim of preparing people for death. At St Mark's it is valid to prepare the user for death because of the finite prognosis of the user. But in a day centre in an old people's home, is it quite as legitimate to prepare users for death rather than living? A real choice would imply that the user would be able to choose to continue at home by having the back-up services to support this decision.

More elderly users of day care in residential homes die – for whatever reason – than their counterparts in social services community-based day centres. Although this study has no evidence about the rates at which people die after they are admitted to residential homes, findings from other studies indicate that moving old people into residential homes is associated with increased mortality and morbidity, particularly if the move is related to meanings of 'loss' for the user (Tobin and Lieberman, 1976). Whether or not loss is modified or exacerbated by moving old people into an environment already known to them through attendance at a day centre is not known. Perhaps it depends, in part at least, on the *meaning* that attendance at the day centre has for them and the subsequent move has for them? In other words, if the experience of day care is constructive and users have a choice about whether they stay at home or are admitted to the same institution, perhaps the feeling of loss may be minimised? This deserves further exploration.

NOTES

1 Eight of the ten staff worked in units in the 'true' interviewing sample. Another two came from a unit added to the interviewing sample as an 'extra' because it was an unusual example of day care, offering a service to people with terminal malignancies However, for the purposes of this survey it was classified as 'mixed', because it also provided day care for adults with chronic physical handicaps: see Chapter 3.8.
2 These two day units were selected as examples because at least half the staff and users of each were interviewed.

REFERENCES

Edwards, C. and Sinclair, I. A. C. (1980) Debate: Segregation versus Integration *Social Work Today*, Vol. 11 No. 40 p. 19–21.
Tobin, S. S. and Lieberman, M. A. (1976) *Last Home for the Aged* (Jossey Bass).

PART THREE

Chapter 16

QUESTIONS OF SATISFACTION

Chapters 4 to 15 indicate that the aims of heads and staff in day units contain themes around which people organise their means and ends. What this implies is that the aims of those in day units are less of a blueprint for immediate or long-term action, than an *understanding* around which the events – and non-events – in day units shape themselves. But we cannot leave the aims of heads and staff without reviewing one further issue. Nearly all the aims look 'inward': apart from rehabilitation, few relate either to the world outside the unit or to the process of putting the user in it. In fact, occasionally staff suggest that the day unit itself is the outside world: as in the case of that aim which strives to keep people out of hospital. Here the day unit is viewed as the same thing as the outside world and the institution such as the mental hospital becomes the setting from which the user should be protected.

On this basis, the aims of staff can be viewed as 'external' (that is, they direct users to the outside world), or 'internal' (in that they confine their vision to the four walls of the day unit) or a mixture of both. With this criterion in mind, there is an imbalance of the 'internal' aim over the 'external'. Only 2 per cent of the aims outlined for the unit by heads and staff might be described as external while over two-thirds can be classified as internal.[1] Contrast the internal aim, mentioned first, with the external aim which follows. Both examples are taken from heads of units for the physically handicapped.

Internal

This centre provides a place with a change of environment from their homes. It gives a change of company; it broadens their scope socially. We give the physically handicapped a sense of well-being here: the centre gives their lives a greater fulfilment by having available various craft outlets for them to express themselves in full.

External

Basically we attend to the needs of the handicapped persons and their families as a whole. We want to discuss with the family about the mortgage, etc., then we try to get the person back into the community so there is no need for this place. We want to cater totally for the individual. One way is to try to get further education for such people in existing technical colleges.

But not all heads and staff could be described as either 'internal' or 'external'. For nearly two out of every ten staff, the aims are 'mixed', that is, an amalgam of both the internal and the external. Then another group – almost one in ten – indicated that they were reconciled to keeping the user inside the unit, but that it was their intention to influence the user's life outside the day unit, for example on evenings and at weekends. If he could be helped to post a letter or go to a shop on Saturdays, something was achieved. This view in particular related to those who worked with the mentally handicapped. A staff member in the day hospital for the terminally ill said: 'We look after people who need companionship and medical treatment. Handicrafts give users something to do and also something to take home and do. This is important as some of them are on their own . . . By making things, they feel useful and are not put on the scrap heap; they get great pleasure from that.'

How does the direction of the aims of day units as seen by the staff relate to what users get out of coming to the day units, if anything? Some got quite a bit, as we shall see, but what is generally missing in their accounts is a commentary on the effect of going to a day unit on their lives outside the unit. Their lives away from the unit must constitute two-thirds of their week if they come every day: more if they come less often. Nevertheless, in reporting what the day unit had done for them, twenty-four of every twenty-five users reported that the influence of the day unit was confined to the day unit itself.[2] Amongst the exceptions, those few users who related the influence of the day unit to everyday life were users found in family centres. A father reported: 'The centre had helped me to work out all my bills and that. Now, at home, we say we'll pay that and then that, and then we'll have a pound or two left over.'

At the other extreme, other users commented on the value of the day unit as a refuge. For example: 'There's a temptation to come here and to isolate oneself from the outside world', said a 30-year-old attending a social services day centre for the mentally ill. 'You can forget economic, political and aesthetic life with friends and others.'

If we accept that most users saw the gains accrued from coming to the day unit as confined to the day unit itself, what things did users say that coming to the day unit had done for them? The point made most often was that coming to the unit helped them by giving users social contacts, friendship, or company with other people. For just under half, the unit influenced their relationships with other users and, for the elderly, the elderly confused, the mentally ill, the physically handicapped, families and offenders, this was the foremost thing that coming to the unit had achieved for them. The following comments are selected at random. First, a 70-year-old woman speaks at a voluntary centre for the elderly: 'This place has enabled me to make friends, to get to know people. I've lived here since I was thirty-eight but I know far more people now, since I've been coming here.'

Or take this middle-aged woman in a day centre for the mentally ill: 'It's helped me a lot here – I'm a person who likes people and mixing with people. I hate my own company. My husband is very introverted and I'm extroverted and if this place shuts down I'm sure I'd land up in hospital.'

The second thing the unit had done for over a third of the users was to make some difference as to how the user felt about himself or herself. According to the second largest group of users, coming to the unit had affected matters such as self-confidence, self-esteem or feeling settled. This is an elderly woman attending a mixed centre for the elderly and children: 'This place has made me feel happier because otherwise I'd be at home all day – it stops me being snappy.'

Or consider this statement retailed by a 21-year-old man who went five days each week to a centre for the mentally handicapped: 'This place has made me feel I could take things at my own pace. I'm very slow at picking things up. People get cross with me but here they understand and know I do my best.'

In short, most users got the most from the personal and interactive aspects of the day unit and for some, of course, both things went together.[3] But a third aspect in the reckoning of users about what the unit had done for them was help in the matter of dealing with time. The way that the staff deal with time is discussed in Chapter 9, but as Chapter 13 indicates, 'signposting' time is a critical function of the day unit for some users too. It is more fundamental a matter than merely relieving boredom because it is a matter of constructing markers to provide a timetable which gives meaning to daily living activities. So a young man in a psychiatric day hospital explained: 'The day hospital gets me up in the morning and occupies my time. Nothing else.'

Said an old man, living alone, attending a day centre for the elderly: 'Coming here passes the time away, just that. While I'm doing that, I get my dinner, that's a good thing. I get my dinner then I'm off again. Everything is quite perfect for me.' Getting up and eating dinner are supposed to be normal events of a day but for some users their function is not that of providing normal routines but of providing *solutions* to the *problems* caused by having too much time.

In summary, the most important three things a day unit offered to most users is a place where one could mix with others, a place where one could promote alterations in one's view of oneself and a place which offered signposts to tracts of time. But what did the users mention least often? First, very few (3 per cent) considered that the unit gave them a role or a part to play, and those who did limited their comments to the ways in which they contributed to the smooth running of the unit. One 17-year-old girl in an adult training centre reported: 'I help Christine in the office. I collect the dinner money and take it to her.'

A second issue, rarely mentioned by users as a feature of what the unit had done for them, was the development of a skill. 'This place has improved my writing', said a 23-year-old in a centre for the mentally handicapped. 'I can enjoy writing now. I could not write my own address but Mr W. showed me how and now I can write my own address.'

Apart from asking what the unit had done for them, other ways of assessing the impact of the unit were sought. Would a user recommend the day unit to someone else in the same situation? Four out of every five would do so. The groups containing the highest proportion of users who would recommend the place to others are the families, the elderly and the mentally ill. These comments are culled from each group.

'Yes, I have recommended it already', said an old lady in a voluntary centre. 'People are so friendly. I have someone to chat to there, there's no need to be alone.'

'Yes, it's a good place to discuss things if you have any difficulty and that', said another in a family centre.

'Definitely', said the user of a psychiatric day hospital. 'Because it's enabled me to have my treatment and continue to live at home. I've just bought a new flat . . .'

'Yes, I would', said a physically handicapped user. 'I think it's good for you, it brings you out of yourself. It helps you to concentrate, occupies your mind.'

A third method of assessing what users thought of the units was to ask whether they enjoyed the time they spent at the day unit. Two of every three users enjoyed 'all of it'. The groups registering this enjoyment were first the elderly, followed by those in mixed centres and then the families.

Three other ways of assessing how users felt about the unit were attempted. The first was simply to ask users if they were satisfied. Eighty-eight per cent of the 888 users were. Those in centres for the elderly, in mixed centres, in family centres and those for the mentally ill contained the higher number of satisfied 'customers'. Second, it seemed of interest to assess not only whether people *said* they were satisfied, but how they sounded when they said it. On this basis, nearly three in four of the users sounded 'positive' when they said they were 'satisfied'.[4]

The third method was to rate whether or not the user had improved. Coming to the unit was an improvement for one in six users. They were enabled to do some activity or had progressed beyond a baseline they defined present at entry to the unit. On the other hand, maintenance, which meant being 'kept going', was the outcome rated for one in two of the users. One in twelve of the users mentioned that the day unit had prevented an event or condition which the user expected to affect him adversely and in these cases, prevention was said to have taken place. And where a user said that the day unit had done nothing for him at all or he indicated that he had deteriorated since coming, a negative impact was rated. This happened for one in ten users.

How can 'improvement' be illustrated? 'Improvement' was thought to have taken place if the user indicated progress had been achieved during the time of day centre attendance. For example, starting from a defined baseline, this user attending a mixed centre made it clear that he had shown an improvement in himself. He commented: 'I've learned a lot more about myself and this has given me a better insight into other people's problems as well. It's helped me to have an interest. Otherwise I would have been around the streets and gone full circle and got depressed again.'

Similarly, this woman attending an adult training centre who suffered brain damage after an accident at birth claimed: 'Coming here has made me stand up for myself. I was always very shy, now I'm not so shy. It's made me more or less able to stand on my two feet.'

On the other hand, other users stated that the unit had maintained them. They indicated that the virtue of the unit was to have kept them going, either personally, socially or physically. One physically handicapped attender put it this way: 'Well, I can't call them all friends here but they are all friendly. I've met different people and this is more pleasant than being at home.'

A user at a day hospital for the mentally ill assessed the day hospital like this: 'It hasn't cured me of mental illness but it helps me to occupy my time. My mental health is still in a quandary and I'm still getting over it. I have attended the doctor and still have to take medications. The drugs help but have side effects that make you shake. The staff are quite nice here.'

For some users, attendance at the day unit had stopped or avoided the occurrence or recurrence of an adverse event or condition which the user would have expected to happen or happen again. An 80-year-old woman at a day centre sponsored by a voluntary agency asserted: 'It gave me something to live for when my husband died three years ago. I think I'd be dead without it.'

A man attending a day hospital for the mentally ill said: 'When I was at home, I used to drink a lot, I got depressed very badly. Coming here has snapped me out of it and I've stopped drinking, so I feel a lot less depressed. I don't feel as lonely as I did, now I have something to look forward to every day. I couldn't have pulled out of it on my own.'

What this chapter indicates is that by every measure used, far more users felt favourably disposed towards coming to the unit than the reverse. But 'how favourably' did, in part, depend on what the users were asked about, as the following list indicates:

- 66 per cent of users volunteered that they had enjoyed 'all of it';
- 80 per cent would recommend the unit to someone 'in the same situation';
- 84 per cent listed at least one thing that 'coming to the unit' had done for them;
- 88 per cent said they were, 'on the whole, satisfied'.

Turning from the statements volunteered by users, to the way researchers rated them:

- 73 per cent were rated as expressing that they were satisfied, in a 'positive' tone of voice;
- 89 per cent were rated as having 'improved', been 'maintained' or as having had an adverse event 'prevented' by coming to the unit.

Table 16.1 User Assessments of Day Units: Rank order

Users' assessment	Mental Handicap[a]	Mental Illness	Physical Handicap	Elderly	Elderly Confused	Families	Offenders	Mixed Centres
				User group				
User enjoys all of it (range: 25–83%)	7	6	5	1	2	4	8	2
User would recommend the place to someone (range: 70–96%)	8	3	5	2	4	1	7	6
User listed something the unit had done for him (range: 83–97%)	6	3	7	1	3	2	7	5
User is satisfied (range: 83–98%)	8	6	3	1	3	2	7	5
Researcher's assessment								
Attendance improved, maintained or prevented adverse event (range: 78–93%)	6.5	3	5	2	4	1	8	6.5
User's tone of voice positive (range: 66–93%)	4.5	8	3	1	4.5	2	6.5	6.5

[a] Scores for the mentally handicapped are calculated on the basis of those able to answer each question.

What this suggests is that over a variety of approaches many more users were favourable about the day unit than the reverse.[5] Table 16.1 lists these different approaches in order. The groups of users with their responses are ranked from the highest (number 1) to the lowest (number 8).

So, on this basis, the elderly were most often the group favourably disposed to the day unit over the range of questions with the users in family day care second. By contrast, the mentally handicapped and the offenders were the least favourably disposed group: for they had fewer users expressing favourable comments over the range of issues than other groups. Even then, it must be remembered that eight out of ten offenders listed something the unit had done for them, although only one in four enjoyed 'everything' at the centre. And although only seven out of ten mentally handicapped users would recommend the centre to someone in the same situation, 83 per cent were 'satisfied'.

HEADS' AND STAFF SATISFACTION

No exploration of attitudes towards a service is complete without a review of what the staff see as rewarding. All heads and staff we spoke to found something satisfying about their job although it is not clear whether this was always sufficient 'trade off' to mitigate the frustration reported in the next chapter.

What defined success? On the one hand, more of those working with the mentally handicapped, the mentally ill and offenders defined their particular success in the light of being able to see 'improvement' in their users. On the other hand, more of those working for the elderly, the elderly confused, the physically handicapped, families and in mixed centres indicated that criteria for success were equivalent to 'maintaining' the users. Although the group of staff which claimed that their success lay in 'prevention' was small, more of those working with the elderly confused, the mentally ill and offenders indicated that success was prevention, for instance, preventing the user's return to an institution such as hospital or prison.

The actual sources of satisfaction and rewards is an interesting and complex matter which can be given only a cursory mention. The source of satisfaction most frequently mentioned by heads and staff was to feel that the unit met the users' 'personal' needs. Half the heads and staff said that this was the reason that they found their jobs satisfying. This was particularly the case for those in units for the elderly and the elderly confused but was less often mentioned by those in units for the mentally handicapped and physically handicapped. Second, having the unit meet the users' 'interpersonal' needs – such as requirements for company and friendship – was nominated as satisfaction by more of those working with offenders and families. But actually a consistently even number of heads and staff in all user groups (about a third) mentioned this. Third, seeing the users develop new skills was satisfying to over a quarter of staff in all groups but

was mentioned more often by those working with the mentally handicapped, the physically handicapped and offenders. A fourth source of satisfaction was a sense of 'helping'. This rather vague idea was mentioned by
over a quarter: in particular, those working with the elderly, the elderly
confused and the physically handicapped. Fifth, just under a quarter
(those working with the offenders, the physically handicapped and the
elderly predominated) saw satisfaction as the discharging of a professional or trades work skill. Sixth was the view that what was satisfying to
the heads and staff is that the unit contribute to the way the user coped
with a role in the community. Staff working with the mentally ill and those
in mixed centres subscribed to this. Equally important to satisfaction for
some was that the job met the staff member's particular personal needs.
This was particularly so for those working with the physically handicapped and the elderly and the least true for those in centres for offenders
and family day care.

These then were the main sources of satisfaction for heads and staff.
Other matters raised less often were the satisfactions accruing from
liaison and teamwork with other staff members (prominent amongst
those working with the mentally ill); the importance of improving the
physical status of users (mentioned particularly by those working with the
elderly confused and the elderly); the pleasure of being able to discharge
users from the unit (seen as rewarding by those working with the mentally
ill); and the autonomy that went with the job (a matter of more consequence to some working in family centres and with the mentally ill). The
gratitude of users was also a source of reward to those working in mixed
centres and with the elderly and the physically handicapped. Giving relief
to relatives was a source of reward mentioned by those working with the
elderly confused.

Did heads and staff get more out of giving to the users than they got in
return? Their remarks about what constituted satisfaction and success
were rated according to whether the staff indicated that their satisfactions
lay primarily in *giving* to the users, or in *receiving* from them. In all user
groups, apart from the elderly confused and offenders, more staff indicated that rewards were in what they received from the users ahead of
what they gave to the users. In other words, four out of ten staff received
something from the users which supplemented their personality ('It
broadens my outlook', 'It makes me happy') or maintained them socially
('It gives me companionship too', 'friendship as part of a team') or it gave
them a feeling of having a niche ('It gives me something useful to do', 'It
occupies my time'). Or, other staff members said that they felt good when
the users were grateful.

What the heads and staff gave to the users was defined rather more
vaguely than what they received. The three out of every ten who were
primarily 'givers' nominated just 'helping', or getting users back to community roles or discharging a particular job skill as ways of giving. But
giving to users and receiving from them was not always one way: a small
group of heads and staff, one in eight, defined their rewards as an

amalgam of giving and receiving. Neither entirely 'givers' nor wholly 'getters', these were, after their own account, called the 'exchangers'.

DISCUSSION

One interesting feature of day services is that both staff and users live at home, or elsewhere, and meet only during the day. Neither the worst evils of 'total' institutions, nor the non-communication described by commentators who observe brief encounters in clinics or area offices are the routine of relationships between users and staff in day units. In day services, the potential of achieving contacts which are satisfying to users and also the staff may be more feasible than either in the 'total' institution (where users are more powerless simply because they cannot leave) or in the clinic or fieldwork team (where repeated research shows that staff and users talk past each other because of misunderstandings and clashes in perspective and class). One of the interesting outcomes in this evidence is that what users and staff independently report as rewarding come down to much the same thing. A consistent area of reward for both related to meeting the personal and interpersonal needs expressed by users.

Many reports on social or health services concentrate either on soliciting the users' point of view or that of the staff. Few are able to review both together. What validity do the views of users and staff have towards evaluating a service? The value of taking a user's view must relate to the recent growth of the consumer movement which has altered in the recent past – and may still influence in the future – the structure of relationship between staff and users. If the user is viewed as 'consumer' ahead of 'patient' or 'client' this gives his views a legitimacy quite different to the position of a recipient of a service defined as 'client' or 'patient'.[6] Client or patient relationships are often predicated on the dependence of the patient or client on the superior skills and knowledge of the staff. This approach does not account for what goes on in day units where four in ten staff admit they get a lot from the unit and its users too, in a highly personal sense. So we cannot view the staff as neutral figures who can view their users' difficulties with olympian detachment, since it is clear that staff have personal needs too.

We sought the views of heads and staff as a corrective to a common emphasis which seeks only the views of the 'top people' of organisations. On the other hand, we cannot assume that the views of heads and staff on their own are an unequivocal mandate for change. The old dictum 'hospitals are run for the staff' is one extreme example. In practice, however, this is not a particular problem in this instance as there is not much conflict between the views of heads, staff and users, either about the rewards they get from the unit or about what they want changed: matters to be taken up by the next chapter.

A third entrant to the assessment of satisfaction is the writer who, by now, one might say, has seen as many day units as she has eaten hot dinners. She has reviewed a census of 290 day units and read the comments of nearly 1,500 heads, staff and users, some of whom she interviewed. In the process she has visited hundreds of day units. In one sense, it is pleasing that the head, staff and users see so much in common. But does this contribute greatly to a desired state of affairs in day services? For example, to leave this book on this note would be to conclude that because most heads, staff and users view the aims of the unit as 'internal' this is desirable. Whilst this may represent the *current* state of affairs, we need to *question* whether this is 'desirable'. Chapter 18 will make it clear that this cannot be regarded as desirable in all circumstances.

It needs to be remembered too that most users of day units must be 'satisfied' to some extent. After all, they still go to the day unit; they do not represent those who have left the day unit because they are dissatisfied. According to heads, more users in units for the elderly (especially in day units in residential homes, in family day centres and units for the physically handicapped) came and then left, because they did not like the unit. (It is worth setting this against the finding that the elderly users and the families were the two groups who were most satisfied.) Leaving the unit because the user did not like it accounted for very few of the overall number of discharges in the previous twelve months but the figures provided are probably an underestimate, and consist only of those users brave enough to impart their unfavourable views to the head or sufficiently in conflict for their dislikes to be known.

So this chapter represents the views of those who are still in the units; those who have not made the ultimate criticism of leaving the unit. Nevertheless, users at all stages, old and new attenders, are represented, some of whom may, of course, have left as 'dissatisfied' users after the research. The unknown question is whether those users left in day units are *really* those who like the day unit well enough to stay, or those with little other social alternative and, perhaps, more pressure on them to come to the unit, either from their families or other agents such as social workers and doctors? These may well be points of some importance to take into account in the future in evaluating the satisfaction of all groups.

The degree to which the satisfaction of users relates to their previous expectations is another interesting question: if a user expected the worst from the day unit before he started and then found his fears unfounded, is he likely to be more satisfied than a user who expects a lot from the unit and who is disappointed? But low expectations followed by a good experience do not entirely explain the attitudes of day unit users, for more of them claimed, albeit in retrospect, to have had more positive expectations about going to the day unit than negative ones.

There are two further difficulties. One is what expressing satisfaction actually means. For a start, most surveys tend to show that high levels of satisfaction exist on almost anything that social scientists care to investigate (Gutek, 1978). Second, does saying that one is satisfied mean that users think that the unit is effective? Or is it that users are acquiescent? By 'acquiescent' one wonders if they weigh up this day unit experience against all possible alternatives and indicate that the day unit is either, at the worst, the best of a bad job, or (more favourably) the best of an available lot? Some users were not acquiescent. They expressed positive and some very negative comments about the unit and still decided they were satisfied. Does this ability to evaluate mean they thought the unit was effective? This applied to a number of the offenders and partly, one suspects, because more staff in their day units encouraged and rewarded expressions of honesty and criticism as evidence of personal growth.

All we know for certain is that most users have given, at the very least, a favourable endorsement of their day units. Others offered favourable and unfavourable views about the day unit almost in the same breath, indicating that it is quite possible to feel satisfied and dissatisfied at the same time. It is probably accurate to point out that enjoyment and satisfaction are not the same thing, since more users express satisfaction than enjoyment with the unit: the offenders are a case in point. This introduces the subject matter of the next chapter because, as we shall see, whatever the implications of expressed satisfaction, it cannot be interpreted as a mandate from users, staff and heads as an endorsement of the *status quo* of day units or as an indication that nothing in day units needs to be changed.

NOTES

1 Of those users able to answer the question, nearly three-quarters described the aims of the day unit as internal.
2 It is impossible to predict the influence that interviewing users away from the unit might have had: interviews at home might have jogged the users' memory about things the unit had achieved in the user's life outside the day unit.
3 Some improvements, such as confidence and friendliness, may well generalise outside the unit.
4 A further 10 per cent were rated as sounding 'neutral' and 15 per cent sounded 'negative'. During training, interviewers were trained to recognise 'positive' from 'negative' and 'neutral' tones of voice from prepared recordings. High inter-rater reliability was obtained on these exercises. The interviews with a stratified sample of 8 per cent of users were observed by a third party, either a researcher or a field supervisor who rated the user's tone in reply to the question of satisfaction. Blind ratings were compared: inter-rater agreement was obtained in 73 per cent of cases. The method used was adapted from that described by Brown and Rutter (1964) who advocated using aspects of speech as an independent measure in an attempt to amplify self-reports about feelings and to report the emotion expressed in the interview.
5 The extent to which these measures tested independent constructs is not known.
6 Researchers who view their respondents as consumers are more likely to consider their account of an event as sufficient in itself. Viewing the respondent as a patient or client – as in much psychiatric or prison research – is likely to have the researcher looking for external measures such as recidivism rates of validity and reliability rather than user opinion.

REFERENCES

Brown, G. W. and Rutter, M. (1966) 'The measurement of family activities and relationships: a methodological study', *Human Relations*, 19, pp. 241–63.
Gutek, B. (1978) 'Strategies for studying client satisfaction', *Journal of Social Issues*, 34, 8, pp. 44–56.

Chapter 17

ROOM FOR IMPROVEMENT

This chapter will present the spontaneous comments of users and staff about the improvements they suggest for their day units. These represent issues which users and staff have recommended as possible improvements for day services. Their suggestions are not a numerical estimate of staff and user opinions, and for information about how many back or oppose a point, the reader should turn to other evidence.[1] The issues discussed in this chapter represent those matters which at least some users and staff felt *very strongly* about. By a happy coincidence, they coincide with some issues the writer would like to be considered as possible changes to day services.

The previous chapter indicated that satisfaction did not necessarily imply agreement with the way things were. Nearly half the users suggested improvements to the units but only one in seven expressed their views as part of a complaint. Likewise, nearly all heads and staff found some aspect of their job at the unit satisfying but, at the same time, eight out of ten found some aspect of working at the unit frustrating. Almost everyone wanted some change to the policy or the practices of the service.

This chapter will, first, explore the content of each 'improvement'; second, comment on the issues the improvements raise; third, summarise a checklist; and fourth, comment on the way other day units have tackled similar problems. The chapter deals with suggestions from heads, staff and users from all user groups and all service providers. This is not meant to imply that all suggestions apply equally – or at all – to each day unit: the reader will need to select his own priorities.

Six areas of improvement have been summarised in Table 17.1. Changes to the programme will be discussed first and reforms to the organisation last, the order reflecting the priorities of the users. Of course, in one sense the dividing line between these topics is very thin – changes to the programme may mean changes to the organisation too.

I Improve the Programme

What improvements would one in every four users and one in every four heads and staff make to the programme? They want to alter (in this order) the work activities, the social programme, the treatment programme, the arts and crafts activities, the schedule of meetings and discussion groups,

Table 17.1 *Improvements to the Unit*

The users say:			*The heads and staff say:*		
1 Improve the:	programme	(25%)	Improve the:	organisation	(41%)
2 " "	users and	(16%)	" "	staff	(37%)
	their regime				
3 " "	building	(12%)	" "	users	(28%)
4 " "	facilities	(11%)	" "	programme	(25%)
5 " "	staff	(8%)	" "	building	(23%)
6 " "	organisation	(2%)	" "	facilities	(23%)

and the education activities. Detailed information about this provision is outlined in Edwards and Carter (1980).

1.1 WORK

Four out of every ten day units provided users with contract and industrial work and the main comment about its content was that it was tedious and boring. Heads, staff and users asked for more variety and scope, a better organised flow of work, and work which had personal significance. Users and staff in units for the mentally and physically handicapped predominated in these complaints.

'Find me different and more interesting work', said a 35-year-old deaf woman, who had spent the previous week packing plastic toys in boxes. 'Doing all the same things get on your nerves. Can't we make the toys, or do something different?'

Another group of users complained less of the lack of variety than about periods of time doing nothing, for there was often no work available. They criticised a management which did not seem to be able to organise the flow of work so it kept people busy. According to a middle-aged man in a sheltered workshop: 'Time drags on quite a lot here. A day seems longer here than when I was at work. It's because there's not sufficient work to do. Mornings are the worst – after lunch the time goes quicker.'

Periods of inactivity were confirmed by some staff who indicated that one function of contract work was to occupy their users. Without this occupation, disorder and disruption were dangers in the unit. 'When you have no industrial work, you just don't know what to do with them when they are all arguing and fighting', said a woman instructor at a training centre. The implication that the function of contract work should be to keep users quiet was argued against by younger staff members and a related issue, that the demands of processing contract work prevented staff from helping the users, was raised. An instructor in a training centre complained: 'I have to spend too much time on gnome production, which means I'm not giving enough time to the lower grades, the ones who are not as capable. It's so overcrowded and the general attitude here is wrong. Very few trainees will even be employed outside. We should be geared to help our people cope with life rather than outside employment.'

Investing the work programme with significance and meaning interested some users and staff. 'If only we could make toys for children or somesuch', mused an ex-offender. 'We could help children in hospital or give some kind of community service to give us a purpose in life.' In this connection, a young, physically handicapped man was interested in the economics of work co-operatives. 'Why can't we work on self-supporting projects?' he said. 'Something to help the NHS would at least benefit society.' Project work was supported by some staff members concerned about the lack of interest and variety in the work. 'Why don't we think of project work?' said an instructor in a training centre. 'Maybe running a small farm or even a project making childrens' clothes.'

For another group of users, the whole idea of contract work was suspect, because they considered that it exploited people with low bargaining power and little social and economic 'clout'. An ex-mental hospital patient in a work centre said: 'It's exploitation, using the ex-mental patient as cheap labour, making them work any length of hours without being paid.' Amplifying this, a physically handicapped user said, 'I could and should get more for jobs, more for outside jobs. I reckon I'm out of pocket at the end of the week. When I take out my travelling expenses, it's not really fair.' This issue was of concern to some staff too. A manager of a sheltered workshop, housed in an old and leaking building, commented: 'Disabled people come here to work in all weathers and with all ailments and earn a very low wage. Some perfectly fit people draw more money from social security for staying home all day.'

Other users criticised the poor teaching of job skills, inadequate supervision of work and lack of individual assessment which might fit a user to a job. A further grievance was that day units did not accommodate users' individual skills or tastes. 'They could have given me something I liked to do', complained a 19-year-old in a 'mixed' industrial centre for the handicapped, 'like working with wood or something.'

Some users resented the lowly payments offered in return for contract work and wanted this changed.[2] Finally, there was feeling by users that work offered by the unit was dead end and that it did not relate to that most common hope expressed by most users, a job 'outside' the unit: 'I thought they would give you help to find a job but they don't'; 'I think it should be more of a job assessment centre where I could be put through certain jobs to occupy me. I'd like to see more industrial training, but they just don't have the money to do it on any scale.'

A COMMENT ON WORK

Fundamental questions are raised by work in day units, yet there has been minimal exploration of its meaning. One important question sidestepped is whether work in day units should parallel the opportunities, choices and variety of work experiences and industrial practices outside.

Of two approaches to this, one could be labelled 'unrealistic' because it assumes that users should have choices. This starts from the assumption that the mentally ill, the mentally handicapped, the physically disabled and the elderly are excluded from the workforce by individual, social and economic constraints outside their personal, social and economic control. Since users cannot be held accountable for their physical or mental handicap, their low education or unemployment, there is no reason why their job opportunities in day units should not parallel the interest and variety of the outside work. Against this, others argue that users who cannot compete on the labour market can only be expected to be given the jobs commensurate with their low economic value. Day units with a work programme adopt this view, since they offer simple manual routine tasks in a factory atmosphere.

The alternative view of work might be defined as an attempt to reinstate the 'craft' ethic against the dominance of the 'production' ethic. This could be viewed also as those things which staff try to get out of their work: in other words, the 'craft ethic' is a view applying to non-manual artistic or intellectual work where the supreme concern is with the quality of the product and the skill of its making (Fox, 1971). The worker (or user) must 'own' the product psychologically, by his skill, blood, sweat and toil. This does not mean the work is always rewarding but the worker sees any drudgery as part of the context because the work is part of the development of skills and of himself as a person. In the 'craft ethic' there is no divorce between work and leisure, the discipline learned is self-discipline. Thus work in day units should cater for the individual user's interests and offer the 'self-actualisation' opportunities that staff claim to get and that work *might* do in the wider society. But few alternatives to simple manual work have yet been explored by day units.

WORK: SOME SUGGESTIONS

(1) Study the pros and cons of user co-operatives: such ventures would meet many of the criticisms and dissatisfactions of the current structure of work in day units. For example, an analysis of a common ownership venture amongst disabled people in South Wales considered its technical and financial problems (Hadley, undated). Morale and involvement by workers and 'staff' (who, in this context, become workers) was high. But its needs to be recognised that such ventures are unlikely to be totally financially self-supporting.

Work: a Checklist

Can You . . .

---

1. . . . provide individual work assessments to determine user interests and capacities?
2. . . . concentrate on learning what users want out of work? It is clear that many users and staff want work to be a more productive personal experience.
3. . . . provide more *variety* and *scope* in work? Encourage more user discretion and allow the users to proceed to learn more complex work skills?
4. . . . improve the *flow* of work and try to reduce the amount of time spent doing nothing?
5. . . . explore the financial risk in starting possible co-operative projects which might be partially self-supporting?
6. . . . provide work with more obvious training functions? Many users want to do work which can be linked clearly to future jobs outside the unit. Contract work, if it is used, needs to be tied to a personal plan for each user.
7. . . . support a public investigation into the present methods of reimbursement for work which takes the question of the economic exploitation of disabled workers, and the disincentive to take the leap from statutory benefits to wages as its terms of reference.?

---

(2) The Maudsley Psychiatric Day Hospital has established its own sheltered workshop, as one outlet for some users from the day hospital (Bennett, 1972).

(3) In Sweden, some disabled non-manual workers are employed on archive work; special schemes developing out of relief work in the 1930s employ workers on clerical jobs. For example, in addition to its ordinary staff employed as guards, craftsman and clerical workers, a museum may have forty disabled people subsidised by government as archive workers. A special form of these are clerical sheltered work settings called 'Office Work Centres' (Eriksson, 1975).

(4) An enclave of mentally handicapped workers established in a small packaging company in the midlands has been a social success for the council and the firm. Its financial repercussions for users are less successful since they cannot be paid above the social security disregard limit (Stanley, 1975).

(5) A local authority day unit for the mentally ill pays users for 'work'. But work is described in the most intriguing way. Users 'work' if they are on the users' committee, if they help to make a video film of the unit, if they do the clerical and administrative work for the unit, if they make leather bags or pottery for the unit's shop or (lastly and more conventionally) if they do contract assembly work for outside

industry. (All these activities except the last would more usually be defined as 'non-work' by most day units).

(6) Community service work is one type of short-term work pursued for younger patients at a psychiatric day hospital. A small number of patients are allocated a certain number of days per week to work with community projects, such as helping with adult literacy schemes.

(7) Consider the commercial production and marketing of an art or craft: this will be discussed at greater length under the section on arts and crafts.

(8) As an interim measure, while the levels of payments to users continue to be constrained by supplementary benefit rules, users could be consulted about the disbursement of monies. For example, one centre of middle-aged physically handicapped users prefer to save its small profits and then to spend them on 'joint' group outings, for example, on a visit to a restaurant, rather than to allow each individual to 'earn' the allowed maximum of £2 per week.[3]

1.2 SOCIAL ACTIVITIES

Although a staff member in a voluntary centre for the elderly said, 'We need more fun in the place', users were clearer than staff about what they wanted from social activities. Three-quarters of the units provided some kind of social programme and users raised two themes for reform: first, more feeling of involvement in social activities, and second, a livelier atmosphere were requested. On the point of more involvement, one patient in a psychiatric day hospital said: 'I think it should be more informal and have more active participation. People should not just watch, but dance. Patients should be encouraged to get out of themselves more.'

Things should be more lively and cheerful. 'People just sit around in twos. The atmosphere is a bit gloomy and there's nothing going on. It's not anyone's fault. It's just a shortage of staff', said a user, again in a psychiatric day hospital. 'There should be more dancing and girls', said a mentally handicapped youth hopefully. Staff were not impervious to the gloom conveyed by desultory social programmes either. A young man, staffing a family day centre, said: 'More social variety would help. I'm a bit bored and the pace is too slow for me.' An occupational therapist in a day hospital said: 'I badly need some new ideas: I go over the same activities time and time again.'

More of those users recommending changes to the social programme were in mixed centres, units for the physically handicapped and the mentally ill. Requests for more outings, more opportunities for physical exercise and a greater range of indoor activities had interesting rationales. For example, the common request for more outings, out and away from the unit, was impelled by two separate motives. First, a need to get outside into the world was mentioned by the elderly and disabled who otherwise were very restricted in their movements. 'Let's try to have trips out', said a 23-year-old man in a centre for the physically handicapped. 'Help us get out of the place for a bit. The staff need it as well; we are all cooped up here together.' Second, a desire for outings to cultural and educational activities was a disguised request for more learning opportunities. Said a 44-year-old woman in a psychiatric day hospital: 'We could have outings sometimes and be stimulated. Let's try something more adventurous than being confined to this community.'

Day units did very little to help their users, often badly handicapped, to discharge surplus physical energy, some users considered. Brisk walks are unfashionable but: 'It would help the younger ones to kick a ball around or play rounders', said a 49-year-old policeman being treated for depression at a day hospital.

'If only there was a swimming pool in the garden for us handicapped', sighed one user, restricted by the fact that the units assisting users to discharge physical energy by sports were adult training centres (although two-thirds of the psychiatric day hospitals offered keep fit or relaxation classes as part of 'treatment'.) 'Little things which are important are ignored here. A punchbag in the gym would be a good way of letting off steam', said one psychiatric day hospital user.

A greater range of indoor activities, whether inside or outside the day unit, was wanted. Trips to the cinema and theatre would be helpful: 'I'd like to go to the theatre but no one has suggested it', said a user living alone who went to a day hospital. Others made age-specific requests for 'entertainments' to visit the unit: concert parties for the elderly, pop groups for the younger mentally handicapped people. There was also demand for puzzles and indoor games and a man confined to a wheelchair commented: 'For folks like me who can't move about there could be more choices of games at tables we could participate in. A round table would help too.'

Underlying all these requests was an impression that users felt that it was up to the staff to initiate new activities and carry them out. Unwritten prohibitions prevented users from usurping staff territory.

COMMENTS ON SOCIAL ACTIVITIES

More careful thought about the repercussions of social and sporting activities is needed. The context is the special limitations imposed on users' lifestyles by disabilities. Once these restrictions are analysed, one might look for activities which demand either a degree of interchange with other people or an accomplishment which involves performing a skill: for example, a card game or a game of table tennis involves some exchange with another person. But watching a film or listening to a visiting concert party does not require this exchange, unless of course a discussion is held afterwards. In the same way, swimming or playing table tennis implies the possession of a skill on the user's part; but listening to records may not. By combining these two elements, the condition of interchange with others and performance of a skill, a unit might develop an index to classify its particular social and sporting activities.[4]

Some day units – especially the day hospitals – consider their commitment to 'treatment' or 'therapy' precludes the introduction of social activities. 'I don't want them to think it's a holiday camp', said one consultant psychiatrist. Occasionally, there was outright antagonism to any activity which might be fun for users: at one geriatric day hospital, the patients were seated at six feet intervals from one another so they could not talk to each other. A fear implicit within some day units which try to achieve a turnover of users is that users will become over-dependent on the unit if the atmosphere is pleasant and the activities rewarding.

Eric Midwinter (1977) has said that our philosophy is that our social and health institutions should be joyless and lacking in fun. If our health and social service programmes had developed from the spirited context of the Victorian music hall instead of the workhouse and asylum, would the same objections to enjoyment apply? Users may be just as likely to cling to units they report as sterile and boring. Limiting the concept of activity to that of treatment, whether medication, ECT or even therapy groups, is a restricted notion which those early Victorians who introduced 'moral treatment' (not moralistic treatment) to the care of the mentally ill would have found prejudiced and narrow-minded.

Social activities ought to draw out the user's interest, develop his skills and therefore his self-confidence, and show a route to taking part in community leisure acitivites, whether a theatre club, a bird-watching class or a yoga group. These comments are not a plea to avoid the sober realities of the users' problems through diets of dancing and games. But a balanced view suggests that there is a time for fun as well as for weeping in day units. One user in a psychiatric day hospital said: 'I think the people working here are too involved. Their attitude is not happy-go-lucky enough. They're too intense.'

Social Programmes: A Checklist

Can You . . .

---

1. . . . discuss ways in which a livelier atmosphere can be developed?
2. . . . investigate how users and staff can get outside the unit regularly? There needs to be a time to relax outside the unit and a time to be stimulated.
3. . . . provide more outlets for users to expend their physical energy?
4. . . . offer more opportunities for users to learn new social skills and for stimulation in their socialising?
5. . . . avoid the staff conveying the impression to users that they are the only ones sanctioned to organise activities?

SOCIAL ACTIVITIES: SOME SUGGESTIONS

(1) One voluntary day centre for old people prepares and stages an annual drama production. This plays in local old people's homes and other institutions.

(2) A psychiatric day hospital organises a weekly visit to the town to the theatre or cinema. Users go in small groups of four to six and find their own way there and back on public transport.

(3) A day centre for the elderly and physically handicapped teaches its members 'how to swim' at sessions at a council pool. A user aged 79 recently gained a swimming certificate.

(4) Some units have elected social committees to plan new social activities. A small budget helps.

(5) Users at one day centre organise a social club for former users one night a week. This has the dual function of offering current members the responsibility of devising a social programme and keeping in touch with ex-users who want to stay in touch and need the partial support of the unit. It also allows ex-users to report on life outside.

1.3 IMPROVE THE TREATMENTS

Physical treatments of various sorts by a doctor, a nurse or therapist were offered in 161 units. Only one day hospital for the mentally ill and one for the elderly claimed to offer treatment alone, without other activities. Basically, what users, heads and staff wanted was more time from doctors, more remedial therapy, more individual time from staff, better supervision of drugs and more information about their condition. These changes of course are not only requested in day hospitals. The criticisms on which they are based are endemic in health services, as the Royal Commission on the National Health Service has shown (DHSS, 1979).

Lack of time and commitment from psychiatrists was a bone of contention with users and staff. 'I dislike the medical side here, because of shortage of time and number of patients', said a 22-year-old married woman with four children. 'There's just not enough time to see the psychiatrist.'

'The doctor could have listened more to my reasons for depression other than just the symptoms', said another.

'I'd like to speak to a doctor more often.'

'There's a lack of support from the doctors.'

Heads and staff also raised the problem of the disappearing psychiatrist: [5] 'If only we had more co-operation from the doctors', said one nurse. A psychologist reiterated: 'One frustration is the lack of consideration of some staff. Consultant autonomy is taken too far: one consultant is always very late for appointments with patients and staff: he thinks he is the only person here with anything to do.'

'I find the lack of routine medical care frustrating', said a nurse in charge of a day hospital for the elderly confused. 'I have to say it: the psychiatrists are not interested in our patients or their welfare.'

Another allied series of observations from users requested more individual time from staff. 'It could have people here that you could turn to without feeling you are putting people out. They could give you a lot more guidelines on how to control or handle what is wrong with you. I don't consider I get any help here except for drug treatment' (this from a depressed 28-year-old single mother at a psychiatric day hospital).

'They need a welfare officer or padre here', said a user in a centre for the disabled. 'They should be more interested in us. They don't understand us.'

Other users indicated that the information dispensed about their condition was less than useful. 'I was here about five weeks before I saw the psychiatrist. Then it was not explained to me fully enough: I did not know what was happening.'

'When we see the doctor, they should spend more time breaking down our problems', said another. 'One can be left so to drift along.'

A few users, again in psychiatric day hospitals, considered their drug supervision to be haphazard: 'In a way, they don't pay enough attention to the effect of the drugs we are taking. They are a bit lax or easy going.'

'I think we should be able to see a doctor when possible after taking drugs', said another. 'It would help one to discuss the after-effects.'

More remedial therapy was a request from old people: more often in geriatric day hospitals – a matter discussed already in Chapter 8. 'Oh, I wish we had more lady therapists', said an old lady with a stroke.

'People with physical afflictions need exercises', commented another, a patient in a geriatric day hospital without any therapists.

'A gymnasium where we could use our arms and legs would make all the difference.'

'It's all voluntary here so you can't impose', said an old lady in a voluntary day centre. 'But there has been talk of a chiropodist coming in the afternoon. I can't reach my feet, so a chiropodist would be wonderful.'

A COMMENT ON TREATMENT

'Changing the treatment' begs difficult questions about manpower and the division of labour and it might just as easily be discussed in the section on 'Improve the Staff'. In the psychiatric day hospital, for example, it raised a particularly thorny issue: that of relations between a discipline such as psychiatry which is imbued with classic notions of professional autonomy and the other disciplines of nursing, occupational therapy, psychology and social work. Yet an organisation like a day unit has to get through a certain human workload each day and this is a task which requires considerable interdependence.

Of course, complaints were not about *all* doctors – on the contrary, staff in geriatric day hospitals seemed to appreciate their co-operative *rapport* with geriatricians. Relatively few consultants were interviewed since few worked as such in the day hospital, as opposed to running clinics. This means that psychiatrists have not been invited to report their views for change as often as their senior nursing colleagues, for instance. However, viewed from the point of view of others, psychiatrists appear to have more difficulty in establishing a role in the day hospital than the geriatricians and some reasons for this are discussed in section V, 'Improve the Staff'.

The request for more remedial therapists is discussed in Chapter 8. There is a complex interaction between manpower training, policies, regional employment patterns and of structuring available manpower while accommodating personal preferences: for example, that some therapists do not wish to work exclusively with old or chronically disabled people. Other reports have looked at these issues more comprehensively, although not in relation to day units (Donald, 1978). One issue in organising services is whether already strained services for hospital inpatients should be diluted to provide remedial staff for day hospitals, domiciliary services and the social services (Partridge and Warren, 1978). Another problem is how gaps and overlaps between therapists and other staff such as nurses should be dealt with. For example, should therapist aides be employed or therapy work diverted on to nurses? Can relatives and neighbours play a greater part in the therapeutic team?

Treatment: A Checklist

Can . . .

1. . . . psychiatrists develop a policy about their role in day services? Some options are discussed in section V.
2. . . . each user have an individual staff member to whom he or she can turn as counsellor and/or liaison officer?
3. . . . each unit consider offering more practical information about the nature of disabling conditions and, where relevant, the impact of drugs?
4. . . . more ways of compensating for shortages in remedial therapy be considered?

TREATMENT: SOME SUGGESTIONS

(1) Some day units have experimented with groups and meetings designed specifically to inform patients (and their families) about their illness, their treatments and possible side effects. This reduces the frequent problem that imparting of information is an *ad hoc* and hit and miss affair. Such groups have been tried with relatives of stroke victims (Mykyta *et al.*, 1976) and parents of handicapped children

(Carter, 1976), and offer opportunities for doctors to be involved in groups.

(2) The Barbican Day Centre (which asks 'attenders' to become 'members' by agreeing a contact between user, staff and centre) allows a user to nominate which member of a staff will be his or her counsellor.

(3) Some ways of compensating for the shortage of trained remedial therapists have been outlined in Chapter 7. Other suggestions involve introducing schemes which include:

(a) group rather than individual speech or physiotherapy;
(b) relatives' groups, so that planned treatments can be carried out at home;
(c) more encouragement of users helping each other. For example, in the Primus Day Centre, discussed in the next chapter, users with speech problems following strokes pair up with more recently afflicted victims to 'hear their new words'.

1.4 ARTS AND CRAFTS

Arts and crafts are a pervasive feature of day unit activities as three-quarters of the units offered some form of arts and crafts to users in the week before the survey. Users of family centres and those in units for mentally ill commented most on the efficacy of arts and crafts, while amongst the staff, those working with the mentally ill and the physically handicapped produced more suggestions for improvement.

User reviews of arts and crafts centred around these matters: the requirement that more users be able to follow individual interests, a view that some programmes were approached in a desultory, aimless fashion, leaving the user feeling under-extended. There were also pleas for better equipment.

Allowing users to pursue more individual pursuits was at odds with the current expectation that users should slot into whatever craft the unit offered. Some users reported little initiative on the part of the staff to find out what a user wanted to do, or what he or she was good at. 'Let the patients do what they are interested in', declared a user at a psychiatric day hospital. 'There are some things that you don't want to do. But I like art and wouldn't mind doing it all day.'

Allowing more individuality was inseparable from the available facilities. 'We need money to increase the facilities here', commented a patient in a psychiatric day hospital. 'For woodwork and pottery there just aren't the facilities for these things.'

'If OT could be in smaller rooms', said another, 'we could all concentrate better. I don't like it all in one place. I know there isn't enough money for separate cubicles and room though.'

Users were left without things to do at times. A particularly notable example of this was the centre where elderly users were asked to knit woollen squares for a quilt, which were then dismantled by the staff after the users had gone, to be knitted by the next batch of users next day. The approach to arts and crafts in many day units was criticised by younger staff with professional art training. One stated: 'There is an unenlightened, old-fashioned approach to arts and crafts here. We desperately need more money and resources.'

COMMENT

Arts and crafts are almost never regarded as paid work in the unit and few units paid users to produce them. Rather, users are expected to pay for arts and crafts materials themselves. Clearly this disparity reduces the possibility that users may regard their arts and crafts efforts as 'work', since one rationale attached to work – wages – is removed. Any comparison between industrial and contract work and arts and crafts is difficult because of different financial and symbolic rewards.

Why offer arts and crafts? If it is not work, is its prevalence in day units a reflection of the recent renewal of interest in crafts? Public dissatisfaction with mass-produced, standardised, machine-made products is well documented: do day units provide users with skills to handmake goods which are marketable?

If this is the intention, there is little evidence that it works, as a mere handful of units sell arts and crafts products and the absence of specialist art/craft teachers (only one in ten of units with arts and crafts have them) suggests that teaching users a skill is a low priority. The actual organisation of arts and craft work in day units, where most users spend very little time at any one activity, militates against the development of specialist skills. Limited sales of arts and crafts suggest insufficiently high standards and/or a lack of enterprise in tapping the appropriate markets.

If arts and crafts are not viewed as work or taught as skills, are they regarded as self-expressive therapy in either the physical or emotional sense? Do activities such as painting or pottery help individual users deal with physical or emotional difficulties? The answer is sometimes yes and sometimes no. One measure of the therapeutic intentions of service providers is the number of trained therapy staff in day units. Under half the units offering arts and crafts employed trained therapy staff, mostly occupational therapists, and very few had trained art therapists.

If arts and crafts are neither work nor skills and only sometimes seen as therapy, what is the explanation for their ubiquitous presence? A plausible explanation may be found in those units which offer both work and crafts. In those units, there is a definite balance of work over arts and crafts in terms of the number of users involved. This suggests that arts and crafts are offered as relaxation from industrial work or that they are offered to certain users as routines to 'fill in' and provide occupation. Some support was given to this because only one of the units who involved twice as many or more users in work over arts and crafts had a trained arts and crafts teacher.

A different criticism of the use of arts and crafts is what has been called the 'fruit salad' approach (Bennett, 1978). This stems from a philosophy of making up a programme which implies that users need variety each day. So the timetable switches users from one thing to another without any chance to develop concentration or continuity, let alone a skill. However, this approach is not implicit in using arts and crafts since the development of a skill requires concentration and personal discipline.

In summary, then, it is easier to suggest what arts and crafts are not doing rather than what they are intended to do, an ambiguity which provides an opportunity to ask whether arts and crafts should have the status of work which may in turn entail arts and crafts being taught as a skill. If this happens, quality control of the product will need to be introduced; although quality control is less of an issue if arts and crafts are viewed as a specific therapy. However, if arts and crafts are regarded as a routine occupation, to fill gaps in the programme, and are supervised by unqualified or uninterested staff, it may not be surprising that the outcome for users is vague.

Arts and Crafts: A Checklist

Can . . .

> 1. . . . . there be a balance between encouraging users to follow individual interests and providing a concentrated and disciplined learning experience? Could some arts and crafts for some users be provided in community settings?
> 2. . . . . more emphasis on employing staff with a craft or community arts skill be explored? Such staff might liaise between a user's defined interests, the day unit and other local arts and crafts facilities, such as the community arts centre, and further education colleges.
> 3. . . . . a relationship between a user's development and arts and crafts be explored? These might include the need to develop a skill, or helping the user to express himself.

ARTS AND CRAFTS: SOME SUGGESTIONS

(1) Community arts centres or regional arts groups may consider the role of such workers to local day centres. This may mean that some users may be able to spend some time each week at the arts centre to use specialist facilities. Another role is to act as a consultant to day unit staff. Examples of the use of such workers and the facilities and activities offered by community arts centres are to be found in a directory of community arts centres (Arts Council, 1976), and a

specialist service, 'Shape', puts professional artists in touch with day units (*Observer* magazine, 1979).

(2) Some units have organised annual public exhibitions of arts and crafts of selected user exhibits.

(3) Some units use local sales outlets. One centre which concentrates on leather work has opened a shop where users sell handbags, belts and sandals. Another takes a monthly stall at a local market.

(4) Some units try to experiment with media. A group of users at a centre for the mentally ill made their own video film to show to newcomers and local social services staff. A centre for the mentally handicapped is finding that some young people can handle photographic equipment and plans that they take photographs of the centre to be used for public relations.

(5) Users in a centre for the physically handicapped, which is user-managed, share their own craft skills with each other.

1.5 MEETINGS AND GROUPS

Meetings and groups in a day unit are contentious, although less so than work programmes. The requests for improvement were for more meetings rather than for less, particularly from those users classed as mentally ill and those in family day centres.

'We should', said a user in a day hospital, 'have, all of us, a discussion with all those concerned with what we do. If we patients could freely chat to these people, then they could find out how we feel. We could all meet here, knots would be unravelled and discussed, we don't get any of that. There are a lot of people who come up with different ideas. This is the kind of therapy we need.'

Those few users who wanted *less* not more groups and meetings did so because they found them boring, frightening or too big (in that order). 'I would do away with some of those meetings and have more physical exercise instead', advocated a patient in a psychiatric day hospital. 'Group meetings, just talking, are boring. You run out of subjects to debate on.'

Others found groups overstimulating. 'In these group meetings, I'm too frightened to open my mouth', said a depressed 26-year-old mother of three in a day hospital for the mentally ill. 'They have plays in the meetings too' (presumably psychodrama). 'I'm too frightened to take part.'

'Monday mornings there's always a big meeting, all in a circle. You always want for a smaller group: you might be able to speak then', said another in a separate day hospital.

The procedures associated with groups were bewildering to some users and not always well explained by heads and staff who had little to say about improvements to meetings and groups. A couple made sharp criticisms of the 'depersonalising' aspect of groups and the ways groups could be manipulated to get users to conform to the rules of the unit. Another point made by some users was that groups could lose their dynamic and degenerate into rituals of repetitive recitation. 'When you have a discussion or a therapy group, you say things that people don't take any further than that. Everyone just takes your problems at face value. But there's a lot more to them than that', a young woman in a psychiatric day hospital said.

COMMENTS

Apart from a meeting between head and users before users start at the unit, few units organise any kind of orientation programme, which makes it appear unlikely that any special introduction to groups or meetings takes place. But a discussion of the possibilities of groups and the ways they run may be of benefit to some users and minimise clashes of understanding about purpose between users and staff.

The present state of leadership of groups in day units is a difficulty. Few units had staff trained to lead groups and there is a strong case for developing more group work expertise amongst staff. The possibilities of training users to share in the running of groups deserves further exploration too. Other experience suggests that mutual aid groups contain powerful therapeutic possibilities (Parents Anonymous London, 1978).

Arts and Crafts: A Checklist

Can ...

---

1. . . . . meetings and groups be prevented from degenerating into rituals and routines as meaningless to users as some contract work? Can groups have targets which are regularly reviewed?
2. . . . . one member of staff in each unit develop expertise in running groups? (Carter, 1976)
3. . . . . therapy groups select their users since not all users cope with therapy in public equally well?

GROUPS AND MEETINGS: SOME SUGGESTIONS

(1) Two or three users may constitute a group. One social services unit for the mentally ill uses co-counselling techniques, a method whereby users counsel each other. At a minimum, users might help each other by planning more adequate introductions to the day unit for new users.

(2) Some day units have experimented with relatives' groups, as a bridge

between the centre and the home. They need careful definition and interpretation. Chapter 10 implies that they are open to considerable misunderstanding.

(3) Some units prefer a group worker from outside the day unit: one who 'visits in' on a sessional basis to take groups. The implication is that there is less chance of groups becoming instruments of control with an external leader. There are advantages in having a person external to the daily activities to whom users can complain about the unit (Carter, 1976).

(4) The same applies to staff. The tensions of working in a confined space with a group of users each day led the Maudsley Day Hospital to introduce an external consultant to work with staff, to discuss concerns about users and working together (Bennett *et al.*, 1976). The potential contribution a clinical psychologist or the clinical social work practitioner attached to an area team might make, could be considered.

(5) Groups with functional purposes are described by the Marlborough Day Hospital. For example, there is a potential leavers' group, and an ex-users' group, the latter held away from the day unit premises (Foster, 1979).

(6) Criteria for selection of psychotic patients into therapy groups in day units are suggested by Stevens (1973).

1.6 IMPROVE EDUCATION

The overlap between social activities, arts and crafts, meetings and groups, with educational classes is rather obvious. User requests were generally for more *formal* education and these came from centres for families, offenders and the mentally handicapped. For staff it was those in centres for the mentally handicapped who wanted more education and this issue has been exposed in Chapter 6.

Users wanted more individual educational help from staff, while staff felt they had no time to give this. 'If only we had more time to spend on individuals', said a staff member in a training centre. There was also a reservation expressed by a few that confining education to formal classes conducted within the four walls of a centre did little to help users transfer their learning to the outside world, a matter discussed in Chapter 5.

COMMENT

Since few users have formal qualifications or job skills, it is important that day units consider their basic educational requirements. For example, the survey interviews revealed that some users, including the mentally handicapped, are unable to read or write. Thus education classes need to be planned around two basic functions: first, around sheer survival and then, second, around what might be termed the 'quality of life' issue. Survival classes teach basic abilities to enhance the survival of the user in the outside world: literacy and numeracy classes, shopping groups and cookery classes. 'Quality of life' interests are extra-curricular to the basic survival kit (things like drama and music classes). Arts and crafts sessions might just as easily have been classified in this section.

Vocational assessment would appear to have value in ascertaining what users can do after they leave the centre. This is a skilled procedure because of the margin for error in the instruments used and educational psychologists and careers advisers need to be involved in assessment and review procedures. An example about how not to assess a user for a day unit was unwittingly provided by a recent BBC documentary film 'Timmy and the Experts'. Timmy was a mongol. Assessment should try to overcome the assertion of vague generalities ('community care is best') and produce individual behavioural and vocational targets. It should not assert moral categories about mixing users ('it's good for young and old to mix together' or 'it's more normal to live in town than the country') over individual preference; nor should it assert the power of bureaucratic 'expertise' over consumer preference.

Education: A Checklist

Do . . .

> 1. . . . day units offer sufficient opportunities for their users to close their gaps in formal education?
> 2. . . . day unit staff pay enough *individual* attention to users' educational defects? Would improved assessment of users' educational activities and deficits help?
> 3. . . . users have the opportunity to repeat classroom learning in trials outside the centre?

EDUCATION: SOME SUGGESTIONS

(1) Most day units, particularly those for the mentally handicapped including those for the elderly, need an adult education adviser. Some London centres employ staff from adult education but each unit needs a consultant to take an overview of the educational needs of users. This issue is discussed further in section VI of this chapter.

(2) At least one mental handicap service has an arrangement with the local college of further education for a small group of mentally handicapped young people to enrol for a special two-year course at the college. About half these users are placed in open employment at the end of the course.

(3) The application of adult literacy schemes to day services is obvious. A few day units have participated in adult literacy schemes, in

particular centres for offenders and a few for the mentally handicapped. Another application is for literate users to be trained as tutors to
illiterate users, an activity which might continue after both have left
the day unit.
(4) Westfield Community Centre is an annexe to a college of further
    education. It has a day centre for the mentally ill, a club for mothers
    and a work orientation centre for disadvantaged groups. In this
    innovation the day centre is removed to the college campus (Lowles
    and Herd, 1977).
(5) A family day unit in a double-decker bus is a place where ethnic
    minority groups can take part in language classes, discuss ways to
    bring up children, and so on.
(6) A young family care centre which recruited user-mothers to work on
    the staff of the centre has referred some of these new careerists to
    teaching and social work courses.

II Improve the Users and their Regime

'Improve the users', said some users and some staff, which meant in
practice that the behaviour of some users should alter, particularly those
in units where users attracted labels of mental disability (the mentally
handicapped and mentally ill): the catalogue of behaviour from which
their peers needed deliverance was fighting, shouting and loud
arguments, tormenting and criticism, moaning and complaining. Such
complaints were, over the range of users, not frequent, but had enough
intensity to imply that an ability to survive others' bad behaviour was
necessary for coping in a day unit. For example, physical fights between
users were reported in some adult training centres. (Physical abuse was
almost never reported between users and staff.) 'A man here hits me',
complained one. 'I don't like John, he fights me', said another.
    Shouting and loud arguments featured in some day units for the men-
tally ill. 'Some of the characters who come here, the men, are antisocial.
Verbal aggression and swearing: it discourages young girls and quieter
young men from coming and even sometimes volunteer helpers', commented a user in a voluntary-run day unit for the mentally ill.
    Some sensitive users in training centres complained of excessive
teasing. 'I dislike it here when the others torment me', said a girl in a
training cente. 'People criticise me a lot and get on my nerves, the boys
mostly', said a 25-year-old woman in another training centre. 'I don't like
the boys here calling me backward and making fun of me.'
    Moaning and complaining about one's disability was a hurdle placed by
some in front of others. 'Sometimes if you listen to the other patients they
make you more depressed', said a user in a psychiatric day hospital. Other
peccadilloes ranged from the abstract ('People here have no dignity') to
the highly personal '(Chuck out the ones who sweat'). These issues

become important to a group of people who spend most of the day, often for years, in each others' company.

On the staff side, most improvements to the users requested by staff fell into an 'if only' category. 'If only they weren't mentally handicapped/mentally ill/physically limited.' For the mentally handicapped, the variation was, 'If only they weren't so backward'. For example, a 55-year-old instructor, a former engineer, complained: 'It's frustrating to teach them something and then to think they know it and then the morning after they don't know it when they can't contain what you've told them.'

For the mentally ill, one variation went: 'If only they weren't so chronic'. For instance: 'One spends so much time with patients, but they know they can get back in here easily. A few tablets and back they come – I just am not getting anywhere', worried an SRN in a psychiatric day hospital. 'The genuinely ill patient is hard to accept: their changes are too slow for me.'

Exposure for hours every day to people who are not always easy to get on with can be stressful and staff cannot always withdraw to the office, the consulting room or clinic when they need a rest. 'Having to repeat things so many times, to be so patient and controlled: you just feel like a bit of chewed up string at the end of the day', said a woman staff member of a training centre.

A second issue was that of wanting the current mixture of users reviewed and altered. Staff had little to say on this subject in this context but the point which emerged from the users' reviews was that people do not want to associate with a user group that they see as worse than themselves. The point that users can derive comfort from users who are worse than themselves if they belong to the same group, but not unless, has been made for the physically handicapped. 'I'm not being cruel but its the atmosphere here . . . they're mentally handicapped and I'm physically handicapped. Now they are two very different things and we should be in separate places.' In similar vein, a few patients in psychiatric day hospitals wanted the 'bad mental cases' removed, leaving only the 'nerve cases' at the day hospital. Some staff made an allied point in suggesting that an effort be made to separate the 'acutes' from the 'chronics'.

A third issue relating to improvements to users' regimes was that some users wanted some individual help from staff, while some staff regretted not having time to give more. Three points were made. First, as we have seen, users wanted more *personal* help. In 'Improve the Programme', users and staff identified 'personal help' as 'treatment' but this was not always the case. 'The staff could have talked more to me at first. I couldn't stand the group therapy and I felt I was being cut off without any help at first. It's better now, though.'

Aside from more personal contact with the staff, other users wanted more strategic planning for the future and expressed disappointment that there was insufficient focus on what would happen after leaving the unit. 'I wish they would help me with my future problem, trying to fix me up with some kind of sheltered work', said a user in a social services day centre for the mentally ill.

The fourth change users suggested was more participation in the formal running of the centre. Suggestions included a programme committee composed of users, a user representative on a management committee and more interest by outside unions in the running of more centres. On the latter one commented: 'The unions should get more involved in centres. Outside managements should too, they could be on the committee. It should be a matter not of law but of standard practice for unions and outside management to be involved in full running of these places. They could set a standard of ability for the people concerned to go back into industry. These are good places.'

Those with actual practical suggestions for more involvement in the programme were few: but there was a diffuse feeling that somehow more participation was needed. One user put it this way: 'They could bring more out of you than they do. They tend to leave you sitting around doing nothing and don't say anything to you. You need to be pushed a bit to do things.' Along similar lines, another woman said: 'We need to have people putting ideas together. They ask you to come and you do but you still don't get anywhere.'

COMMENTS

Changing the position of users in day units revolves around one fundamental issue. As background, construct a mental map of a day unit, with a hierarchy which extends from the manager or head at the top, down through the staff to the users who are conceived of as being at the bottom. But what would happen if the hierarchy were reversed? Or flattened? Half the day unit heads and staff claim to encourage participation but most of this is at the level of encouraging users to help with the chores around the unit. A few day units have user committees but, in practice, these do not appear to work very well. This is, perhaps, because the current pattern is to invite participation without affecting the distribution of power in the unit. The French students' wall poster seen during the student–worker confrontation of 1968 described participation without power in this way:

(in English) 'I participate, you participate, he participates, we participate, you participate . . . they profit.' Quoted by Arnstein, S. (1969) 'A Ladder of Citizen Participation', *Journal of the American Institute of Planners*. July, Vol. XXXV No. 4, p.216–24.

Staff in each unit might attempt to rate the unit by the degree of involvement the unit provides for users on the ladder shown in Figure 17.1. For example, some users and staff have made the point that their unit does not allow participation. In the middle of the ladder are levels of participation where users are allowed a muted voice. But most have a long way to go

Figure 17.1

(Adapted from Arnstein (1969))

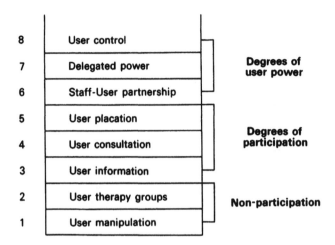

8	User control	
7	Delegated power	**Degrees of user power**
6	Staff-User partnership	
5	User placation	
4	User consultation	**Degrees of participation**
3	User information	
2	User therapy groups	**Non-participation**
1	User manipulation	

before their units offer degrees of user power, since doing chores around the units and helping with contract work were two largest user definitions of participation.

Two further points. It is, of course, probably impossible for users to increase their power unless the heads and staff in the unit already participate fully in the unit themselves. The relationship between the staff and head office will be examined in section VI. Second, in units where most users are long term and where the issues of staff versus user power may be more crucial, it may be easier to introduce self-management (an example is given in Chapter 18) than in those units with a fast turnover and more emphasis on staff expertise. In these circumstances it may not be practicable to turn the unit over to the users. But more experimentation is needed on how to involve users in short-term units as a practice run for returning to everyday life.

SUGGESTIONS

(1) Users in 'long-term' units can manage their units themselves – see the next chapter for an example of a unit for the physically handicapped. But some voluntary units for the elderly operate on a user self-management basis too.

(2) The Barbican Centre, primarily for offenders and the mentally ill, has a staff member whose job it is to deal with issues connected with users leaving the centre. This staff member is an ex-offender: it is considered vital that this member of staff understands what the

Improve the Users and their Regime:

A Checklist

---

1. Is there a case for users setting rules for behaviour in the unit to extend peer pressure on 'difficult to manage' users?
2. Is it possible to mix user groups only with the prior agreement of users?
3. Is it possible to offer more personal help to users? Specifically, users ask for (a) more individual discussion of their here-and-now problems and, (b) more concentrated examination of their future after they leave the day unit.
4. Is it possible to improve the involvement of the users in the running of the centre, both by more participation in the formal structure and more actual engagement of interest?

---

experience of leaving the security of a unit means (Barbican, 1978).

(3) User-run centres seem to suggest that the subjective meaning of user-imposed rules is more acceptable than externally imposed constraints. Thus to have users define criteria of unacceptable behaviour and their penalties may constrain potential trespassers 'out of bounds' with more feeling of personal responsibility (Barbican, 1978). ('What we need is more discipline here', said an offender at a day training centre!)

(4) Some centres have employed ex-users as care staff. This has happened at Langtry Young Family Day Centre, where former users of social services have joined the staff (Brill, 1976).

(5) A specific contract is made between a member and staff at the Barbican Centre. The agreed focus of the work and the time this should take is specified and reviewed weekly by user and counsellor. This method is now used in certain psychiatric day units such as the Marlborough Day Hospital (Foster, 1979).

III Improve the Building

Most requests to improve the building came from those in units which were not purpose built. The first point was the need to upgrade the internal environment: users of sheltered workshops, in particular, criticised poor temperature control, too much noise, poor ventilation, insufficient attention to safety, and draughty buildings. One sheltered worker said: 'This isn't a good place to work in. It's too dirty. The building itself is ropey. It rains in. It's cold in winter, too many draughts.'

Poor working conditions were mentioned less often by staff. Staff comments concentrated on suggestions for improved amenities, such as wider corridors, bathrooms, canteens, and so on. 'We need a bathroom desperately', said an instructor in a training centre. 'How do you deal with trainees who are incontinent and need a bath or shower?' However, the biggest amenity sought most often by user and staff was more space. Overcrowding was seen by both users and staff as an inhibitor to developing new activities. One-room day centres came in for particular criticism. 'Space is our problem', said a nurse in a day hospital for the elderly. 'Everything is virtually done in one room. Moving furniture every time you want a different activity or lunch is no fun.'

Complaints were not resolved entirely by shifts to new purpose-built buildings. Some handicapped people, in particular the blind, found their new setting unsympathetic and disorientating. One said, 'I don't like having to come to a place so far out in the wilds and having to be shut in all day. The old factory in town was central: you could get home to dinner or go into town.'

One issue on which users were more sensitive than the staff (as adjudged by the higher proportion of user comments) was the attractiveness or otherwise of the interior of the day unit building. 'Brighten the surroundings', said many users. Shabby or drab walls and dirty toilets were the two specific bugbears: and many of these criticisms came from those users in psychiatric day units. 'Doing the place up to make it more cheerful would help. Have some music around too.'

'Make the lunchtime social centre more comfortable; chairs, easy rather than sitting and staring at each other around the wall. The dining room is in the old building and it gives you a very institutional feeling. Some older ward patients are there and I feel very institutional.'

Users with physical handicaps were opposed to dirty facilities but often qualified their complaints with an understanding reference to the national economy: an issue of doubtful relevance in these cases: 'It's dirty, but not so bad. I suppose you have to expect it in a place like this.'

'The toilets in the basement are a disgrace. It's not kept half as clean as it could be.'

'It's as much as you can expect, with the country being in the state of finance it's in, I suppose.'

COMMENTS

Aside from requests for adding specific amenities such as bathrooms, the main deficiencies in the buildings were 'nuts and bolts' items (such as asking for toilet doors which shut properly, more cleanliness, or more visual attractiveness). These issues should not be dismissed as trivia as they are clear indications to users of the way their services treat them: significant issues of morale. The celebrated case of the Paddington Day Hospital where patients protested to the area health authority that the graffiti-laden, faeces-covered interior of the day hospital made it appear that they were part of a bizarre experiment is an extreme example of the interaction between physical conditions and low morale (Herbert, 1976). Day units in this project were less spectacularly filthy, but nevertheless, protests about shabbiness came from users rather than staff, confirming perhaps that because staff had their own washrooms, toilets and staff rooms to escape into, the impact of unattractive surroundings was muted.

Some of the oldest buildings offered some of the most imaginatively adapted environments. For example, one day hospital housed in a nineteenth-century mental hospital had turned a former cell with thick walls and barred windows into a 'graffiti room'. Painted yellow, furnished with foam rubber and punchbags, overwrought patients could attack their staff or their spouses in fantasy by scribbling messages on the wall or pummelling the punchbag. The same building was decorated with collages made by groups of users, posters, wallcharts and tropical fish. Staff and users contributed to this decoration and the morale of both was high.

The inescapable implication is that new buildings are not essential, although there may be standards of human decency and comfort below which staff and user morale cannot be resurrected. In one local authority day unit, staff and users interviewed protested strongly that the only suitable fate for the unit was to raze it to the ground. Complaints sounded surrealist: 'Get rid of the building. The last manager had field mice in this room to feed his snakes. The room was alive with mice and has only just been cleaned. There are gas leaks everywhere.'

There must be a level at which conditions become so unacceptable that staff and user inertia develops. If there isn't the space, why bother with new activities? If there isn't a bathroom, is it easier to allow a mentally handicapped user to stay incontinent? If it is an extremely long walk to the toilet, what is the point of habit-training for toileting the elderly confused? It is hardly an original point but architects and administrators could learn more about the use of buildings from regular discussions with staff and users.

At the same time, the implicit assumption of staff and users is that day unit activity needs to be confined to the building. We noted that the absence of purpose-built facilities for the elderly tended to relate to a slightly higher usage of outside community facilities. A similar point has been made in relation to adult training centres (Curtis and Edwards, 1977). Over-provision of facilities can assist to make adult training centres into self-supporting island communities. The provision of sophisticated working and dining accommodation, vast changing rooms and shops may be counter-productive if it protects users from everyday living outside the centre. Eating in a cafe at lunchtime, buying sweets in a shop, having a drink in a pub, using the local swimming pool are all less likely if facilities are over-provided at the day unit.

What seems important is to develop a domestic scale of building which allows relationships between users and staff to flourish in comfort. One imaginative training exercise would be to send advisers, consultants and heads to a unit in a different area to play the role of user. 'Taking the role of the other', as the sociologists put it, means being able to live in their conditions, too.

Improve the Building: Checklist

How Can ...

---

1. . . . day unit policies take account of user views of the attractiveness of the building? Users are sensitive to shabby, drab surroundings.
2. . . . staff introduce minimum amentities for servicing a particular user group: for example, bathrooms for incontinent users?
3. . . . staff and users take responsibility for making minor improvements to the unit?
4. . . . new buildings contribute to user morale? The suitability of the site and the degree of accommodation they offer a particular handicap are crucial issues.
5. . . . adequate space be developed to work in? This issue is paramount to staff and users.

SUGGESTIONS: THE BUILDING

(1) An adult training centre housed in an old hall compensates for its lack of a lunch room by taking trainees in groups to local pubs and cafes.

(2) Another unit for the mentally handicapped has its headquarters in an old house with lots of small rooms. This allows small groups called 'home bases' to develop for basic daily activities including lunch and tea. Users and staff brew their own in the same 'home' group.

(3) A centre for the elderly confused sited in an unpromising conversion in an inner city building has a glamorous Hollywood bathroom. Fit for a film star, it is aimed at nudging failed memories to recall 1930s movies. More important, it also allows the staff to perform potentially undignified tasks of bathing and toileting in conditions of maximum dignity.

(4) One centre has communal toilets for users and staff, to overcome the implication that users are second-class citizens. But it is appreciated that staff can need their own territory too. Two comfortable, quiet rooms are provided, one for users and one for staff and each is out of bounds to the other.

(5) Allocating a small annual budget to staff and users to spend on decoration and internal facilities is one way of encouraging those who use the building to take responsibility for it. It was found, for example, that second-hand sofas were more acceptable to users than smart new furniture in one family day centre.

(6) Not all day units need to be housed in a building. A probation service uses a boat as a focus for community service and a social services department uses a narrow boat as a day facility for children and young people. A mobile day centre, a 'centre' for the elderly in a

motor van (Kaim Caudle, 1977) and two double-decker buses used as family centres are other useful developments.

IV Improve the Facilities

The facilities in this instance are the meals, the transport to and from the unit and the hours of opening of the unit. More users wanted improvements to the meals, the transport and the hours, in that order, while the concern of staff was to alter the transport, the hours and the meals, in that order.

Users' complaints about the meals centred on the lack of variety, the poor quality of cooking, the sloppy serving and certain misgivings about the standards of hygiene adhered to in their preparation. As we have already seen in Chapter 6, nearly all elderly people were satisfied with most aspects of their food: most complaints came from offenders and users of day hospitals for the mentally ill. Staff rarely pronounced on the food: in the case of day hospitals for the mentally ill, perhaps because they ate in a separate dining room.[6]

The second concern to users and by far the largest to the staff were difficulties with transporting the users. Frustrations were either that transport was inadequate (a complaint coming most often from units in health authorities) or non-existent (a problem with voluntary and some social services units). Some social services units with disabled members made an additional point: more transport would mean that they could do more outside the four walls of the unit with their users.

A third issue – but not a large one – was the question of the opening hours of the unit. As users saw it, two separate matters were involved. There was, first, the number of days the unit was open. But there was also the matter of the number of days the user was allowed to come. Most users in family centres wanted to come more often than the one or two days a week allocated them, while some older people suggested an extension of the hours of the unit into the evening hours.

COMMENTS

If food equals love, some day units appear unloving. It needs to be remembered that British mass feeding, from motorway cafes to British Rail, does not have an outstanding international reputation. Does this excuse poor standards in day units? It is ironic that those lunch services attracting least complaint were staffed by volunteers. (It is also true, of course, that their users may feel less able to complain.) One potential role for the WRVS might be to act as a culinary watchdog for local food services in order to draw up a kind of Day Care Good Food Guide. Deficiencies might be reported to social services committees and community health councils.

Transport appears to be deteriorating by the month. Many units have been forced to restrict their transport because the oil crisis has led to shortages and increased prices of petrol, an effect which will reduce the supply of volunteers willing to use their own cars. Local voluntary organisations seeking a new role might explore the possibility of providing a transport service for disabled users, which might, amongst other things, take them to their day unit, regardless of service provider. Such services could experiment with either a 'dial a bus' basis or a voucher system. This would allow NHS ambulance transport to revert to emergencies and widen the context in which transport is seen as a need for the disabled, within an ethos of establishing priority use of a scarce resource.

The numbers of hours per week a day unit offers its users will also become a matter of priority. For example, on the assumption that day unit provision of the late 1970s and 1980s is unlikely to match the growth of the previous fifteen years, the question of 'who uses' day places may become problematic. The predicted growth in the numbers of old people may swamp the current provision of the day unit places. Extensions to the hours the day unit operates are feasible, but these should not be done by diluting the staff–user ratio, unless this is achieved within an agreed context of offering more opportunities for self-management to users.

The Facilities: A Checklist

Can Day Units Offer . . .

1. . . . an improved meal service? This would, in statutory sponsored day units particularly, include more choice, dignity and hygiene in meal preparation and service.
2. . . . transport to connect day unit users with the outside world? Adequate planning needs to be done on the transport needs of potential users first, based on the degree of disability.
3. . . . to review the existing number of hours the unit is open and the number of 'days' allocated each user?

SUGGESTIONS

(1) Staff and users rarely eat together, which reduced an important potential aspect of community.[7] If the staff ate with the users, the food might well improve! The centre for the mentally handicapped which organises its meal-serving in a home base has been mentioned.
(2) Transport. Each area needs a working group to consider its future transport needs and to allocate priorities for user groups *across* the current boundary drawn between service providers. The severely physically disabled might be a first priority.

In rural areas, more thought could be given to the obvious economy in taking the day unit to the users. The travelling day hospital for the mentally ill in Dorset and the mobile caravan for the elderly in Sunderland are examples (MIND, 1975; Kaim Caudle, 1977).

(3) Hours. At present, the hours of opening of the unit depend on the availability of staff: but this may not be an appropriate future assumption for the maximum use of an expensive purpose-build resource. In a social services unit for the mentally ill when staff posts were frozen, the staff decided to work with the users for four days a week only and to set apart the fifth for staff meetings, planning and staff training. The users' committee, given a small budget, organised the programme for users for the fifth day. The same principle could be extended to evening and weekend usage.

V Improve the Staff

Altering aspects of staffing the day units was of concern to more staff than users. More staff saw the main change required as that of getting extra staff into the unit; while more users wanted alterations to current staff attitudes. This second matter will be discussed first.

A minority of users pointed out that they felt that a few staff members had adverse attitudes to users or showed little interest in them, and the groups commenting on adverse attitudes were those with physical handicaps, the mentally ill and the mentally handicapped. The following comments come from people in the middle age groups in units for the physically handicapped. The first three comments come from local authority centres and the fourth from a 'voluntary' centre:

Although we are physically disabled, we are treated as if we are mentally disabled.

I had to take some tablets last week, and I used a glass with water that I had previously used with tea. The instructor thought I had helped myself to an extra cup of tea, and he told me off. I was surprised that a man of his intelligence should carry on so. He went through me like a dose of salts.

Various members of staff like to keep us down. They give us no feeling of confidence in ourselves. They do everything for us: we are capable of doing more for ourselves. Some like to lord it over us.

At times, we're treated like school children instead of adults. We're called out to go to lunch and we have to queue to get our tablets. I think it is childish.

Other unhelpful staff attitudes were 'bossiness' (in units for the mentally ill), and infantilisation of users (in units for the mentally handicapped). Bossiness is illustrated by this comment: 'It's the way we get treated at dinner time. If we go in too early they shout "Get out, get out" – male and female nurses. The inpatients get preference and we take what is left. That makes you feel so inferior. All the scraps and bits are left for us . . . and if you try to help someone else they tell you off, if you wait for someone else's food.' (From a 58-year-old woman in a day unit for the mentally ill, who felt depressed and said she usually had trouble expressing her aggressive feelings.)

Being infantilised can be frustrating. A 62-year-old recent entrant to a centre for the mentally handicapped who had managed the house alone for twenty years after her mother died was recently admitted to a hostel and training centre: 'The staff treat you like school kids here – they keep calling your names out and telling you to be quiet at lunch. I don't like the way they treat you here.'

Adverse attitudes to users by a few staff were confirmed by other staff. More awareness of the need to change staff attitudes was expressed by those working with the mentally ill and the mentally handicapped. Less often a staff member working with the physically handicapped spoke up, as this example demonstrates: 'The manager here, I just don't like his attitude to the members. He treats them as if they were stupid, and doesn't give them the opportunity to make any decisions. I don't think he understands their problems. He is too dogmatic.'

The most common opinion from the staff was that the main improvement needed was to have more staff, particularly more direct service staff. Those working with the elderly confused, the families, the mentally ill and the mentally handicapped expressed the rationale that more staff would allow more time to be spent with individual users, a matter on which, as we have seen, users feel positive too.

'Less clerical work would give more time for myself to become more involved with the patients.' (Charge nurse in geriatric day hospital. Her comments highlight the fact that of requests for extra 'back-up' staff, most were for extra clerical backing.)

'It would be really nice to have more staff. When you first come, you feel you would like to be able to talk to them, and they haven't much time; they have to be with the group in general. When a member of staff was away, the place almost fell apart, it was very noticeable. They had to cope with their administrative work.' (User in a psychiatric day hospital.)

Finally, some heads and staff working in psychiatric day hospitals regretted the lack of involvement of their consultant psychiatrists which they interpreted as due to lack of interest or too much work. Very few staff expressed a need for improved staff training or supervision, but it needs to be remembered that seven out of ten staff wanted more in-service training and nearly five in every ten wanted a basic qualification or a further qualification.

COMMENTS

Are more direct service staff required, or is it a re-examination of staff tasks that is needed? This is an open question. However, heads, in particular, appear to spend time on clerical and administrative duties ahead of working with the personal or social care of users. This investment of time in the 'housekeeping' of the unit may be consistent with increased management demands for better records, efficient ordering of meals and stores, and for effective use of expensive resources such as transport. But if what the sociologists call 'pattern maintenance' in the unit – keeping it ticking over – takes priority over talking to users, there is a case for more adequate back-up in more units by administrative or clerical officers which may, in turn, reduce the requests for more direct service staff.

One radical question is whether 'pattern maintenance' of the unit might become the task of users themselves, particularly in units where the turnover is low and most users long-term. A self-management system, such as that to be described in Chapter 18, calls on user commitment and responsibility and invests routines with the significance of keeping the unit alive. There are, of course, many fears about letting handicapped users take personal responsibility which are connected with adverse staff attitudes. These are expressed in Arthur Kopit's play 'Chamber Music' set in a mental hospital ward where patients formed a committee. The staff treated this as a therapeutic diversion for the patients rather than a responsible exercise in democracy. Essentially pessimistic, the play ends with anarchy among the patients indicating that disordered users cannot be trusted to act as adults. Such attitudes can subtly creep into day units.

In all, only one in twenty users wanted to improve any aspect of the staff. And more positively, users gave clear definitions of the two characteristics they valued most highly in staff members. Half the users considered social skills in the staff to be essential: an ability to be friendly and to be a good mixer, to like people, and to have an affinity with them, an ability to be sociable. The characteristic mentioned by a second group was an ability to communicate with users. This included being able to listen, being a suitable person to confide in, being able to feel the user's predicament, and being able to communicate a sense of confidence and achievement to a user. For some users, these characteristics overlapped. Although the staff considered these two dimensions to be of importance too, they emphasised cognitive knowledge, an ability to organise and 'life experience' as desirable attributes more often than the users.

Although nearly two-thirds of the users considered the staff needed to be trained, it was not clear that they felt that essential qualities could be inculcated by training. They are not alone in this: the degree of correspondence between training and behaviour on the job is one of the most perplexing issues facing educators and trainers.

The lack of involvement of consultant psychiatrists has been noted. Whether this is due to an excessive workload is not known, but it is interesting to compare the psychiatrists with the geriatricians. On the one hand, geriatricians are comparatively new entrants to medicine, still determined to establish themselves and succeed. On the other hand, psychiatrists are an older occupation with a longer history of isolation from working with others inside and outside medicine. Perhaps psychiatrists have a stronger sense of déjà vu: most psychiatric 'reforms' can be said to have happened before (Alldridge, 1979). Further, the psychiatrist may have a more difficult problem than the geriatrician in defining his legitimate territory. He may, on the one hand, view his job as dealing with a strictly organic notion of mental illness, 'allowing' the other staff to get on with 'the rest'. On the other hand, if committed to the importance of either social or psychological factors in mental illness (or both) he will need to establish a *modus vivendi* with non-medical staff (who may in some cases, have had more substantial training in the social or psychological factors connected with mental illness than the psychiatrist). He will need to decide whether to adopt a role as leader of the day hospital staff or whether he should be an equal colleague in a collegial team. Alternatively, he may 'opt out'. The disappointment of some staff and users in psychiatric day hospitals is that some psychiatrists appear to have chosen the option of 'opting out'. Certainly two psychiatrists writing recently have characterised medicine as a hit and run profession (Bentovim, 1974; Kushlick, 1975).

On the other hand, perhaps heads and staff in geriatric day hospitals expect less of geriatricians than those in psychiatric day hospitals do of psychiatrists? Whether or not this is the case, expectations are created, simply by attaching consultant psychiatrists to day units; expectations which are not present in non-medical settings within social services departments and voluntary agencies dealing with mental illness. More needs to be known about the way such expectations relate with a contribution to the day unit by each discipline. In the interim it might be said that psychiatric patients are not the only group in psychiatric day units with role problems!

Role problems are also raised by the way that heads and staff deal with a user's feelings of stigma. A critical clash of focus exists between some handicapped users and some staff members. A handicapped person in a day unit might assume that the day unit staff will not label him as 'deviant' in the same way as the less well informed layman or the public, but he is unprepared for a response which appears to be central to the behaviour of some staff, which neither accepts or rejects, but suspends both by reacting with neutral detachment to the handicapped person. To justify this 'affective neutrality', as some sociologists call it, from a medical or psychological point of view is easy: handicap needs to be abstracted from everyday life and classified into a frame of reference. The search for a cause for the handicap, determining the treatment to be supplied and arriving at an estimate of the prognosis are major issues to staff. On the surface, this allows the staff to be morally neutral, objective and value free. But to be neutral and value free seems artificial to the user and indicates a lack of personal involvement and an absence of concern and warmth. 'The central feature of the stigmatised person's situation in life is a question of what is often vaguely called acceptance' (Goffman, 1963). The user wants acceptance to be directed mainly at himself, not his handicap. He may find acceptance of his physical or mental limitations difficult and sometimes impossible. By contrast, the detached staff member who accepts the handicap ahead of the person is viewed as uninvolved and unconcerned. As one user in a centre for the mentally ill said: 'The way the job for the assistant manager in the local paper was advertised was badly phrased. Psychogeriatrics they called us and I'm only 56!' Another blind user said: 'The way we feel is not understood by the management. We like quiet because we have to concentrate more on what we are doing but they don't seem to understand this.'

One least attractive and most described feature of 'institutionalised' institutions is staff authoritarianism. In day units, users reported staff authoritarianism less often than they praised staff for being helpful, but when it is present, authoritarianism is unpleasant. Countless investigations show that authoritarianism relates to the structure of an organisation as well as the personalities of its members: one crucial issue is that one small group (the staff) has power over another less powerful but larger group (the users). The structure of the day unit will be discussed in section VI but one problem is the degree to which staff take up the conventional role within the day unit which means, in practice, a dominant position. One mentally handicapped user said: 'They just give you orders all the time. It makes you want to leave.' Abandoning the hierarchy in favour of a structure which views professional and bureaucratic knowledge as just one kind of knowledge, neither intrinsically superior or inferior, at times helpful and at other times inappropriate, is an alternative staff attitude. This alternative would regard users as partners with staff members, a view reinforced by changes such as the rise in the consumer movement. By contrast, traditional staff–user relationships based on the mutual acceptance of the superior knowledge and authority of the staff leads to inevitable social distance between the user and staff, and discrepant expectations about the behaviour of each.

In general, the very act of training for an occupation reinforces a stance of the superiority of professional wisdom over lay insights. (Staff in day units have yet to identify those particular areas of their intervention where dominance might be justified on the basis of an expected outcome rather than on the basis of custom.) So if some staff adopt a collegiate role in a day unit with users, while others do not, this might bring them into some disagreement and conflict with their colleagues and with superiors with more traditional views. There were examples of this, particularly in units for the mentally handicapped. Alternatively, units which try to 'impose' non-hierarchical ways of working on the staff can produce problems too. (For an account of a day unit where this happened see Carter, 1976.)

Can a staff member, without a handicap, really be accepted by users with handicaps? Some handicapped people consider that 'true' acceptance of each other is only possible by others in the same predicament: that is, true acceptance is only possible if the other possesses what has been called the distinct datum of one's own experience.[8] But 'acceptance' offered by staff needs to be understood as acceptance of a different order. It is based on the ability to 'take the role of the other': essentially attempting to put oneself in the user's place, without claiming to 'be' the other; a subtle but fundamental distinction. Those who can do this have been termed the 'wise': those whose job makes them privy to the secret life of stigma (Goffman, 1963). If they are sympathetic, users can give them a measure of acceptance, a kind of courtesy membership in the clan.

The Staff: A Checklist

Is It Possible . . .

---

1. . . . to improve the attitudes of a minority of staff? In particular, attitudes which belittle users need to be discouraged. More identification about how it feels to have a disability would help.
2. . . . that more favourable staff–user ratios would allow individual staff and users to spend more time talking together?
3. . . . to introduce more back-up staff and volunteers.

SUGGESTIONS

(1) One London borough day care section organises regular 'exchange of skills' meetings, so that staff from one day unit can share new skills from each other. These might include: the use of video, principles of co-counselling, the art of batik or principles of planning the food.

(2) Regular auditing and discussion of staff progress is achieved in another area. Targets for certain standards of performance are defined and transfer to another job is suggested if staff cannot develop the requisite competence.

(3) At another day unit for the mentally ill the users accompany staff on those visits out of the unit which explain the unit's work: they give part or sometimes all of the presentation. This allows users to get across *directly* the point of how it feels to be both a user and a handicapped person, providing more powerful and less oblique learning for the audience than the same points would, mediated by staff.

(4) Some units have an external consultant who visits regularly to discuss staff attitudes to users and to challenge practices to users which can

easily pass unnoticed (Bennett *et al*., 1976). Whilst in social services departments, at least, this may be a potential role of advisers, certain prerequisites are necessary, namely, an understanding of each of the following areas: the sociology of organisations, the dimensions of stigma, the dynamics of change and the functioning of groups.

VI Improve the Organisation

Would a rose by any other name smell as sweet? In other words, do the improvements already suggested for the day unit, which involve the programme, the users, the buildings, the facilities and the staff, inevitably improve the organisation? To some extent, yes, but so far the improvements have centred on what goes on *in* the day unit, neglecting its structure in relation to its sponsoring authority, its resources, or other organisations right outside the day unit.

Improving the structure of the day unit is the next issue. Few users made a point about this, although many of the comments on earlier matters such as the programme could be construed as mandates for changing the organisation. After all, most users are likely to be less knowledgeable about the unit than, say, the heads and, unless they are very long stayers, they are unlikely to have had the same exposure to hierarchy and its values. So turning to the heads' and staff views on the structure, we consider first their opinions about central management.

Most day units are parts of large organisations, as Chapter 2 indicates. If absence of criticism is a valid indicator, staff of area health authority day units are rather less critical of their central management than social services departments. While one in ten health heads and staff interviewed wanted improvements in relations with their central managements, three out of ten of those interviewed in social services units wanted changes, and most of these were in units for the mentally handicapped. In the view of heads and staff, 'head office' were out of touch, uninterested and demonstrated lack of leadership and indecisiveness (in that order). Health service staff added an addendum: 'head office' was also slow.

Being 'out of touch' meant to heads and staff that senior officers in the social services department lacked a detailed understanding of the tasks, the work flow and the crises points in the unit, which led them to misjudge some situations. The impression given was that management decisions about day units were taken without a detailed understanding of the nature and the content of the task and that those in day units, particularly heads, reacted by thinking of head office as impediment rather than ally. The converse was that many units were left to struggle with decisions with (as they saw it) little support and back-up. 'My senior officers at times display a complete lack of understanding of our situation. For example, the fact that we are unable to cope with certain groups of the mentally handicapped', said a manager of a training centre.

Lack of interest was another complaint: 'I think the employing authority could take more interest in our centre. They come once a year but there's a lack of interest; they don't want to know us. They didn't even know one work centre had shut down. More support from our top bods would help', said an officer in a local authority day centre for the mentally ill.

Four out of every ten social services units for the mentally handicapped, the elderly, the physically handicapped and the mentally ill had not been visited by the director of social services. In the previous twelve months one-third of the same group had not been visited by their assistant director. Over half had not been visited by even one area director. In fact, since only seven out of ten units had been visited by a social services committee member in the previous twelve months, local politicians appear to demonstrate more personal interest in day units than their senior officers. Health units were equally lacking in visits from District Community Physicians and Area Medical Officers, but we have no information on how often the Area Nursing Officer visited the unit and this would be a more relevant measure.

A second point was a request (from some staff rather than heads) for improved management *within* the unit. This ranged from the most common point, the need for better communication between staff, to complaints about the restricted degree of delegation of work from the head. There were few differences in the proportion of comments made by staff in the health as opposed to the social services units. The basic request was for better-run staff meetings – although a small group found current staff meetings frustrating: 'Just inquests', said one staff member cryptically.[9]

A third group wanted to do away with the hierarchy altogether or to reduce it and its arch-ally, red tape. 'Admin', 'red tape', 'the number of memos and stats', 'clerical work', were bones of contention. Few said how this might be done or what might replace the hierarchy; an exception was a staff member in a social services unit for the mentally ill:

Remove the hierarchy. I find it frustrating that I can't stand up to the hierarchy here. If I want to talk or comment, I can't go to the top, I have to go to the head. If we removed the hierarchy, we could all take out some time for administration. Things like petty cash could be administered more easily if it could be divided between us so that if I wanted to I could buy cream buns for my users. We could be responsible for our own money and not have to beg. We could use money as a means of interaction with the users so they could make choices for themselves: what to spend on lunch, whether to buy buns, whether to save it or put it towards equipment.

The second request was from heads and staff for increased resources: money and time were the two most often mentioned. Money was wanted largely for more amenities mentioned in section III of this chapter. Time was wanted to increase the output of the staff, either for treatment or 'to do the little things' – such as writing letters for old or disabled people. This matter has already been discussed. On the subject of allocating resources, the day unit is not the same thing as the building, as this head of a psychogeriatric day unit indicates:

> If only more was invested in personnel and ideas, not capital expenditure. This doesn't only apply to day care. Too much is spent on buildings like old people's homes, residential establishments which leave much to be desired. If there was more investment in the personnel end of day care they would have kept people out of the homes. The council is far too concerned with physical environments alone. They are too interested in the merits of wall-to-wall carpeting, instead of what can be done to improve an old church hall. The purpose of all resources is after all to improve the quality of life of the users.

There was another requirement, that links outside the unit be improved, both with outside services and the families of users. First, the outside services. Those most commonly referred to were (in this order): field social workers, general practitioners, domiciliary services, remedial therapists and special schools. The purpose of better liaison was to achieve a better understanding by outsiders about the nature of the day unit: there was a feeling that few understood the nature of day units. 'There is little understanding forthcoming from agencies outside the hospitals, for example, the [local] Department of Health and Social Security whose actions often seem designed to torpedo our therapeutic programmes', said a social worker in a day unit for the mentally ill.

The other reason given for improving relations with outside agencies was not so much to educate the outside world as to improve the knowledge and skills of day unit staff and heads. 'If there was more exchange and liaison with other facilities, we could supplement each other, for example, use each other's facilities. There is very little co-operation with outside bodies. They [head office] need to invest more in personnel and buildings, not in capital expenditure.'

Better liaison was wanted with the families of the users, particularly from those working with the mentally handicapped, the elderly confused and the physically handicapped, and Chapter 10 expands this. 'It's no good teaching one to light a gas stove if their parents say they can't do it at home', said an instructor in a training centre.

Relatives were said to be overprotective and unwilling to reinforce any learning the user achieved at the unit, as well as sometimes showing lack of insight into the user's problems. Few staff commented on productive, constructive relations with families: if a social theorist from another planet were examining the day units, he would conclude not only that relations between staff and families were almost non-existent (except in the case of family centres), but that the family was also the genesis for the users' lack of progress. But since only one in every ten heads reported that day units had more than monthly contact with most users' families, one in ten never had any contact, and six out of ten saw families only at an annual occasion like a Christmas party or irregularly in a crisis, this judgement appears to be based on a lack of appraisal about how users get on with their families.

COMMENTS

At present, some day units are like island communities: isolated, rather self-sufficient, stoical. In good weather there is intermittent contact between the island and the head office on the mainland over a rather muffled radio receiver but it is clear to the islanders that not all messages are received or interpreted correctly by recipients. So supplies from the mainland come intermittently and usually in the wrong quantities. For example, head office is likely to send a boatful of umbrellas across the narrow but rocky straits which divide the island from the mainland. This frustrates the islanders enormously because what they were really asking for, they now realise, was life rafts so that they could go to the mainland themselves to meet head office. But it is not only that the reception on the radio receiver is poor, and that the mainland operator insufficiently tuned in. The islanders now recognise that their formulations of messages are vague and capable of two or even three interpretations. Meanwhile head office, unable to concentrate on learning about its offshore islands, had moved on to deal with more readily visible action. With urban aid, crises, emergencies, casualties, sections and admissions, head office is more at home in the field or community than on an offshore island.

The islanders call a meeting. They recall that they were not founded to live on an offshore island but in a suburb. Their genius was the sheer ordinariness of their original aspirations: a magna charter which offered a bridge between home and work, or hospital and home. Yet somehow the community has got itself on to this rocky, barren island with few outlets and not many chances to escape.[10] The mainland, and particularly the suburbs, are normally covered by fog . . . The islanders decide to build bridges . . . .

In the view of the heads and staff in day units, there is little consensus with central management about what shared understandings underpin the action in day units. Leadership is a concept rather unfashionable within the social sciences (and possibly within all Britain at present). But one aspect of this which applies to day units is the need for senior officers to switch from an over-reliance on formal authority and to develop sapiential authority instead. Authority based on wisdom and knowledge rather than on formal bureaucratic procedure would be more acceptable to the day units. At the same time, heads need to develop more skills in communicating with their staff and to extend their influence outside the unit to those which might include their bureaucratic superiors. More work done on priorities within the unit then translated upwards might give 'head office' clearer messages about priorities and areas of investment. The same applies to communicating with strategic outside agencies and families of users.

There is very little concept of accountability for the quality of performance in the day unit at present and to make this a central notion might be one method of dealing with the day unit's structural problem of isolation. In a personal and psychological sense, we have seen that many heads and staff feel accountable fundamentally to their users, in that the users' satisfactions become theirs. But this lacks translation to an accountability formulated in organisational terms. Currently accountability is construed as the formal and hierarchic performance of red tape rituals rather than a way of improving the service to users.

One issue which needs serious thought is whether the unilateral formal accountability which most day unit staff have to their heads of units is appropriate? Clearly, users cannot be given more say in the running of their units until staff consider that they have a voice in running the place, too. Thus, complaints about the red tape and hierarchies within the unit need exploration, particularly within the adult training centres. Hierarchies, of course, are not the only way of arranging the work of a day unit: there are other ways of working which do not rely on centralised authority and chains of command. Rather, other methods rely on an integrated pooling of skills, democratic decisions and willingness to share tasks across a skill boundary. Called variously the arena model (Hunter, 1971) or the polyarchy (Algie, 1970), and discussed elsewhere in application to other areas of health and social services, these methods of organisation are rare at present in day units; other than those examples described in Chapter 13.

One of the difficulties of introducing more participative ways of working in the unit is the incipient clash which can result between the hierarchy outside the day unit (based on bureaucratic principles) and the hopeful collective inside the day unit (based on democratic principles). In the health service, hierarchies and their application are more complex: with consultants responsible to themselves (Chapter 2), nurses responsible to their 'Salmon' structure and others such as remedial therapists having a complicated system of accountability, say, to the Head Physiotherapist or her equivalent, the consultant and, in a vague way, to her colleagues in the day unit. The multi-disciplinary approach has a different set of problems in developing participation than a day unit based purely on hierarchical organising principles like a social services unit, but some examples of a democratically-run day care service in local authority are given by Archer (1979).

Is the present system of accountability to a chain of command above and beyond the day unit in statutory day units or voluntary agencies appropriate for such highly programme-centred organisations? For example, in a structure which is perhaps unique, one London social services department day care section reports not only to the social services committee but also to the leisure committee of the council. The idea that the aims of day units can be influenced by the beliefs and services offered by a particular management structure is an interesting one and deserves more exploration. In the same way it may be logical to consider the possibility of dual accountability for centres for the mentally handicapped to local education services as well as local social services; of day units for the elderly confused to health and social services. However, new accountability structures should not be imposed by central fiat: they are essentially the result of local reviews and local decisions, for they involve taking decisions about the direction of *that* day unit for *this* group of users.

If dual accountability is pursued and day units develop more diverse aims and programmes, this does not overcome the problem that the present lines of accountability are too long and remote. How can a Director of Social Services visit a day unit regularly when he has over 100 establishments to visit? The present problem may be not just that he does not take an interest but that the present hierarchical structure may produce the expectation in the day unit that he will do so and should do so. Thus day units need to consider a system of delegated accountability to which they can relate laterally rather than hierarchically. Each unit need its own management committee composed of representatives of staff and users. Other groups representative on the committee would be those representing the outside agencies most important to the unit, whether field social worker, clinical psychologist or DRO. There may also be a place for incorporating representatives of the families of users. In social services departments, the day care hierarchy needs to be represented and also the elected members, perhaps as chairman of the unit committee. In the health service, area specialists in nursing and medicine need representation as well as the relevant district and community health council. Reflecting the multi-disciplinary nature of the NHS, chairmanship of the unit committee might be based on a rota basis.

Day unit management committees need to report to one or more appropriate local authority committees but day units in the health service pose a more difficult problem because whether or not a day unit is an area or district resource is unclear. The district seems more an appropriate locale but it is a moot point whether the unit should report to the district management team or the closest thing a health district has to a show of local democracy, the community health council.

The purpose of considering changes to the organisation is not to inflict yet another organisational reorganisation on a relatively *ad hoc* and unsystematic set of services as the reorganisations of health and social services of 1971 and 1974 did. Rather, changes to the structure of day units should seek to maximise opportunities to be flexible and locally responsive. In other words, changes to the organisation need to be incremental and local rather than surgical and national. (Indeed, what could be more *radical* in reorganisation of public services in Britain at present than incremental local changes?)

The Organisation: A Checklist

How Can ...

---

1. ... senior officers develop a more detailed systematic understanding of the day unit task?
2. ... heads of some day units develop middle-management skills which promote clear methods of communication with and between staff? How can some heads of units tackle the question of delegation of the work?
3. ... day units reduce what is considered to be an over-reliance by the head office on hierarchy and red tape?
4. ... head office re-evaluate the priorities of spending? More amenities in buildings and investment in personnel are advocated ahead of purpose-built centres.
5. ... better links with agencies outside the day unit be developed? These might educate outsiders about day units and also help staff to use outsiders' skills.
6. ... links with the families of users be improved?

SUGGESTIONS

(1) One example of dual accountability is provided by the day care section of a London borough which is accountable to the leisure committee as well as the social services committee. Day units who care to use this dual connection (to take the young family care day services as an example) incorporate an extra dimension in their day care. In the young family care centres heads and staff are not only out to create a therapeutic setting and to train their users, but also to give them a good time, entertain them, encourage them to use recreational facilities and to have a good laugh. Likewise the services for the elderly in this area have a close connection with the adult education services. They not only provide practical services for therapeutic ends but they believe they can teach the users new things: swimming, Spanish and sculpture.

(2) One user-managed service for the physically handicapped has a management committee which contains the users' committee and a member of the day care advisory staff. They meet quarterly and report to the assistant director of social services. This is reported in the next chapter.

(3) One London borough, concerned about its lack of turnover in day units and the stated tendency of outside workers to 'dump' their clients in day units, now makes a contract between day unit, social worker or other responsible worker and user. This is formulated at

the time of the user's entry to the day unit and specifies the tasks and responsibilities of all parties.

(4) These suggestions have covered user and staff recommendations about changes in day units and in the organisations running them. However, there also needs to be attention to the inco-ordination[11] between day units for the *same* user group sponsored by *different* service providers in the same area. For instance, local planning teams should pay attention to the potential *duplication* of services for the mentally ill (Chapter 3.4), the *discontinuous* services for the physically handicapped (Chapter 3.3) for which the Employment Services Agency needs to take some responsibility, and the *incoherent* services for the elderly (Chapter 8).

NOTES

1 For example, only a quarter of the staff and users mentioned 'improvements to the programme' as their suggestion for improvement. But when then asked directly if they wanted changes to the present programme, nearly all staff did. A detailed outline of the programmes offered is provided by the ancillary text (Edwards and Carter, 1980).
2 A quarter of users who had done work in the previous week found the payments unfair and a further 30 per cent found them only 'moderately fair'.
3 This ceiling has now been raised to £4 per week.
4 This matter is discussed in more detail in Edwards and Carter (1980).
5 Nearly one in every three nursing officers in day hospitals for the mentally ill (29 per cent) commented on the lack of involvement of their medical colleagues. They interpreted lack of support as the doctors being 'too busy' or as 'lack of interest'. See section V of this chapter.
6 There is an anomaly in the fact that users in the health service get a free lunch, whilst those in social services and voluntary agencies usually pay.
7 The convention in area health authorities which precludes staff and users eating together applies to many day hospitals. Although there is a risk of the abuse of food by staff (such as stealing food intended for patients: DHSS, 1969) these practices are unlikely to be transferred to day units, particularly if users are asked to pay a nominal amount for lunch in all day hospitals. (At present only the staff pay for lunch.)
8 For a discussion of the differences between empathy and sympathy, see Scheler (1954).
9 Only a quarter of the heads reported that their day units had a weekly staff meeting. Twice as many health-sponsored units had staff meetings as social services units.
10 One theory about this is that the community was left stranded on the island after a day outing when petrol ran out ...
11 Inco-ordination practices were first discussed by Martin Rein (1970).

REFERENCES

Algie, J. (1970) 'Management and organisation in the social services', *British Hospital Journal*, LXXX, p. 1245.
Alldridge, P. (1979) 'Hospitals, madhouses and asylums: cycles in the care of the insane', *British Journal of Psychiatry*, 134, pp. 321–34.
Archer, C. (1979) 'The therapeutic community in a local authority day care programme', in R. D. Hinshelwood and N. Manning (eds). *Therapeutic Communities: Reflections and Progress* (Routledge & Kegan Paul).
Arts Council (1976) *A Directory of Arts Centres* (Arts Council of Great Britain).
Gloucestershire Probation and After Care Service (1978) *The Barbican Centre*

Now (unpublished; available from the Barbican Centre, 1a Barbican Road, Gloucester.)

Bennett, D. H. (1972) 'Principles underlying a new rehabilitation workshop', in Wing and Hailey, op. cit.

Bennett, D. H., Fox, C., Jowell, T. and Skynner, A. C. R. (1976) 'Towards a family approach in a psychiatric day hospital', *British Journal of Psychiatry*, 129, pp. 73–81.

Bennett, D. H. (1978) Personal communciation.

Bentovim, A. (1974) 'Treatment, a medical perspective', in J. Carter (ed.), *The Maltreated Child* (Priory Press).

Brill, J. (1976) 'Langtry Young Family Centre: a method of intervention', in M. R. Olsen (ed.), *Differential Approaches in Social Work with the Mentally Disordered* (British Association of Social Workers).

Carter, J. (1976) 'Parents' meetings in a hospital day centre', *Child: Care, Health and Development*, 2, pp. 203–12.

Curtis, J. and Edwards, C. (1977) *The Environment of the Adult Training Centre: A Critical Appraisal* (Medical Architecture Research Unit, Polytechnic of North London).

Department of Health and Social Security (1969) *Report of the Committee of Inquiry into Allegations of Ill-Treatment of Patients and other irregularities at the Ely Hospital, Cardiff*, Cmnd 3975 (HMSO).

Department of Health and Social Security (1979) *Royal Commission on the National Health Service*, Cmnd 7615 (HMSO).

Donald, B. (1978) 'Professions auxiliary, supplementary or complementary to medicine', *Health Trends*, 10, pp. 5–9.

Edwards, C. and Carter, J. (1980) *The Data of Day Care* (National Institute for Social Work, London).

Eriksson, S. (1975) 'Organising clerical sheltered employment', Conference Paper No. 14, *International Seminar on Sheltered Employment*, British Council for Rehabilitation and Remploy Ltd in Association with the Vocational Commission of Rehabilitation International, Guildford, England, September.

Foster, A. (1979) 'The management of boundary crossing', in R. D. Hinshelwood and N. Manning (eds), *Therapeutic Communities: Reflections and Progress* (Routledge & Kegan Paul).

Fox, A. (1971) *A Sociology of Work in Industry* (Collier Macmillan).

Goffman, E. (1963) *Stigma* (Pelican).

Hadley, R. (undated) *Rowen, South Wales* (Society for Democratic Integration in Industry).

Hebert, H. (1976) 'Hospital's methods may do harm', *Guardian*, 5 October.

Hunter, T. D. (1971) 'Arena or amoeba: managing the health care network', *The Hospital*, April, pp. 113–15.

Kaim Caudle, P. R. (1977) *The Sunderland Mobile Day Centre* (Help the Aged).

Kushlick, A. (1975) 'Some ways of setting, monitoring and attaining objectives for disabled people', Research Report No. 116, Paper presented to a conference on The Handicapped – Towards Independent Living, National Committee on Residential Care, Brisbane, Australia, 19–21 June.

Lowles, K. and Herd, C. (1977) 'Joint provision for disadvantaged groups', *Social Work Today*, 8, 29, p. 113.

Midwinter, E. (1977) 'The professional–lay relationship: a Victorian legacy, *Child Psychology and Psychiatry*, 18, pp. 101–13.

MIND (1975) 'Hospital goes to market. Dorset's travelling day hospital', *Mind Out*, 11, June.

Mykyta, L. J., Bowling, J. H., Nelson, D. A. and Lloyd, E. J. (1976) 'Caring for relatives of stroke patients', *Age and Ageing*, 5, p. 87.

Observer magazine (1979) 'Arts for all', *Observer*, 25 November, p. 85.

Parents Anonymous London (1978) 'Can we help you?' presentation at Second International Congress on Child Abuse and Neglect, London, 12–15 September.

Partridge, C. and Warren, M. (1978) *Physiotherapy in the Community* (Health Services Research Unit, University of Kent at Canterbury).

Rein, M. (1970) *Social Policy* (Random House).

Scheler, M. (1954) *The Meaning of Sympathy* (Routledge & Kegan Paul).

Stanley, R. (1975) 'Working in industry – enclaves', Conference Paper, *Internal Seminar on Sheltered Employment*, op. cit.

Stevens, B. C. (1973) 'Evaluation of rehabilitation for psychotic patients in the community', *Acta Psychiat. Scand.*, 49, pp. 169–80.

Chapter 18

————◆————

GETTING IT TOGETHER

THE CENTRE WITH THE VELVET CURTAINS

The Primus Club[1] is a social services day centre for the physically handicapped in a residential area of Stockport, near Manchester, in north-
west England. It meets in a former health clinic with orange painted walls
and high windows. The windows are hung with the kind of long, green,
velvet drapes seen in Sunday newspaper colour supplement advertisements, displaying antique furniture, Sanderson wallpaper and good
taste. The curtains confirm that twenty-five disabled people who meet
there each weekday have choice and purchasing power.

When the assistant director of the social services department announced to the forty prospective incumbents of the new day centre for the
physically handicapped that they could run their own centre, the response
was quizzical and suspicious. Where was the catch? As the managing
committee of disabled members of the centre see it now, the catch was a
lot of hard work and worry. But the rewards? 'Well, you do go home at
the end of the day quite worn out', confirmed one committee member,
confined in a wheelchair, but radiating energy. 'But it's marvellous to
think what the place can do for people, how it makes them start living
again. Today, for instance, we had to decide the following . . .' And an
agenda was rattled off: would the club hire a television set for Wimbledon
fortnight and, if so, could the expense of a colour set be justified? Are
members co-operating with a recently made group rule that they should
be ready and dressed when the centre transport bus called for them at
home in the morning or else be left behind? The proposed bus trip to
Fleetwood Port: was it reasonable to use up such a lot of petrol, given the
oil crisis and council finance cuts? Had the quarterly electric light bill
been paid and how was the new treasurer progressing: was he 'sharing' his
job with committee members more effectively than his predecessor?
What assessment would be made about the students currently on
placement in the centre?

Most centre members are middle-aged, with acquired disabilities, such
as arthritis and strokes. Most need help, or at least aids, to talk, walk or
toilet themselves. The members elect a management committee from
amongst themselves annually and the committee then runs the centre.
Accountable to the local authority social services committee via the

assistant director of social services, the committee pays the bills, controls the budget and hires and fires the staff. One member of the social services day care advisory staff also sits on the committee and the assistant director is *ex officio*.

The members decided that the basic activity at the centre should be craft work: they make crafts, sell them, the proceeds build up the amenity fund, and then, rather than paying individuals for their work each week, the group 'rewards' itself every now and then. Last week, for instance, the members had a big evening out in the restaurant of a local 'good food' hotel. The crafts done at the centre are simple handicrafts, such as crocheting and basketry, usually known already to the members themselves. They teach each other, although the local authority can make a handicraft instructress available as a consultant.

The care staff employed to work in the centre are accountable to the user management committee, which functions in place of a head of centre. The committee has had to learn the diplomacy of industrial relations: for instance, how to persuade the cook to provide the menu the users would like. Some committee members have experience to contribute from their past work background, but not all: the backgrounds of members are very mixed.

And the velvet curtains? Well, they were important early in the life of the new day centre. The council put up its regulation curtains and, in its first trial of strength, the committee sent them back. A committee man explained through his dysphasic speech that he could get velvet material at cost price from the textile firm he had worked for before his stroke. Then what did the curtains mean? Well, he explained, durability for a start, they'd last for years. Also they look classy, not cheap. They're individual, too; other places don't have them. And above all, the members chose them.

The green velvet curtains are a parable about the members of the Primus Club. Although disabled, the members are canny. Like the green velvet curtains, the members of the committee can be considered as both durable and classy. The curtains signify their individuality and choosiness.

The Primus Club is one unintended consequence of this research project. One question of a report of the pilot study circulated in 1975 was why 'new careers' ideas and self-management had apparently never been tried amongst disabled people. One person set out to examine this question in earnest[2] and the Primus Club is the result. Although the Primus Club staff and users have not been studied in the same way as staff and users discussed in the previous chapters, it is obvious that the way the Primus Club is organised is a change to the *status quo* represented in this book.

One theme implicit in the previous chapter and this, is that change is possible in day services. Cynics will comment that it is more feasible to start a new day centre with progressive ideas like the Primus Club, but what about changing the views of heads, staff and users in this book who represent, of course, thousands of existing services? These doubting Thomases are right: changing existing organisations is probably not as easy as starting new ones. Even once a reform has taken place, it is not easy to sustain, when the first flush of enthusiasm has worn off. Further, sometimes organisations do not maintain reforms after the departure of a charismatic reformer. Organisations do tend to revert to old bureaucratic habits. These unpalatable facts are, perhaps, responsible for the pessimism of some social researchers about changing things, because the assumption is that, once changed, reforms in organisations are not long lasting.

To explore the dynamics of potential change in day units is beyond the brief of this project, but this book will conclude with comments on possible factors which might be explored by those committed to improving day units. Two examples will be given of older day services which have changed radically in recent years.

GOING SOMEWHERE?

Until recently, the Metropolitan District of Stockport, near Manchester, had one training centre for the mentally handicapped in an old building, near some mills in a cleared area of town. Fifteen years old, this centre with ninety places was a traditional one: on entry to the foyer, corridors separated 'Boys' from 'Girls' (although in recent years both sexes have met at lunch and worked in integrated workshops). The staple activity was industrial contract work of a simple variety; there were long periods in between work, when trainees had nothing to do; instructors were remote from trainees and desultory and inconsistent attempts were made at offering 'formal education' to a few trainees in a rarely used education room in the centre. The manager was 'old school', a tradesman retrained as a teacher for the mentally handicapped.

A few years ago, Stockport decided to build a second training centre, an elaborate purpose-built centre in a different part of town to the old centre. By 1975, however, the combination of local authority cash cuts and new information from the day care research project made the assistant director of social services explore other alternatives for his new service. Two assumptions developed. First, in the future, the mental handicap day services of the area should concentrate on producing plans for people, not providing places in centres. Second, plans for people imply the development of specified points of entry and exit for the people. (You cannot work with a 'place' towards exit from the day unit, but you can work with a person.) So planning for places, a mechanistic exercise on paper, was replaced by planning for mentally handicapped people. The first step was to collect information about the people the service needed to serve. Then it was clear that not all mentally handicapped people needed places in day units, although most needed some kind of protected care by the day. So a new type of day service emerged, providing fewer places in units than there were mentally handicapped people in the area. The focus of the day service shifted from filling a certain number of places in centres to planning for the relevant people of the area.

So, plans for a new purpose-built centre were scrapped. A former convalescent hospital, an old country house in beautiful grounds, became the base of what would have been a new centre. As Chapter 17 has noted, Poise House organised itself in small rooms around six home bases, each staffed by two workers. Workers were recruited because each had at least one, and sometimes two, skills to give mentally handicapped people. The recognised qualification was one skill, recruited along with others, but more important was the ability to impart skills to users without preconceived notions of their supposed limitations.

A programme was organised; the basic concept was that each user, however retarded, needed the emotional security of a 'home base', but at the same time needed the chance to move out and explore a new world of skills. One main job of the head of centre became that of co-ordinating a highly complex programme for each user in particular and the centre in general. So from the home base each day, each user moves to a skill area, within his ability level. Language, dressmaking, bakery, photography or self-care are some skill options: the ability range of the users in the centre is very wide, so in practical terms, programmes range from tooth-cleaning to using the light meter on a camera. The idea is that the user should explore in a concentrated and directed way the skills offered within the centre and maximise these before moving on to learn other skills in or out of the unit.

At the same time, other alternatives for users were being developed by the day care advisory staff. A two-year course for a small number of mentally handicapped young people was commenced at the local college. Twelve young people at a time now attend college for two years and at the end of the course some move to open employment whilst others return to the work centre, now housed in the old training centre. All previous contract work from local industry has stopped: work contracts are now accepted only on grounds of their commercial viability or their training value. (In other words, a boring contract may be accepted if it pays well, but not unless.)[3] Within the work centre, users are allocated to particular contract work projects, while others work for a 'flying squad' (an at-the-ready group which can rush out to rescue local commercial concerns who need emergency manpower). A third group works as part of a self-contained horticultural project, which started on the gardens of Poise House but is developing into a self-contained work group, which hopes to work in the council's parks and gardens. Developing this kind of self-contained project and starting new projects, such as a woodwork project which will pay more attractive rates than social security, is one proposed way of overcoming the problem of work for trainees who will need sheltered work. Another possibility is to develop a day centre club for middle-aged mentally handicapped people who need some shelter during the day but who do not need to work all the time: this may develop along self-help lines.

Thus, mentally handicapped people in Stockport now have a service which provides a series of graduated stages, with entries and exits at a number of points. They move in and out of the service, go back and forwards. This is a similar plan to the Maudsley Day Hospital's day programme for the mentally ill described in Chapter 9, which provides a rehabilitation ladder for both short-term and long-term users, contingent on a user's progress and his personal conception of time. The Stockport plan, still experimental, is providing ladders (in the plural) rather than one ladder, partly in an attempt to offer work diversity and also partly because less is known, in practical terms, about the outcome of 'habilitation' ladders for the mentally handicapped than 'rehabilitation' ladders for the mentally ill.

What points about change in day units can be derived from this example? First, there was the belief that change is possible. Second, there was an impetus to change from the world outside the day service. In this case, the cash crisis led to re-evaluating the need for an expensive new building and this coincided with a new group of ideas about day services. Third, there was a leadership committed to implementing improvements. Fourth, there was the capacity to develop a suitable structure to take the strain of the incremental changes. Fifth, there was the understanding that the calibre of the new people appointed to work in the services was fundamental. Sixth, there was a commitment to involving and informing the staff and users of the changes. Seventh, there was a willingness for the leaders to examine and review the 'nitty gritty' of the day unit and then devolve alterations to sectional leaders. Finally, and quite important, all these issues were grappled with simultaneously, but over a time span of three to four years. What this meant was that, although the changes were radical in conception, they were implemented at the pace of the workers and at the degree they could tolerate. At the same time, it was recognised that change needed to proceed on a number of fronts at once: there was no point in incremental change (encouraging the mentally handicapped to sugar their own tea) while ignoring the need for change to the structure (metaphorically barring the exit doors to centres).

Another project producing changes by exploiting all these factors, is the family centre project at the Brotherhood of St Laurence, a voluntary agency in Melbourne, Australia, which has for many years run a social work service for poor families by tradtional methods: social casework (psychological support) and material help (piecemeal and *ad hoc*). In the early 1970s, the Brotherhood reviewed its services over several generations. Recognising that it had achieved little for chronically deprived, 'multiproblem' families, the agency decided to close down its 'treatment' service to families and to explore the use of self-help and mutual aid (Liffman, 1978). (But self-help was not interpreted as a matter of withdrawing services and leaving the families to pull themselves up by their bootstraps. This was recognised as technically impossible, for these poor families had no 'boots' – Perlman, 1968.)

The agency became a family centre along the lines described in Chapter 3.6, with an interesting programme, bulk shopping, camping facilities and an informality and blurring of the distinctions between staff and users. One component of the new centre philosophy was that poor families need money on a stable, continuous basis. Thus a guaranteed minimum income subsidy, composed of a family and rent supplements, was given to members of the family centre by right over the three years of the project. Also, increasing participation in the centre was developed by the sixty families. In effect, the families mounted the rungs of the participation 'ladder' outlined in Chapter 17. Family members became indigenous staff workers and took on management committee posts. This was not done without anxiety and upheavals amongst the professional workers, whose contribution gradually became redundant over the period. In the third year, the increasing power of the families in the programme led to the eventual removal of the professional workers from the Council of the centre and, unexpectedly, unseated the indigenous staff workers on the Council too! Removing all paid workers from the Council (a consequence accompanied by considerable breast-beating) left the centre controlled by the users, who then decided to open up the centre to outsiders as a new agency. So the result was the Action and Resource Centre, a service for poor people run by poor people.

As David Donnison points out, the Brotherhood of St Laurence family centre project did not invent solutions which can be mass produced elsewhere, since not every agency will provide resources for sixty families over several years (Liffman, 1978). On the other hand, over several generations – and in the short term too – chronically poor and disorganised young families consume disproportionate volumes of routine agency time and resources (Goldberg et al., 1978; Oliver and Cox, 1973). The Brotherhood of St Laurence family centre project gives many pointers to the potential of day services for so-called 'problem' families when they are treated, not as problems, but as persons with potential: a model which can be applied to other user groups too.

What do new day schemes for the mentally handicapped in Stockport, England have in common with multiproblem families in Melbourne, Australia? The first and rather obvious point is that both the mentally handicapped and 'multiproblem' families are, in professional terms, regarded as 'difficult to work with'. Neither offer riches for the aspiring practitioner who wants a fast cure or a quick solution. Nevertheless, both projects exploited similar sets of factors to produce changes. First, there was a belief by the leaders of both projects that change was possible. Second, there was a stimulus for change from the outside. At Stockport, the stimulus was overcrowding in the old training centre, a need for a new service, the end of the 'growth' era, a new pressure about economy, and a set of ideas from a research project. At the Brotherhood, the outside impetus for change was a vague set of ideas circulating from the American poverty programmes about self-help, and an ethos of reform inculcated by the Whitlam Labour government in Australia. Although each project operated within a different set of political, economic and social circumstances, both contexts favoured change.

Third, a belief in change was accompanied by action, exemplifying the biblical dictum in organisational terms that faith without works is dead. Both projects had done a lot of homework. Stockport knew who its mentally handicapped persons were, now and for the next ten years. The Brotherhood knew its multiproblem families and their characteristics well. Change was based on a detailed appraisal of the actual problem, rather than a naïve opportunism culled from sociology texts. So rather than waving magic wands and issuing *ex cathedra* statements, the leadership viewed change as a consequence of persistence and endurance. For example, discussion and training programmes were organised in both agencies to get a consensus about change by all groups to be affected. As well as arranging training for staff, Stockport held meetings for the families of the mentally handicapped users. Some meetings produced far from predictable results (the families of the mentally handicapped were far from positive initially about the new plans and this led to modifications). The meetings were aimed at democratic consensus, rather than imposing preordained decisions by fiat. Next, each project had to develop a new organisational structure. Although the new structure was quite different, it was not (like the reform of the new national health service) created arbitrarily and imposed overnight. The structure was introduced by negotiation and persuasion over a time span.

Fifth, new staff appointments were made on the basis of an appraisal of what the users needed rather than what the practitioners were trained to offer. The Brotherhood decided that income maintenance and development of survival skills was more vital to multiproblem families than the insight developed by casework. Stockport saw continuing education leading to a job as more crucial for mentally handicapped people than a place in a training centre. The repercussions of this were that both projects concentrated on the assets rather than the deficiencies of their users. Both projects saw the importance of the centre as a setting where co-equal relationships between staff and users could flourish. In the language of the research trade, both projects were interested in the instrumental (skill) and the affective (feelings) dimensions of the changes they introduced. This, in itself, meant that the leaders of the project paid detailed attention to the everyday issues: the 'nitty gritty' was not ignored while they defined their focus as the structure. Yet, at the same time, leaders were prepared to develop a structure which offered considerable autonomy to staff and users to implement change.

FACING THE FUTURE

Much has been written about change and how to achieve it, and the classic literature on organisations can be seen in the light of balancing the organisational tensions of change against conservatism. For those who would rather see day units set within the context of the bureaucracies from which they spring, this book can only constitute a first step which indicates that there is a tension between maintaining the *status quo* and seeking improvements. Others in the future may want to redefine this problem in theoretical terms; in the view of this writer, this final chapter, which has pointed the way to change, has tried to bridge the gap between theory without praxis on the one hand, and praxis which discounts general principles on the other.

This book cannot provide more that the first word on day services. Predictions for the future would probably be more accurately made by an astrologer than a social researcher. Recent upheavals have already affected the social beliefs and the resource base of services and the Britain in which this project ended is politically, economically and socially different to the Britain in which the project began.

That being the case, it would be insensitive and unwise to claim that day services are a 'solution', that they are a universal panacea, that their potential is unlimited. This has happened in some institutions in the century past and in the community care of this: and unjustifiable claims turn sour and leave a disconsolate pessimism in their wake. Further, this book has resisted the temptation to erect 'grand theories' or monolithic philosophies to account for the creation of day services: such baroque confidence being out of keeping with the sober and straitened spirit of the age. Aside from that, the reader will have seen the tension between regarding day care as a system and a disparate set of component parts. Strictly speaking, it is less of a system than an approach. Building a system means developing plant and places. Building an approach means aiming to develop practical steps to implement the aims already referred to – and other – in the different user groups of day services. Therefore, such theory as there is in this book, hopefully arises from the data of each user group. This 'grounded' or practical approach to theorising is an approach similar to the opinions expressed by the shepherd in Shakespeare's *As You Like It*. On philosophy, the shepherd said:

> I know the more one sickens, the worse at ease he is and that he who wants money, means and content is without three good friends; that the property of rain is to wet and fire to burn, that good pasture makes fat sheep, and that a great cause of the night is lack of sun. . . .

If change needs to be about practice, this has repercussions for the aims of day units too, because the aims need to be about the people in day units as well as about the day units themselves. The aims in day units need to encompass the methods used as well as the ends, and to be related to the jobs of the staff as well as to the aspirations of the top people. The next job is to try to close the gap of rhetoric between aspirations and routines, and other workers have shown how this might be done (Kushlick, 1975).

It would be foolish to disagree on either philosophic or practical grounds that the future of day services is, at least in part, tied up with the future of the economy. For example, if unemployment is merely a short-term crisis, its impact on the development of day services is likely to be only marginal. But if unemployment in Western societies is the long-term result of the decline and fall of certain production industries and markets, its implications for day services are more profound. Long-term crises will fall doubly on the unskilled and disabled members of a community, so the view that day care is an interregnum between acquiring a disability and subsequent employment will have to be reconsidered. This is a long way from the truth now, particularly in units for the mentally and physically handicapped, and increasing unemployment will exacerbate the problem.[4] Will day units become a larger and larger reserve for the rejects of the contracting employment market? Or can day services demonstrate a potential creative function as alternatives to conventional unemployment? This may not interest governments committed to restoring capitalism and market mechanisms. But day units might be involved in developing new technologies which need long-term investment in people as well as capital. This notion is a long way from the stop-gap job creation schemes advocated in recent years.

Genuine job creation on a long-term basis needs to develop new technological innovations, such as solar energy, which will create jobs rather than eliminate them. For example, there is a place for developing new technologies to restore the environment destroyed by the repercussions of the last industrial revolution, and other aspects of job creation that come to mind are the needs of the human service industry – for example, planning for the explosion in numbers of the elderly and confused elderly people in Western societies expected a decade from now. All these aspects of job creation could be the subject of technical innovations which are simultaneously labour intensive and long term. As we have seen, current government measures which encourage public and private enterprises to employ disabled people are not likely to be much use if conventional employment does not *need* more manpower (Windschuttle, 1979).

At the time of writing, however, the future of employment and the role of public services is problematic. But one important lesson from the past appears to be that it is not social changes in themselves, but the attitudes which accompany them, which are critical to the survival of reforms. For instance, during the nineteenth century, when many new reforms and ideas were introduced to the care of mentally ill in asylums, optimism was high (in the view of some, too high). Then came a changed set of economic and social circumstances: overpopulation, unemployment, new scientific beliefs and technologies. Faced by new social conditions, optimism amongst social reformers ran out of steam and was replaced by pessimism. This became a negativism which indicated that nothing could be done for the mentally ill. The lesson from this for day services in a period of social change is, perhaps, not to lose the belief that improvements are possible, but not to get carried away! After all, even that strange pessimist, Ecclesiastes, depressed enough to conclude that there was nothing new under the sun (not even day units), would acknowledge through his frustration and negativism that there was a time and a place for everything. In the light of his cyclical perspective, perhaps the past decades have been the time for planting and the time for building day services. Now there is an opportunity to consider change: or, as Ecclesiastes put it rather more figuratively, for pulling down and breaking up. So this book has provided the opportunity for reflection on the future direction of day services, an activity which has, at times, induced pessimism. Yet for the future, we can be optimistic about the potential of day services, which is as yet unfulfilled.

NOTES

1 All units referred to in this chapter only, are given proper names, not pseudonyms.
2 Robert Lewis, Assistant Director, Stockport Social Services Department.
3 The problem of paying users adequately for their work has not been overcome, however.
4 One interesting feature of the examples of this chapter is the way that those projects committed to maintaining disabled users in the long term are doing so by releasing the users' capacities to look after themselves. This may, in the long term, be cost-effective care.

REFERENCES

Goldberg, E. M. *et al.* (1978) 'Towards accountability in social work: long-term social work in an area office', *British Journal of Social Work*, 8, 3, pp. 253–87.

Kushlick, A. (1975) *Some Ways of Setting, Monitoring and Obtaining Objectives for Disabled People*, Research Report 116, Health Care Evaluation Team under the auspices of the Medical Research Council, Department of Health and Social Security, University of Southampton, Wessex Regional Health Authority (Paper presented to Conference on The Handicapped – Towards Independent Living, National Committee on Residential Care, Brisbane, Australia, 19–21 June).

Liffman, M. (1978) *Power for the Poor: The Family Centre Project, an experiment in self help* (Allen & Unwin).

Oliver, J. and Cox, A. (1973) 'A family kindred with ill-used children: the burden on the community', *British Journal of Psychiatry*, 123, pp. 81–90.

Perlman, H. (1968) 'Casework and the case of Chemung County', in G. E. Brown (ed.), *The Multi-Problem Dilemma: A Social Research Demonstration with Multi-Problem Families* (Scarecrow Press).

Windschuttle, K. (1979) *Unemployment* (Penguin).

PART FOUR

Appendix I

METHODS AND PROCEDURES

PART ONE: METHODS

In the first part of this appendix is a synopsis of the methods of the survey. A skeleton of the decisions taken about procedures will be reviewed within the time available for the survey. In the second part of the appendix, some of the constraints on the project of a more intellectual nature will be discussed. These include the degree of commitment to traditional scientific method and a discussion of the degree of confidence a reader might have in the results. A much more detailed account of the techniques of sampling, interviewing and other technical matters can be found in the technical volume (Edwards and Carter, 1980).

Year One, Month One
At the beginning, the total asset of the day care project was a flimsy file containing some correspondence between the Joseph Rowntree Memorial Trust and the National Institute for Social Work. There were some newspaper articles about psychiatric day care along with an odd article and one or two names and addresses. Five years later the assets of the day care project had swollen to over 1,700 questionnaires, six filing cabinets and a four foot high stack of computer printout.

During the initial period references about day care were reviewed. The information this yielded was subsequently published in *Adult Day Care: Selected References*, by the National Institute for Social Work.[1] Information about day care was sought from practitioners, administrators and day units and different parts of the country were visited. The principal researcher joined, as an observer, a working party holding discussions about a possible new training for workers in day care (the Certificate in Social Service) at the Central Council for Education and Training in Social Work. Staff appointments were made – a research assistant and secretary joined the team. Some theorising about the position and significance of day services was spelled out in discussion papers.

Year One, Month Six
During the pilot stage of the project a small study was held to attempt to assess what information should be collected from whom and how this might be done. It had been decided to meet all ranges of people in day units; that is the attenders, the staff and those in charge.

Embryonic versions of questionnaires were tested out in three areas of the country, north, south and metropolitan, for a fortnight. After discussions with fifty-three staff and thirty-six users and an analysis of their comments and replies, the scope of the study was defined more precisely. A report of the pilot study was circulated.

Year Two, Month One
The brief was to try to review all day services for all groups of people. This meant persuading a number of statutory authorities and voluntary agencies that their ostensibly specialised and separate services had something in common with each other. Not all organising bodies held this view. It was necessary to contact, discuss and persuade day services under varied sponsorship to co-operate with the study. The health service, via area health authorities, local authorities through social services departments, voluntary organisations of a number of shapes and sizes and a miscellany of other statutory agencies,for example, the probation services, agreed to be part of the study.

'Across the board' sponsorship uncovered the myriad of people attending day services outlined in Chapter 1. Some sponsors argued that this smorgasbord of services had little in common. Others were aware that tradition, arbitrary administrative definitions and recurrent departmental reorganisations meant that an attender might, by luck as much as design, fall into the catchment of one day service as much as another. For instance, services for old people were operated by health, social services and voluntary agencies, but they rarely offered the attender a choice. So, for that matter, were services for the psychiatrically disturbed.

Some commonalities of day services seemed to be disguised by the language used to define each scheme. Thus some attempt was made to reach common definitions and to reduce the language barriers which were a construct of a particular professional approach. These are described in Chapter 1.

Year Two, Month Three
The next problem was to work out how to go about selecting representative areas of the country for the national survey. A detailed account of the technicalities of sampling is found in Edwards and Carter (1980). Thirteen areas of the country based on local authority boundaries were selected at random, with certain 'stratification' factors guiding the sampling process. Thirteen authorities, 11 per cent, were selected as the smallest number of authorities in England and Wales which would adequately gross back to a national picture of day services. Three stratification factors were introduced, namely, region, type of authority and population. These factors and the sampling process are described fully elsewhere. The thirteen areas were:

Area		Estimated Population
London boroughs	Innerborough	171,600
	Outerborough	330,600
	Northborough	230,800
	Westborough	166,800
Metropolitan districts	Coaltown	295,700
	Steeltown	558,000
	Cottontown	227,500
	Cartown	199,600
County councils	Southshire	1,002,900
	Eastshire	577,600
	Northshire	916,400
	Welshire	389,200
	Midshire	505,900

Total = 5,572,600

(OPCS, 1977)

Year Two, Month Four

By this time the aim was to commence the fieldwork of the project within two months. The aims of the survey were defined: these are outlined in the Introduction at the beginning of the book.

The detective work phase of the survey, which meant locating every single day unit in the thirteen areas, was started. In most areas there was no central reference point for statutory authorities and voluntary agencies with this information, so this was not a straightforward job. Local newspapers, noticeboards and job advertisements were read assiduously before 291 day units were located and mapped in the thirteen areas. (Three day units were missed until after fieldwork, but considering the absence of central information on day services the search was reasonably successful.) The 291 units in the thirteen areas constituted the *census* sample.

The next task was to approach the appropriate professional associations to ask for their good will towards the study. Then each director of social services and area medical officer and the heads of voluntary agencies needed to be visited to explain the study. Once their agreement was obtained it was important to contact all those in charge of day units to explain the study. Because we were unable to visit all the units in the census sample, 157 units were selected for interviewing. These 157 units were selected by another stratified random sample. This time the relevant stratification factors were the user group and the service provider. For the three largest user groups – the elderly, the mentally ill and the physically handicapped – we set a ceiling of three on the number of units to be visited in each area. In the case of the mentally handicapped a ceiling of two units per area was set. This is because these services were invariably provided by the local authority and also because a recent survey gave information about these units (Whelan and Speake, 1977). All the units provided for the other minor user groups (for example, families, elderly confused, offenders, mixed groups) were included. No sampling was necessary because their overall number was so small. So this is how the 157 units in the interview sample were selected.

In each day unit the head was always interviewed. All the staff and users were eligible to be interviewed but three staff members and six users were selected at random from those eligible. A meeting was held for heads of day units within a certain area. As well as communicating details about the project at this meeting, a set of random numbers helped select staff and users for interview.

Meanwhile further decisions had been made about what questions would be asked and to whom. A personal questionnaire to be answered by the staff and head of day units was developed, along with questions for the users of the day unit. The questions are listed in Edwards and Carter (1980). The questionnaires contain a number of 'open' questions and the technique of the interview allowed the possibility of addressing the user in language familiar to him.

It was also decided to carry out a limited series of observations in units visited by the researchers and to talk to administrators of services. A telephone questionnaire about the policy and administration of day services was directed to senior administrators in each of the thirteen health and social services authorities. Observations were made in seventy-three units, not randomly selected.

Year Two, Month Six
Tenders had been called for an external research agency to carry out the interviewing on the project. In the event, Research Services Ltd were commissioned. A 'dress rehearsal' pilot study was conducted with interviewers from this agency in Cambridgeshire and from this experience we evolved an extensive manual for interviewers and plans for a two-day briefing period to be attended by each interviewer. Techniques for selection of interviewers developed. It was imperative that the interviewers met certain strict criteria, because of the likely variety of respondents. This ranged from highly specialised professionals to extremely handicapped people with impediments in hearing, sight, comprehension and speech.

For the next six months the day services project became peripatetic as thirteen areas of the country were covered. All interviews took place in the day units themselves. Finally, interviews took place in 154 day units, with 888 users and 559 heads and staff members. This represented interviews with one head, three staff members and six users in each of the 154 day units. Of the 290 day units, 276 returned their postal questionnaires. In short, the response rate was as follows:

276 postal questionnaires	95% (response rate)
148 heads	refusals 1%
411 staff	refusals 2%
888 users	refusals 5%

Several points might be made about the interviews. Many ideas were gleaned from other studies, especially consumer studies and research about particular user groups. A number of existing measures (such as the Community Oriented Programs Environment Scale (Moos, 1974), Child Management Scale (King *et al.*, 1971) and the Index of Incapacity (Sainsbury, 1973) were adapted, tested in the pilot study and used to inform the design of certain questions.

Several features of the questionnaires can be mentioned. First is the method used for tapping a particular time sequence in the respondent's memory. Many studies (Cartwright, 1963); Mechanic and Newton, 1965; Brown and Rutter, 1966 have commented on errors in data collection due to the memory lapses of respondents and have tried to illuminate the process involved. Mechanic and Newton (1965) suggest that many of the problems can be summarised by the saliency rule: that is, events further away in time and of less importance to the individual tend to be forgotten. So a decision was made to collect information from respondents only about events in the week previous to the interview wherever feasible. Thus recall would be improved and the time span for memory would be the same for everyone. The week before the survey was chosen because of its closeness in time and because most day units in the pilot seemed to schedule activities on a weekly basis.

Second, staff and users were viewed in day units as co-partners in the project instead of 'subjects' wherever possible. In designing the three questionnaires, the criteria for inclusion of a question was that it be of direct relevance to the people in day units or designed to enlighten an issue of importance to them. A limitation of this was that a question had to be applicable across the range of user groups and service providers before it was included.

Considerable work has been done on the influence of various types of questioning procedures on the responses received (Richardson *et al.*, 1965). Any individual question on a standard interview schedule can be described as 'closed' or 'open'. 'Closed' questions are those which have predetermined lists of responses into which all responses should fall. They include questions which can be adequately answered in a few words. Closed questions usually can be coded by the interviewer before the next question on the schedule is asked. But by contrast open questions call for a longer and less structured response from the respondent and no espected categories of response are specified. Participation is generally encouraged by open questions and it is assumed that if interviewers are not forced to polarise the answers of the respondents into predetermined categories, they can more accurately record the true emphasis of what is said to them. At the same time, open questions allow respondents to fully develop and express their ideas. It is clear though that open questions depend very largely on the interviewer's ability to probe and extend the respondent's views. In an effort to develop the probing skills of the interviewers involved in the project, part of the briefing held for them was devoted to improving their interviewing skills. A section of the manual prepared for the interviewers repeated and reinforced the material covered in the briefings.

In the pilot study most questions were administered in an 'open' form, composing what Richardson calls 'conversation with a purpose'. The respondents supplied facts and insights about day care, based on their own experiences. From these answers, coding frames were generated for those closed questions to be included in the final questionnaires. All 'closed' questions were given a code of ☐ Qualified Answer (for Yes/No questions) (or ☐ Other) to accommodate respondents whose responses did not fit into the predetermined categories. However, where possible 'open' questions were used in the main stage interview schedules.

Another difficulty had to do with the set wording and order of questions. The wording of questions and the order in which they are given is generally fixed in advance in survey interviews. Richardson has argued that although standardised questions are accepted survey technique, acceptance is not the same thing as effectiveness. Standardised questions are based on the assumption that respondents have a common vocabulary and that questions have the same meaning for each of them. Thus standardised questions assume that the respondents have similar personal characteristics, similar education and similar intelligence. In this survey we faced unique difficulties of interviewing a very disabled population. The respondents also came from a wide range of ages and from different cultural and even dialect backgrounds. Experience in the pilot study suggested that it was difficult to select words which meant the same to everyone and that a standard question might go unanswered, for instance, by mentally handicapped people for whom an average question might be outside their range of cultural experience.

To reduce these difficulties a fairly unorthodox procedure for this type of survey was adopted. Interviewers were asked to reword specified questions in terms which made the question understandable to the respondents. They were asked to record the final wording which elicited the response which they recorded, so that the project staff could check the deviation from the prescribed wording. For example, the question 'What kind of accommodation do you live in at present?' might sometimes get a puzzled look from a young mentally handicapped person. But if the question was put in a form which tapped the respondent's own experience (for example, 'Where do you live?' A. 'With Mum and Dad'. 'What do they live in?' A. 'It's a house', and so on), an adequate response was often elicited.

Questions where deviations from prescribed wording were permitted were marked on the schedule with an asterisk. Because some questions needed to be compared with the staff responses, we did not allow deviations from prescribed wording on these occasions. Allowing the interviewers to take a less mechanical role in the interviewing gave them a better opportunity for obtaining the participation of their respondents. Of the two possible forms of bias, over-involvement and under-involvement, we decided that the former was preferable to the latter.

Year Three, Month One
Editing the questionnaires in an effort to eliminate clerical mistakes made by the interviewers or by the respondent is often regarded as a routine task (Moser and Kalton, 1971). The first edit for completeness might be regarded as routine but two other important checks, for accuracy and uniformity, often require a degree of judgement and skill if the respondent's meaning is to be preserved.

The project staff plus three specially trained part-time social science graduates edited the three schedules. A list of additional codes was constructed from a sample of questionnaires. Each questionnaire was edited completely by one person and then checked by another, in contrast to editing a section at a time. Editing the questionnaire as a whole meant that the relationship between responses to different questions could be noted and inconsistencies detected. Even with these precautions, editing was not faultless. Further errors needed to be corrected following the machine editing procedure done by computer.

Year Three, Month Four
Coding the questionnaires is classifying the answers of 'open-ended' questions into categories. The list of possible categories of response for any given question is called the coding frame. Most descriptions of coding procedures tend to disguise their imprecision. In fact, the correspondence between question response and coding frame is extremely *ad hoc* or improvised (Cicourel, 1967). Even when carefully instructed, coders are likely to be guided by 'common sense' or 'folk notions' of what was intended by both the answer to a question and the rules of the coding frame. The very construction of coding frames generates meanings imposed on the data by researchers. Procedures to quantify data are often divorced from the social reality of everyday communication and life experiences which they intend to describe.

We cannot claim to have entirely overcome these difficulties, but we did try to remain very close to the data. Usually coders of survey data have played very little part in interviewing but we found it essential for the project staff to be involved fully in interviewing and coding.

The procedure used to develop each coding frame for 'open' questions was as follows: a random sample of 15 per cent of all questionnaires was extracted and their main themes listed. After discussion, a provisional coding frame was produced to reflect first the answers as they stood and second the purpose to which the data would be put in analysis. The sample of questionnaires was coded by one of us and the reliability of the coding was checked by another, who recoded the sample 'blind'. If good agreement resulted, the coding frame was finalised. If the agreement was 80 per cent or less the code was revised and the procedure repeated until good agreement was achieved. The questionnaires were then coded by one of the two people who did the original coding. Regular checks for accuracy and agreement were carried out.

This was one attempt at what Webb *et al.* have called 'triangulation' (Webb *et al.*, 1966). Another measurement method of an unobtrusive nature was the ratings of the user's tone of voice in the interviews with users, as a parallel measure to a question about satisfaction. Sometimes the use of records can supplement survey data and improve their quality. This was attempted during the pilot study but failed. First, access to records involved particular problems concerning confidentiality. Second, availability and quality of records was unpredictable. Third, record-keeping systems were not standardised so any prediction of the time required for collection of data from them was unreliable. Thus for a project whose budget and time were strictly limited such a technique was not feasible.

No attempt was made to encapsulate the attitudes of our respondents into attitude statements and scales. Attitude scales tend to force respondents into highly polarised positions which do not reflect the ambiguity or uncertainty of their roles or activities. Even if one could avoid this, which is doubtful, we felt that discrete statements of attitudes imply fixed and externally ascertainable values. Also, the relationship between attitudes and behaviours is so problematic (Cohen, 1966) that description of attitudes is of little value in understanding behaviour and social relationships.

Year Three, Month Seven
The data went to the computer and this chronology was written. It reads rather smoothly in retrospect and leaves out most of the upheavals and mishaps which seem to be attracted to a national survey like a magnet. The purpose of outlining a date-history of a research project is to remind readers that there is nothing finite about the results of such a survey: the outcome is achieved by wrestling with extremely practical problems and imperfect decisions in the muddy and by no means distinct context of everyday life.

Part II: Constraints

In fact, there is no longer agreement that social surveys are sensitive forms of social inquiry. Surveys in the 1970s have to take into account some trenchant criticisms (Cicourel, 1964) some of which oversimplify the problems and dismiss social surveys because they apply such rigid technologies. The rationale behind the day care survey is rather complex and has at least attempted to face some of the common criticisms of surveys.

The purpose of what follows is to discuss the following questions:

First, to what extent is this national survey of day services a descendant of the established tradition of social surveys?

Second, to what extent has what is usually called the scientific method been adopted, in preference to alternative methods of measuring day services?

Third, what confidence can one have in the results? In other words, how do we know that we have measured what we think we have measured? For instance, how do we know that we have measured what happens in day units as distinct from what people tell us happens?

THIS SURVEY IN PERSPECTIVE

First, then, to what extent is this national survey a descendant of the established tradition of social surveys? In Britain, there is a research tradition which uses the social survey as the primary method of social investigation. This tradition has its roots in the social inquiries carried out at the end of the nineteenth century and the beginning of the twentieth century. Of course, there have been other traditions where the accumulation of 'social facts' has been used as evidence of social problems or social conditions. One obvious example is the literary tradition where the method used by novelists such as Charles Dickens and Mrs Gaskell was to present 'real' social events as fiction. Mayhew's account describing London, its streets and the occupations of its populace in *London's Labour and the London Poor* is rather more documentary in tone but uses imaginative reconstructions where necessary. Another tradition is that of using the Parliamentary Select Committee as a method of collecting facts. For example, the history of the treatment of the mentally ill of the nineteenth century can almost be constructed from the evidence collected by these inquiries (Jones, 1955). Some of the questions asked in such inquiries are still being asked in surveys today.

By the end of the nineteenth century, social surveys attempted to quantify their results. Take the seventeen-volume survey of poverty of the streets of London by Booth (1891). This was followed in 1901 by Seebohm Rowntree's classic study of households in York, where a house-to-house inquiry revealed the frequency and nature of poverty in that city (Rowntree, 1901). Booth imposed an order on the nature of poverty in London streets by means of ranking the streets according to certain criteria. Rowntree constructed standards of minimum family needs in respect of food, clothing, fuel and rent by constructing a 'Poverty Line'. He also attempted to define primary and secondary poverty and in doing so drew attention for the first time to the 'cyclical' nature of poverty. Mark Abrams (1951) considers that the ensuing enthusiasm for local surveys was greatly enhanced by the discovery by Bowley at the London School of Economics of sampling techniques. The basic techniques of the survey as a form of social investigation were the result of the cumulative work of these three men. Their contribution was the collection of information by interviews with those being studied, the application of quantitative definitions to 'loose' material about such things as poverty, and the collection of information by using a sample instead of a total population (Abrams, 1951).

Enthusiasm for surveys related a good deal to various changes in social thought in the second half of the nineteenth century and the early twentieth century. The 'discovery' of the social survey coincided with, first, a readiness by those in authority to promote the material welfare of a society, and second, a recognition of the fact that social affairs could be susceptible to human control. Third, there was the development of skill in the quantitative assessment of cause and effect (Abrams, 1951). A fourth reason might be added to this catalogue: the development and diffusion of thinking after Darwin led to the view that social information could be subject to the same classificatory procedures as the natural and physical sciences.

Large numbers of social surveys were carried out between the two world wars. After the Second World War, social survey techniques lent themselves readily to market research surveys and to public opinion polls. Their use was extended by government as a tool for what Abrams calls social engineering – the planning and building of physical environmental conditions aiming to maximise human welfare. He considered, writing in 1951, that the social survey provided Britain with an analysis of poverty which saved her from violence and revolution and set her on the road to economic democracy.

This rather large claim implies that there is some reason for considering that the social survey developed out of a specific social period as a research tool of social optimism. Thinkers in this period, from Beatrice Webb to Mark Abrams, assumed that the issue was one of collecting the 'facts', the implications of which would be self-evident to rational intelligent experts. Regardless of their beliefs, men would inevitably accept the facts as pointing the way to the adoption of particular social policies.

In the late 1970s we do not share this confidence. We are aware that there is a huge gulf between the collection of information and the influencing of social and political outcomes. The view that human affairs can easily be changed for the better has come under attack from a variety of sources. Many have reasonably questioned whether gathering data and reporting on them leads to the right outcome – or indeed to any outcome at all. For example, Rowntree's insight into life cycle poverty has been reinforced and elaborated by researchers for nearly eighty years, but there is still no clear consensus about the way in which economic, political and social interventions should tackle this problem. It is an open question whether the apparently more sophisticated measurement 'hardware' of latter day researchers has achieved more clarity about appropriate social interventions than the descriptive accounts of the early social surveyors. Some critics have even argued that resources put into the American 'poverty' research sponsored in the 1960s achieved more for the researchers than the poor. The group of people set up financially were middle class researchers.

Such criticisms need to be faced and provide a challenge for researchers perpetuating survey research. Day services are brand new territory for researchers to explore and a national survey can hope to provide a taxonomy of description and analysis for future work. Day services are also relatively new. For that reason and also because of certain reservations about trends in traditional survey methods, perhaps this survey has more in common with the survey conducted by Rowntree in 1899 than with many current surveys.

SURVEYS AND SCIENTIFIC METHOD

That social data can be collected, classified and quantified in the same way as information in the physical sciences is a view which has been strongly attacked. Scientific methods may suit many of the quantitative concerns of an industrial society, but they do not deal adequately with human problems of a less quantifiable nature. Critics of the traditional scientific method have probably been strongest within the discipline of sociology but the debate about the relevance of the scientific method and what is called 'the positivist approach' has spread to other disciplines such as political science and psychology. The current doubts, controversies and clashes about method in sociology should not be regarded as an internal parochial debate, says Pahl, but as an essential seedbed from which new growth in social theory might develop (Pahl, 1974).

What is usually meant by the 'positivist approach' in social sciences involves three main assumptions (Giddens, 1974):

(1) That the procedures of natural sciences can be transferred to social matters without any difficulty.
(2) That certain laws of generalisations can emerge from research analysis.
(3) That the knowledge of social research is available for practical application. This knowledge is value free because the observer is objective and detached. The knowledge is a tool which should be used to make the world a better place.

An interesting scheme of beliefs developed by Martin Rein has been valuable in thinking about research (Rein, 1976). The first scheme, the *value free* position, has already been introduced as the 'positivist' approach. Rein suggests that the positivist approach can be criticised not because it is wrong but because it is incomplete. It accepts as 'given' what is most problematic – the values surrounding and interacting with the so-called facts. Instead of accepting that the measurement of social events is inextricably tied up with the values attached to them, positivist knowledge claims to go beyond ideological bias and subjective outlooks because it claims to be founded in controlled observation and logical analysis. 'Normative' and 'factual' issues must be separated from each other because neutrality about values is a condition of claiming to be objective. 'What this means is that [it is assumed that] methodological problems faced by social scientists are no more or less insoluble than those faced by physical science, that the epistemological assumptions of the social scientist need to be no different . . . the logic of his explanations must be the same' (Ryan, 1970, p. 15).

However, Rein suggests that there is an alternative way of thinking to the positivist approach. This alternative suggests that human life differs essentially from the subject matter of natural science, because it has a meaningfulness which is denied natural phenomena. So the activities studied by the social scientist are different in kind, as well as being of a different complexity to those studied by the natural scientist. To discuss social life we must encompass concepts of what people intend and plan to do and try to uncover the everyday meanings that human beings attach to their lives. This approach goes beyond attempts to establish causal regularities in research and in turn creates some difficulties. Although research is still agreed to be an empirical inquiry, the respondent and the social scientist can give two different accounts of the same situation, leaving it difficult sometimes to see how these accounts can be reconciled. This is an obvious problem for some because the question of 'whose' account should dominate becomes a difficulty. But the positivist researcher does not need to concern himself with such issues because the canons of his beliefs are that he is an impartial neutral observer. But for the researcher who, in Rein's terms, regards himself as *value committed*, an explicit moral dilemma results.

The value committed approach ascribes that a researcher may acknowledge a humanist commitment, in the sense of being committed to attempting to develop an understanding of the qualities distinctive of human beings and their construction of symbols and meaning. A day unit, for example, is created by human action. The staff and users in day units *create* their own environment by interpreting and giving meaning to their surroundings. If social facts have an intrinsic human meaning, interpretations need to be grounded in the meaning such events have for the respondents. This approach makes the status of this survey relative, since one survey cannot provide the one objective account of day unit life. Instead it is but one particular interpretation of social reality.

Third, there is the *value critical* approach. According to Rein, a critique of methods and values at every stage of the research process is necessary, because the actual analytic procedures in themselves contain all sorts of values. The value critical approach is a relatively doubtful and uncertain position, accepting neither the claim to pure science of the value neutral approach nor the humanist leanings of value commitment. While accepting that facts and values are inextricably welded together, it is considered inevitable that ethical and moral judgements will need to be made and choices exercised in any research. For example, choices are adopted even in measurement. Why ask some questions and omit others? Why neglect factors considered 'too hard to measure' in a national survey (like the quality of staff and user 'engagement') when they may be more critical to understanding a day unit than other more feasible measurements?

Further, the value critical approach wants to submit the *goals* and *practices* of research to critical review. For example, the value critical approach would question a possible research conclusion which, say, suggested expanding day services, by scrutinising the values that this suggestion implies. Thus a researcher who adopts a value critical position needs to take his own commitments into account when he examines social events. This is difficult to do, but perhaps less arrogant than the certainty of the positivist researcher of his objectivity.

This survey owes a partial debt to each of these approaches. The value free approach has made it possible to approach day units in a systematic, orderly way. The value committed approach reminds us that the information collected in day units is actually about human beings, who are capable of giving meaning to their own existence. The value critical approach takes a critical and examining approach to beliefs about research. It also implies that social research is less about accuracy than overcoming problems of error. Researchers too have biases and they are part of the research scene. There is no such thing as a 'pure' collection of interview data.

These three approaches, as Rein points out, are in conflict with each other over a period of time. In practice, we found that one approach was more important than another at different points of the project. But the other two approaches provided a kind of dialectic against which our procedures and approaches at every point of the process could be evaluated.

CONFIDENCE IN RESULTS

One of the most fundamental problems a social researcher faces is how he knows he has measured what he thinks he has measured? This problem can be discussed from several viewpoints, but two have been selected for particular emphasis. The first is the organisation of surveys themselves. Those who have organised a survey will be conscious that the organisations which carry them out approach in many ways the classic 'type' of a bureaucracy. In a survey, as in a bureaucracy, tasks are organised on a regulated basis and then sub-divided into jobs organised by the function they are to perform. The tasks are allocated hierarchically and work is done under supervision by control from the top. There are clear technical 'rules' specifying the way in which the work should be conducted. Each task is done by different people, so in a typical survey, for instance, coding and interviewing is usually done by different people. It is possible to make a strong case against the impersonal and functional discreteness of the way surveys are organised (Cicourel, 1967). We tried to overcome these criticisms, by the project staff remaining very involved in interviewing, editing and coding procedures and by refusing to allow these jobs to be controlled by the external survey organisations.

Second, the technical concepts of reliability and validity qualify the relationship between the questionnaires and the variables that they are intended to measure. Reliability, for instance, reflects the extent to which the same results would be obtained during repeated trials of the questionnaire when all other conditions were held constant. This is an almost impossible condition to fulfil during a survey of this kind. Validity, probably a much more crucial concept, affects the nature of the relationship between the questionnaires and what they set out to measure. When we ask questions of an abstract nature (such as 'What are the aims of this day unit?'), we need to know whether the answers to questions are indicators of these abstract concepts. This particular problem is known as construct validity and it arises 'whenever no criterion or universe of content is accepted as entirely adequate to define the quality to be measured' (Cronbach and Meehl, 1955).

One of the most perplexing problems of validity faced in the day care project is how we can have any certainty that what people *say* happens in day units has anything to do with how they *actually* behave. If the method had encompassed both interviews and parallel observations, our confidence could have been higher. If we had interviewed and observed what was interviewed we would have 'triangulated', as Webb suggests, by producing at least two independent measures of the same thing. So has the survey managed to capture what happens in day units?

This question itself contains several assumptions which could be examined by the value critical approach. First, it is questionable that a day unit consists of words (on the one hand) and deeds (on the other) which should measure up. The everyday reality of day services may be more complex. It is not that the 'realities' of day services are deeds while words are the window-dressing. Rather, any day unit can be studied from the point of view of 'impression management' (Goffman, 1959). A 'team' of 'performers' co-operate to present to an audience a given definition of a situation. 'Backstage' performances are both words and behaviour which take place only between team members, whereas 'frontstage' performances are words and behaviour reserved only for a public view.

But 'frontstage' information is no less real than 'backstage' information. What is important is whether or not the data is composed of both types of information. In order to do so we would need to identify what Goffman calls 'teams', who work together. Sometimes 'teams' may consist of staff only: sometimes staff and users may form 'teams' without the head. For instance, in one day unit staff and users said they were only allowed to talk to each other at lunchtime. But in another day unit staff said they separated from users at particular periods of the day, for instance, at lunchtime.

In retrospect, we discovered that our sampling militated against the construction of a detailed picture about the 'teams' in day care. On the other hand the random selection of respondents probably raised the probability that we have collected 'backstage' information. Whilst sociometric sampling based on close contact or affinity (Coleman, 1959) may have demonstrated the teams in day care, the random sampling of respondents was an implicit threat to those day units which wanted to show the researchers only frontstage performances. Thus because day units did not control the way respondents were sampled, we know that backstage views were voiced in the interviews. For example, in one day unit a head emphasised throughout the interview his concern and involvement with all his users. But the randomly selected staff and users stated that the head discriminated continually against one user group (the physically disabled) and favoured the other group (the mentally ill). So the head's 'frontstage' performance was not sustained by any other team members. When the head complained later about the intrusiveness of the interviews it was possible that he was more upset at the successful penetration of his own frontstage performance.

So we cannot assume that interviews with the staff offer frontstage information while the users offer backstage information. Although familiar with the writings of Goffman who predicts a split between the views of staff and users we did not always find this to be the case. The degree to which staff and users hold similar and different views has been spelled out.

There is a different problem, which relates to the question of how far we can trust the data. This pertains to the method of relying almost exclusively on a user's account of his or her disabilities and limitations, both physical and mental. It might be argued that our confidence could be higher if we had arranged for independent assessments of the 888 users by a physician or a psychiatrist. This is an extremely complex matter, beyond the scope of this appendix. The view a researcher takes on this matter can be related to his or her position in Martin Rein's scheme. A researcher who sees himself as 'value free' will inevitably want to have independent assessments, simply because he considers the assessor to be objective while the respondent is not. A researcher more inclined to the 'value committed' school will consider that a user's view of his or her condition is so loaded with subjective meaning, that he is not entitled to impose an external or independent view on it.

In practice we fell somewhere between these two postures. There were practical reasons why we could not provide independent assessments by doctors. The first was a question of budget limitations; the second, a matter of organisation and training. It is well known that so called independent assessments of clinical status can vary a great deal too. Observers from different disciplines – and even the same – use different criteria for reaching a diagnosis or assessing a performance. This has been demonstrated in fields of physical and mental health. It has also been shown that with training and practice, a group of persons can be trained to apply the same criteria (this was in fact a method we used with the interviewers). But we did not have the resources to extend this technique to encompass the provision of independent assessors. We also considered that to use the staff of the day unit, or the family of the user, or even the records (if they existed) as either a supplementary or a third party account of a user's condition was to introduce unknown biases.

There is, however, some encouragement to be derived from recent studies of interview surveys with handicapped people, which suggest that when compared with a doctor's assessment of the condition, the patient's view is reliable (Warren, 1976). A recent study by Michael Warren concluded that the information given by the patient will be reliable, in so much as it refers to broad disease groupings. The information will, however, be deficient (rather than inaccurate) in relation to specific diseases. As his study assessed mental as well as physical disorders, this is reassuring.

Finally, a comment on the attitude the researchers tried to bring to this survey. There is a world of difference between *evaluation*, which may imply at times adverse criticism, and *cynicism*, which implies an endemic doubting of human sincerity and merit. We considered that we owed our respondents evaluation, but not cynicism. Cynicism, a fashionable twentieth-century posture, is a stance to which social scientists, particularly sociologists, are particularly prone. At times cynicism becomes nihilism: most often when researchers stereotype their respondents. Paradoxically they often do this while they criticise their own respondents for stereotyping other social groups! (So if day unit staff should stereotype the users, it does not help the process of evaluation if we, as researchers, in return stereotype the staff.)

To escape cynicism some personal commitment to one's respondents is necessary. But the commitment needs to be balanced by evaluation. That is why this project faces a continual creative tension between the value critical and the value committed approaches. Perhaps we can have confidence in our results without demonstrating absolute congruence between words and behaviour. It is important to have penetrated frontstage and backstage regions in order to provide a description of day unit life.

NOTE

1 National Day Care Project (1978) *Adult Day Care: Selected Readings* (National Institute for Social Work, 5 Tavistock Place, London WC1H 9SS).

REFERENCES

Abrams, M. (1951) *Social Surveys and Social Action* (Heinemann).
Booth, C. (1891) *Labour and Life of the People*, Vols. I–XVII (Williams & Norgate).
Brown, G. W. and Rutter, M. (1966) 'The measurement of family activities and relationships', *Human Relations*, 19, pp. 241–63.
Carwright, A. (1963) 'Memory errors in a morbidity survey', *Milbank Memorial Fund Quarterly*, 41, pp. 5–24.
Cicourel, A. V. (1964) *Method and Measurement in Sociology* (Free Press).
Cicourel, A. V. (1967) 'Fertility, family planning and social organisation of family life: some methodological issues', *Journal of Social Issues*, 23, 4, pp. 57–81.
Cohen, P. (1966) 'Social attitudes and sociological enquiry', *British Journal of Sociology*, 17, 4, pp. 341–52.
Coleman, J. S. (1959) 'Relational analysis: the study of social organizations with survey methods', in A. Etzioni (ed.), *Complex Organizations: A Sociological Reader* (Holt, Rinehart & Winston).
Cronbach, L. J. and Meehl, P. E. (1955) 'Construct validity in psychological tests'. *Psychological Bulletin*, 52, pp. 281–302.
Edwards, C. and Carter, J. (1980) *The Data of Day Care* (National Institute for Social Work, London).
Giddens, A. H. (ed.) (1974) *Positivism and Sociology* (Heinemann).
Goffman, E. (1959) *The Presentation of Self in Everyday Life* (Penguin).
Jones, K. (1955) *Lunacy, Law and Conscience 1744–1845. The social history of the case of the insane* (Routledge & Kegan Paul).
King, R. D., Raynes, N. V. and Tizard, J. (1971) *Patterns of Residential Care* (Routledge & Kegan Paul).
Mechanic, D. and Newton, M. (1965) 'Some problems in the analysis of morbidity data', *Journal of Chronic Diseases*, 18, pp. 569–80.
Moos, R. H. (1974) *Evaluating Treatment Environments: A Social Ecological Approach* (Wiley-Interscience).
Moser, C. A. and Kalton, G. (1971) *Survey Methods in Social Investigation* (Heinemann Educational Books).
Pahl, R. E. (1974) 'Sociology's conflicting tradition', *New Society*, 30 May, pp. 504–6.
Rein, M. (1976) *Social Science and Public Policy* (Penguin).
Richardson, S. A., Dohrenwend, B. S. and Klein, D. (1965) *Interviewing: Its Forms and Functions* (Basic Books).
Rowntree, B. Seebohm (1901) *Poverty. A Study of Town Life* (Macmillan).
Ryan, A. (1970) *The Philosophy of the Social Sciences* (Macmillan).
Sainsbury, S. (1973) *Measuring Disability*, Occasional Papers on Social Administration No. 54 (Bell).
Warren, M. D. (1976) 'Interview surveys of handicapped people: the accuracy of statements about the underlying medical conditions', *Rheumatology and Rehabilitation*, 15, pp. 295–302.
Webb, E. J., Campbell, D. T., Schwartz, R. D. and Sechrest, L. (1966) *Unob-*

trusive measures: Non-reactive Research in the Social Sciences (Rand McNally).

Whelan, E. and Speake, B. R. S. (1977) *The National Survey of Adult Training Centres in England and Wales* (Manchester University, Hester Adrian Research Centre).

Appendix II

INDEX TO TABLES

*Prepared by Carol Edwards**

* These tables are extracted from the companion document, *The Data of Day Care* (Edwards and Carter, 1980). The tables and much of the information in the companion document were prepared by Carol Edwards with the assistance of a grant from the Department of Health and Social Security.

Table 1 Number of Day Units in the Census Sample

Which Service Providers Sponsor Day Units for Different User Groups in the Census Sample?

Day Units × Service Provider / Day Units × User group	SSD Centres	AHA Day Hospitals	Voluntary Centres	Other Statutory Units: Education Authority	Probation Service	Remploy	Employment Services Agency	DHSS	User Group TOTALS
Mentally Handic.	48 (50)	—	2 (2)	1 (1)	—	—	—	—	51 (53)
Mentally Ill	8 (8)	31 (32)	1 (2)	—	—	—	—	—	40 (42)
Physically Handic.	28 (28)	1 (1)	15 (17)	—	—	5 (5)	2 (2 + 1[a])	—	51 (53 + 1[a])
Elderly	Resid.: 16 (16) Non-Resid.: 19 (19)	31 (31)	43 (45 + 1[a])		—	—	—	—	109 (111 + 1[a])
Elderly Confused	2 (2)	9 (9)	—	—	—	—	—	—	11 (11)
Families	1 (1)	—	4 (5)	—	—	—	—	—	5 (6)
Offenders	—	—	1 (2)	—	2 (2)	—	—	(1[a])	3 (4 + 1[a])
Mixed Units	4 (4)	—	2 (4)	—	—	—	—	—	6 (8)
Service Provider TOTALS	126 (128)	72 (73)	68 (77 + 1[a])	1 (1)	2 (2)	5 (5)	2 (2 + 1[a])	(1[a])	276 (288 + 3[a])

Note: The number in brackets represents the number of day units known to exist in the sample authorities. The difference between the number in brackets and the adjoining number represents the number of day units from which a postal inquiry was *not* returned.

[a] Three units in the sample authorities refused to participate in all parts of the national survey.

Table 2 *Number of Day Units in the Interview Sample*

Which Service Providers Sponsor Day Units for Different User Groups in the Interview Sample?

Day Units × Service Provider / Day Units × User group	SSD Centres	AHA Day Hospitals	Voluntary Centres	Education Authority	Other Statutory Units: Probation Service	Remploy	Employment Services Agency	DHSS	User Group TOTALS
Mentally Handicapped	24	*	2	1	*	*	*	*	27
Mentally Ill	7	21	2	*	*	*	*	*	30
Physically Handicapped	13	1	11	*	*	3	2+1[a]	*	30+1[a]
Elderly	12	10	13+1[a]	*	*	*	*	*	35+1[a]
Elderly Confused	2	9	*	*	*	*	*	*	11
Families	1	*	5	*	*	*	*	*	6
Offenders	*	*	2	*	2	*	*	1[a]	4+1[a]
Mixed Units	4	*	2	*	*	*	*	*	6
Service Providers TOTALS	63	41	37+1[a]	1	2	3	2+1[a]	1[a]	149+3[a]

Note: Units for the elderly confused, families, offenders and mixed units were included in the interview sample by a census rather than a stratified basis.

* Units of this type did not exist in the census sample.

[a] Three units in the sample authorities refused to participate in all parts of the national survey.

Table 3 Date of Opening of Units

In What Year Did Day Units in the Census Sample Open?

Date of Opening	Ment. Hand. SSD N=47	Ment. Hand. Oth. N=3	Ment. Ill SSD N=8	Ment. Ill AHA N=31	Ment. Ill Vol. N=1	Phys. Handicapped SSD N=25	Phys. Handicapped Vol. N=11	Phys. Handicapped Sh.Wk.[a] N=14	Phys. Handicapped ERCs N=2	Phys. Handicapped AHA N=1	Res. SSD N=16	Non-res. N=19	Elderly AHA N=31	Elderly Vol. N=43	Eld. Conf. SSD N=2	Eld. Conf. AHA N=9	Fam. N=5	Off. N=3	Mix. N=5	All Units Total N=276 %
pre-1950	1	1	—	—	—	1	—	3	—	—	—	1	—	—	—	—	—	—	—	2
1950–1959	1	1	—	3	—	3	1	2	2	—	1	1	—	3	—	1	—	—	—	7
1960–1964	7	—	—	3	—	1	4	1	—	—	—	—	4	3	2	—	—	—	—	8
1965–1969	9	—	1	6	—	5	3	2	—	—	1	5	7	4	—	4	1	—	—	16
1970–1972	9	1	3	10	1	2	1	1	—	—	7	3	11	11	—	—	1	1	1	24
1973–1974	6	—	2	4	—	4	—	2	—	—	3	2	5	8	—	3	2	2	1	15
1975–1976	11	1	2	4	—	5	1	1	—	1	2	7	3	13	—	—	2	2	3	22
No information	3	—	—	1	—	4	1	2	—	—	2	1	1	1	—	1	—	—	—	6

N = Number of units in the census sample whose heads responded to the postal inquiry.

Note: Only one response could be given by each head.

[a] Included are one sheltered workshop for the mentally handicapped (opened in 1972) and one for a mix of user groups including the physically handicapped (opened in 1969).

Table 4 Size of Day Units and Established Number of Day Places in Day Units[a]

Type of Day Unit	Units in the census sample: Small (1–29)	Med. (30–59)	Large (60–99)	V.Large (100+)	No info.	Total units	Places Range	Places Mean	Units in the interview sample:[a] Small (1–29)	Med. (30–59)	Large (60–99)	V.Large (100+)	No info.	Total units	Places Range	Places Mean
Day Units for the:																
Mentally Handicapped (Ment. Handic.)																
provided by:																
Social Services Departments (SSD)	2	7	17	21	—	47	23–175	97	2	2	9	11	—	24	23–175	99
Others	2	1	—	—	—	3	10–36	19	2	1	—	—	—	3	10–36	19
Mentally Ill (Ment. Ill)																
provided by:																
Social Services Departments (SSD)	3	5	—	—	—	8	20–50	33	3	4	—	—	—	7	20–50	33
Area Health Authorities (AHA)	9	17	3	2	—	31	6–100	40	8	9	1	2	—	20	17–100	40
Voluntary Agencies (Vol.)	—	—	1	—	—	1	75	75	—	—	1	—	—	1	75	75
Physically Handicapped (Phys. Handic.)																
provided by:																
SSD	3	11	7	4	—	25	15–200	61	2	3	4	3	—	12	15–200	70
Vol.	5	3	3	—	—	11	11–80	38	2	2	2	—	—	6	18–80	43
Sheltered Workshops (SW)[b]	2	3	6	2	1	14	15–150	68	1	1	4	1	1	8	24–150	74
Employment Rehabilitation Centres (ERCs)	—	—	—	2	—	2	100	100	—	—	—	2	—	2	100	100
AHA	1	—	—	—	—	1	20	20	1	—	—	—	—	1	20	20
Elderly (Eld.)																
provided by:							6–14 day pl's in homes with 24–55 pl's								2–14 day pl's in homes with 36–55 pl's	
SSD in old peoples homes (Resid.)	16	—	—	—	—	16		12	3	—	—	—	—	3		14
SSD other sites (Community-based)	5	5	6	—	—	19	12–120[c]	56[c]	3	2	3	1	—	9	12–100[c]	53
AHA	15	15	1	—	—	31	10–70	30	2	7	1	—	—	10	18–70	37
Vol.	11	5	—	4	19	43	12–200	51	4	1	—	1	6	12	12–200	52

[a] The heads of seven units which participated in the interview sample did not return the postal inquiry and therefore are not included in this section.
[b] Sheltered workshops include one mental handicap unit from the census sample and one mixed unit from the interview sample.
[c] The number of users attending was used as an estimate of the number of places in cases of missing information.

Table 4A–5A Size of Day Units and Number of Users Attending Them

Type of Day Unit	Established No. of Day Places in Day Units – Units in the Census – Interview Sample						Places		No. of Users Actually Attending Day Units on Postal Inquiry Day – Units in the Census – Interview Sample						Users	
	Small (1–29)	Med. (30–59)	Large (60–99)	V.Large 100+	No. info.	Total units	Range	Mean	Small (1–29)	Med. (30–59)	Large (60–99)	V.Large 100	No. info.	Total units	Range	Mean
Day Units for the:																
Elderly Confused (Eld. Conf.)	5	5	—	—	1	11	16–50	28	9	1	—	—	1	11	14–32	22
Families (Fam.)[a]	4	—	—	—	1	5	4–9	6	5	—	—	—	—	5	4–6	5
Offenders (Off.)	1	1	—	—	1	3	15–30	23	3	—	—	—	—	3	4–21	11
Mixed User Groups (Mix.)	1	1	2	—	1	5	13–65	45	2	1	2	—	—	5	11–78	45
Total for All User Groups:																
In the Census Sample	85	79	48	40	24	276	4–305	—	127	67	56	15	11	276	4–168	—
In the Interview Sample	44	39	26	22	11	142	4–292	—	68	33	28	10	3	142	4–168	—

[a] The numbers of places given for family centres are for parents, not including children.

Table 5 Size of Day Units and Number of Users actually Attending Unit on Postal Inquiry Day

Type of Day Unit	Units in the Census Sample:						Users		Units in the Interview Sample:[a]						Users	
	Small (1–29)	Med. (30–59)	Large (60–99)	V.Large (100+)	No info.	Total units	Range	Mean	Small (1–29)	Med. (30–59)	Large (60–99)	V.Large (100+)	No info.	Total units	Range	Mean
Day Units for the:																
Mentally Handicapped (Ment. Handic.) provided by:																
Social Services Departments (SSD)	6	10	23	8	—	47	11–168	70	3	4	11	6	—	24	11–168	77
Others	3	—	—	—	—	3	5–22	12	3	—	—	—	—	3	5–22	12
Mentally Ill (Ment. Ill) provided by:																
Social Services Departments (SSD)	5	3	—	—	—	8	5–35	23	4	3	—	—	—	7	5–35	22
Area Health Authorities (AHA)	16	13	2	—	—	31	4–94	32	12	6	2	—	—	20	8–94	33
Voluntary Agencies (Vol.)	—	1	—	—	—	1	50	50	—	1	—	—	—	1	50	50
Physically Handicapped (Phys. Handic.) provided by:																
SSD	8	9	7	1	—	25	9–86	42	4	4	4	—	—	12	9–86	42
Vol.	7	3	1	—	—	11	7–60	27	4	2	—	—	—	6	7–46	27
Sheltered Workshops (SW)[b]	3	4	5	2	—	14	10–116	55	2	2	3	1	—	8	21–116	57
Employment Rehabilitation Centres (ERCs)	—	—	2	—	—	2	68–75	72	—	—	2	—	—	2	68–75	72
AHA	1	—	—	—	—	1	9	9	1	—	—	—	—	1	9	9
Elderly (Eld.) provided by:																
SSD in old peoples homes (Resid.)	16	—	—	—	—	16	6–14 day places in homes with 24–55 places	10	3	—	—	—	—	3	12–14 day places in homes with 36–55 places	14
SSD other sites (Community-based)	10	4	5	—	—	19	10–94	40	5	2	2	—	—	9	10–67	35
AHA	19	11	—	—	1	31	6–48	25	4	6	—	—	—	10	16–43	31
Vol.	14	7	9	5	8	43	8–149	51	4	1	2	3	2	12	10–149	43

[a] The heads of seven units which participated in the interview sample did not return the postal inquiry and therefore are not included in this section.

[b] Sheltered workshops include one mental handicap unit from the census sample and one mixed unit from the interview sample.

Table 6 Ages and Sex of Users

Ages and Sex of Users Interviewed

User Questionnaire –
Question Sixty-One

Age	MH M (N=85)	MH F (N=83)	MH T %	Mentally Ill SSD M (N=21)	SSD F (N=18)	SSD T %	Mentally Ill AHA M (N=55)	AHA F (N=71)	AHA T %	Mentally Ill Vol. M (N=10)	Vol. F (N=3)	Vol. T %	SSD M (N=27)	SSD F (N=44)	SSD T %	Vol. M (N=18)	Vol. F (N=25)	Vol. T %	Phys. Hand. Sh.Wk. M (N=46)	Sh.Wk. F (N=7)	Sh.Wk. T %	ERCs M (N=12)	ERCs F (–)	ERCs T %	AHA M (N=1)	AHA F (N=5)	AHA T %
16–19 yrs.	24	11	21	—	—	—	1	—	1	—	—	—	—	—	—	3	2	11	—	—	—	1	—	8	—	—	—
20–29 yrs.	32	30	37	4	1	13	13	14	21	4	—	38	6	5	15	5	5	23	4	—	8	4	—	33	—	—	—
30–39 yrs.	8	13	13	6	6	31	17	11	22	4	1	31	2	4	8	5	2	16	7	1	15	2	—	17	1	—	17
40–49 yrs.	4	8	7	5	3	21	4	10	11	—	—	—	2	5	10	—	—	—	10	—	21	4	—	33	—	1	17
50–59 yrs.	5	8	8	1	4	5	12	19	25	1	1	8	6	9	21	—	1	2	17	3	38	1	—	8	—	3	50
60–64 yrs.	2	3	3	—	—	—	7	8	12	1	—	8	8	6	20	1	1	2	8	1	17	—	—	—	—	1	17
65–69 yrs.	—	—	—	1	2	3	—	5	4	—	—	—	—	3	6	—	2	7	—	1	2	—	—	—	—	—	—
70–79 yrs.	—	—	—	—	—	—	1	2	2	1	1	8	1	6	8	2	7	20	—	—	—	—	—	—	—	—	—
80 yrs. or more	—	—	—	—	—	—	1	—	1	—	—	—	2	4	8	1	5	14	—	—	—	—	—	—	—	—	—
No info.	10	10	12	—	—	—	—	2	2	—	—	—	—	1	1	1	—	2	—	—	—	—	—	—	—	—	—
Av. age in years	28	33	31	42	48	46	42	47	44	36	54	41	51	55	53	39	57	48	48	53	49	35	35	35	35	54	52

M = Males,   F = Females,   T = Total
N = Number of users in the interview sample by sex

Table 6A Ages and Sex of Users (Cont.)

Ages and Sex of Users Interviewed

User Questionnaire –
Question Sixty-one

	Elderly															Family Centres			Offenders			Mixed Units			Totals		
	Resid.			SSD Non-resid.			AHA			Vol.			Elderly Confused														
Age	M (N=3)	F (N=15)	T %	M (N=14)	F (N=43)	T %	M (N=23)	F (N=38)	T %	M (N=24)	F (N=55)	T %	M (N=18)	F (N=40)	T %	M (N=3)	F (N=26)	T %	M (N=19)	F (N=5)	T %	M (N=10)	F (N=20)	T %	M (N=389)	F (N=499)	T %
16–19 yrs.	—	—	—	—	—	—	—	—	—	—	—	—	—	—	—	1	3	14	4	1	21	2	3	17	36	21	6
20–29 yrs.	—	—	—	—	—	—	—	—	—	—	—	—	—	—	—	1	13	48	6	—	25	1	2	10	80	71	17
30–39 yrs.	—	—	—	—	—	—	—	—	—	—	—	—	1[a]	—	2	1	7	28	4	1	17	1	—	3	59	44	12
40–49 yrs.	—	—	—	—	—	—	—	—	—	—	—	—	—	—	—	—	2	7	4	2	21	—	2	7	34	32	8
50–59 yrs.	—	—	—	—	—	—	2	2	7	—	—	—	2	3	9	—	—	—	3	—	8	—	1	2	13	20	12
60–64 yrs.	—	—	—	—	1	2	2	6	13	5	5	13	2	2	7	—	1[b]	3	1	—	8	2	—	7	37	41	9
65–69 yrs.	—	1	6	1	4	9	4	3	11	4	8	15	4	6	17	—	—	—	—	—	—	2	2	13	20	40	7
70–79 yrs.	2	9	61	2	7	16	12	15	44	11	22	42	6	16	38	—	—	—	—	—	—	2	8	33	44	110	17
80 yrs. or more	1	5	33	8	23	54	3	12	25	4	20	30	3	10	22	—	—	—	—	—	—	—	2	7	17	66	9
No info.	—	—	—	3	8	19	—	—	—	—	—	—	—	3	5	—	—	—	—	—	—	—	—	—	11	17	3
Av. age in years	78	78	78	75	74	74	72	74	74	73	76	75	69	74	73	26	30	29	32	47	35	48	58	55	46	52	52

a This 39-year-old man attended a psychogeriatric day hospital which shared a building with a day hospital for patients in their 20s with acute mental illness. The staff felt the services available in the psychogeriatric day hospital were more appropriate to his needs than those of the day hospital. He was also the only user attending a unit for the elderly confused who lived with his parents – in this case, his mother.
b This woman of 60 attended a family centre because she was bringing up her two grandchildren as a 'single parent grandparent'.
M = Males, F = Females, T = Total
N = Number of users in the interview sample by sex

Table 7 Number of Days per Week Users Attend Day Units: Users' View

Number of Days per Week of Users' Attendance (the week before the interview)*

User Questionnaire —
Question Eighteen

No. of attendances in the week before interview	Ment. handic. (N=168)	Mentally Ill			Physically Handicapped					Elderly								Total N=888	%
		SSD (N=39)	AHA (N=126)	Vol. (N=13)	SSD (N=71)	Vol. (N=44)	Sh.Wk. (N=53†)	ERCS (N=12)	AHA (N=6)	SSD Resid (N=18)	SSD Non Resid (N=57)	AHA (N=61)	Vol. (N=79)	Eld. Conf. (N=58)	Fam. (N=29)	Off. (N=24)	Mx. (N=30)		
One Day	2	1	10	1	10	7	—	—	—	9	12	15	29	4	11	1	3	13
Two Days	6	4	20	1	16	8	—	—	—	3	11	30	6	15	6	1	9	15
Three Days	3	7	24	2	7	1	5	—	1	2	7	9	7	15	4	3	1	11
Four Days	15	2	20	5	3	5	1	2	—	—	4	3	8	6	2	5	—	9
Five Days	114	22	44	1	30	18	46	10	4	1	20	1	23	12	2	9	14	42
Six or Seven Days	—	—	—	2	—	—	1	—	—	—	—	—	1	1	—	4	—	1
User Not in Unit the Previous Week	1	1	8	1	5	5	—	—	—	2	3	2	5	—	4	1	3	5
No Information	27	2	—	—	—	—	—	—	—	1	—	1	—	5	—	—	—	4
Average no. of attendances in the week before interview	5 days	4 dys.	4 dys.	4 dys.	3 dys.	3 dys.	5 dys.	5 dys.	4 dys.	2 dys.	3 dys.	2 dys.	3 dys.	3 dys.	2 dys.	4 dys.	3 dys.	4 dys.

* A half to less than a day counted as a full day   N = Number of users in the interview sample
† Included are the users of one sheltered workshop for a mix of user groups including the physically handicapped.

GLOSSARY

Census sample: The census sample is all day units for adults located within the thirteen sample areas of the country. Information collected by postal inquiry forms the information of the census sample. There were 291 units in the census sample and information was provided by 276 of these (95 per cent).

Day unit: A day unit is a form of communal care which has 'care givers' present in a non-residential or non-domiciliary setting for at least three days per week, and which is open four to five hours per day.

Direct service staff: See Staff of the unit.

Head of the unit: This is the person who has overall charge of the day-to-day running of the day unit. He/she may be known by a number of names within his/her own unit, e.g. manager, officer-in-charge, sister-in-charge, charge nurse, organiser. (In a few units it was necessary to select a head amongst several members of a multi-disciplinary team who shared this responsibility. In these cases, the team was asked to nominate one person to act as head for the purposes of the study.)

Interview sample: This is a sub-sample of interviews of persons in the day units of the census sample. Units for the elderly, the mentally ill, the mentally handicapped and the physically handicapped were selected by rules defined in Edwards and Carter (1980). All day units for the elderly confused, for families, for offenders, and mixed centres were included for persons selected in the interview sample. From *149* selected units, interviews came from *148* heads, *411* staff and *888* users.

Postal Questionnaire: This is the written schedule of questions addressed by post to the head of each unit in the census sample.

Sample areas: The thirteen areas were selected by a stratified random sample to represent the local authorities in England and Wales. As local authority boundaries were co-terminous with area health authority boundaries in most instances, local authorities were used as the sample areas.

Service provider: The statutory or voluntary organisation which was responsible for providing the services in a given day unit was called the service provider. Examples are local authority social services departments, area health authorities and old peoples' welfare associations.

Staff of the unit: Unless otherwise specified, staff refers to the 'direct service' staff of the unit. These are the people who work in the unit and who have direct contact with users within the unit. Examples are: instructors, nurses, doctors, care assistants, therapists and volunteers. They include people who are employed to work on a full-time, part-time or sessional basis, or who work as volunteer staff and are unpaid. They also include workers seconded to the unit (for example, social workers in a day hospital seconded by a social services department). Certain workers normally classified as support staff could be included as direct service staff at the head's discretion if they came into enough contact with users. So a cook who also spent time playing bingo with users might be included as a direct service staff member.

Staff questionnaire: This is the interview schedule of questions addressed to heads and staff.

Support staff: Support staff back up the work of the direct service staff of the unit.

Usually they do not have direct contact with users within the unit. They may include secretaries, kitchen staff, caretakers, drivers, and so on. Support staff were not sampled for interviewing.

User group: The administratively defined label specifying the group of users for whom a given day unit catered; usually a given administrative definition.

User questionnaire: This is the interview schedule of questions addressed to users when they were interviewed.

Users of the unit: This is the name adopted by the national survey for the people who attend the day unit on a regular basis over a space of time. Within particular units, they may be called clients, patients, members, trainees.

INDEX

in mixed centres, 116
in sheltered workshops, 233–6, 239–42
see also employment

work centres, 2, 3
   see also adult training centres; sheltered
     workshops

For Product Safety Concerns and Information please contact our EU
representative GPSR@taylorandfrancis.com
Taylor & Francis Verlag GmbH, Kaufingerstraße 24, 80331 München, Germany

www.ingramcontent.com/pod-product-compliance
Ingram Content Group UK Ltd.
Pitfield, Milton Keynes, MK11 3LW, UK
UKHW021426080625
459435UK00011B/177